THE
NEW
MILLENNIUM
DIET REVOLUTION

Keith DeOrio, M.D.

with Robert Dursi, C.N.M.

Copyright © 1999 by New Millennium Medicine Institute

Published by Prominence Publishing, 219 Broadway, Suite 295, Laguna Beach, CA 92651

Library of Congress Cataloging-in-Publication Data

DeOrio, Keith. The New Millennium Diet Revolution: combines ancient and modern dietary technology into a four part strategy for the new millennia/Keith DeOrio, M.D., with Robert Dursi, CNM.

Includes bibliographical references and index.
ISBN 0-966882-0-0-8

10 9 8 7 6 5 4 3 2 1

Printed in the United States of America

DEDICATION

Dedicated to my beautiful wife Adele,

our son Jordan,

my brother Todd and

my loving parents Don and Norma.

Thank you for your unconditional love and support,

without which I could never have attained my dreams

or completed this book.

ACKNOWLEDGEMENTS

I would like to express my gratitude to my family, friends, colleagues, and patients who inspired and supported me to write *The New Millennium Diet Revolution*. I appreciate the endless encouragement and faith everyone shared with me during this literary quest.

I am especially grateful to Don DeOrio, Mark and Tina Armijo, Gary Klingsheim and Julie Dahl for all their attention to detail, persistence and long hours. This book would have been impossible without your help.

Special thanks to Karen Harris for her artistic talent and to Martin Zucker, Sheryl Rose, Peggy Rogers, Sarah Hinman, Ron Nicklaw and Mike Riley for their editing expertise, going well beyond "the call of duty."

Lastly, thank you to my family and friends who tolerated my absence through many events while I worked on this project. My sincere thanks to everyone.

Table of Contents

Introduction

For many people, eating the right food, following the right diet, maintaining the proper weight, and staying optimally healthy is an enormous puzzle they never seem able to solve. If you are one of those people, this book will show you the way. The New Millennium Diet is a comprehensive program that helps to explain and demystify the puzzle, breaking it down into four major pieces. These pieces combined will provide you with the understanding and the guidance necessary to reshape your diet, your body, and your health.

The New Millennium Diet is a four-in-one program. It contains each of the four pieces of the puzzle as units to be understood and incorporated into your meal planning. The units are these:

1. Blood type,

2. Macronutrient balance,

3. Yin and Yang energy,

4. Avoidance of hidden toxins in foods.

No other dietary plan has ever attempted to bring all these factors into one complete approach. I believe that no dietary plan can call itself complete unless it does so. These are the four steps to effective eating and effective dieting.

As you read the book, I don't want you to feel overwhelmed with the amount of information, some or all of which may be new to you. Take it nice and slow. You may find it easier to adopt the elements of the diet one at a time rather than trying to adopt all of them at once. Do whatever is easy for you. You may first want to incorporate your own individual blood type–specific diet. Once you have done that, then you can move on to the next element: balancing your macronutrient intake of protein, carbohydrates and fats. Then you can continue refining your diet by adopting Yin and Yang principles, and then finally honing your shopping skills so that you eliminate foods with hidden toxins. I certainly recommend that you go for the maximum effect and try to incorporate all these elements. But if you can't, don't be discouraged. **You will reap huge benefits with each level you master.**

The New Millennium Diet is much more than just a weight loss program. It is a holistic program that not only enables you to shed unwanted weight and fat, but really elevates you to the highest level of health. You will look better and feel better. That's what thousands of patients have told me who have followed the program. And that's what their medical tests consistently indicate as well — better health.

Many of my patients have previously been treated by excellent, caring physicians at leading medical centers. They have undergone highly advanced treatments, but yet, they felt they were not making enough progress toward better health. I sincerely believe that the reasons are multi-factorial. However, diet is a very significant reason which is often poorly addressed at most leading medical institutions.

Within a short period on this program, patients experience significant improvement. It has helped individuals with arthritis, diabetes, heart disease, lupus, mental diseases, depression, alcoholism, PMS, candida, and chronic fatigue. The program slows down aging and the appearance of wrinkles, liver spots and spider veins, which are unsightly signs of the degeneration process at work. The program succeeds where other methods fail, I believe, because it enhances and balances the body's natural defenses and healing mechanisms, allowing you to effectively combat the influences that lead to ill-health and disease. With this program, you are likely to experience a level of health that you haven't experienced for years. The New Millennium Diet promotes maximum well-being, peak physical performance, mental sharpness, and increased sexual vigor. It takes you from where you are, no matter how sick you are, and raises you to better health.

As a medical and holistic physician, my professional interest in health, wellness and nutrition, as well as personal illness, has led me to seek a superior dietary program. Over the last 20 years, I have studied and experimented with numerous dietary plans and have not found one that totally fit my concept or standards for a complete diet. Ultimately, I combined my research with the experience gained from seeing more than 10,000 patients to develop the New Millennium Diet which is presented in this book. It is a plan that integrates ancient wisdom with the advances of modern science. It is the culmination of years of clinical experience and exhaustive research, a personal effort to develop the best, most complete, and most workable dietary plan for people interested in achieving total wellness of body, mind, emotions, and spirit.

The New Millennium calls for new knowledge and a departure from the endless fad diets and nutritional plans promoted during the 20th century. In recent years, there has been a great increase in the number of diets being promoted. We have witnessed everything from low protein–high carbohydrate to low carbohydrate–high protein, along, of course, with low-fat diets. The problem is that these plans may work for some people, but they do not work for the majority of people. If they are not working for most people, then something has to be wrong. You have likely tried some of those plans and found they did not meet your hopes and expectations about weight loss, appearance, and health. I believe that the New Millennium Diet will be the answer for you and millions like you who strive for greater well-being and the opportunity to reach your full genetic potential in life.

I have set up the book in three parts. I call the first the "ready" part. The information contained here unfolds the four key elements for a successful diet — eating blood type–specific food, balancing your macronutrients, applying Yin and Yang principles, and avoiding foods' hidden toxins. These are elements that are absolutely essential for you to achieve your proper weight and maintain it, to look good, and to feel good. It is important to understand these elements as a background to understanding the reasoning behind the New Millennium Diet. The concepts I introduce may not be totally new to you. However, you will see that I have made certain modifications, based on my research and clinical experience. These alterations allow my dietary concept to have universal effectiveness, and be useful to all individuals, regardless of race, gender, culture, blood type, or level of physical activity.

Part One "readies" you for the diet. Part Two puts you in the "set" mode. Here, I briefly review the material we have covered to keep it fresh in your mind. Then, I explain how to individualize the diet. There are a few simple calculations you have to make in order for you to tailor the diet to you personally. They are simple. I will guide you through the process so you can easily figure your individual requirements for protein, carbohydrates and fats.

Part Three is the "go" section. You have learned how the diet works, what the components are, and what your individual requirements are. Now you pick the appropriate chapter — based on your blood type — with information and lists of foods and recipes for your optimum meal planning. You will need to know your blood type in order to follow the New Millennium Diet. You may already know it. If not, you can obtain the information through a simple blood test at your doctor's office or through a home test you can order directly from ProSana. Refer to the end of the book. The last chapter in Part Three is for patients with candida. So many of my patients have this common problem, I decided they needed special attention. In this chapter you will find all the New Millennium guidelines geared to the special needs of the person with candida.

The Roots of the New Millennium Diet

My dietary concept has its roots in the monumental work of Weston A. Price, D.D.S. and his landmark book *Nutrition and Physical Degeneration*, published in 1939. This book has been reprinted five times because of the great truths it contains about the relationship between diet and health. It is definitely recommended reading. If you are interested, you can obtain the book through the Price-Pottenger Nutrition Foundation in La Mesa, California (Phone: 800-366-3748).

In 1930 Dr. Price, a dental researcher, set off on a worldwide investigation to confirm his belief that the modern-day diet caused dental decay. The best approach to make this determination was to research groups of people isolated from modern civilization and who were living predominantly on the indigenous foods of their region and culture. The search took him to tribal Africans, Arctic Eskimos, North and South American Indians, Australian Aborigines, Pacific Islanders, Irish fishermen, and numerous other communities scattered around the globe.

Dr. Price's investigations not only confirmed his theory on diet and dental decay, but also uncovered important revelations about diet and health in general. He found high immunity to serious infections among peoples isolated from civilization and living in accordance with the traditional diets handed down from preceding generations. He found more than fourteen different tribal dietary approaches. Although the diets were significantly different from one another, they each provided a sufficient amount of nutritional sustenance to generate strong immune systems and overall disease resistance.

The diets of these tribal groups were based on various food sources including seafoods, domesticated animals and game, while a few were based on purely dairy products. Some contained almost no plant food. Others featured a variety of fruits, vegetables, grains, and legumes. All of the diets contained some form of animal product. Most of these groups cooked their foods, while others ate their foods raw. The diversity of the diets reflected the geographical location, the cultural makeup, and the genetic heritage of the individual group. However, as long as the group was able to consume a diet similar to their ancestors, Dr. Price found that dental caries and other types of diseases were rare.

The most important element these variant diets shared was that they consisted of predominantly whole foods collected in their local regions. There was absolutely no "civilized" food, such as white sugars or flours, pasteurized or skim milks, canned or frozen foods, or any type of refined or hydrogenated vegetable oils.

Analysis of these primitive diets showed that these diets contained at least four times the level of minerals and vitamins, and ten times the amount of fat-soluble vitamins, as the typical American diet of the day. Dr. Price believed that the fat-soluble vitamins were the key components of these primitive diets. These nutrients facilitated the absorption of the other proteins, minerals, and water-soluble vitamins. Insufficient fat-soluble vitamins would prevent the absorption and assimilation of the minerals even if such minerals were present in high concentrations.

Dr. Price found that when isolated groups began to consume a "civilized" diet of refined and devitalized foods, the incidence of problems soared. He found more children with facial deformities, more birth defects, more tooth decay, and greater susceptibility to infections and chronic diseases, as well as psychological imbalances typically leading to criminal and deviant behavior. When these groups returned to their traditional diets, he found that these problems ceased to occur in the following generations.

The information Dr. Price collected from studying these primitive groups of people substantiates three important points I have emphasized in my New Millennium Diet.

> **Point One:** The blood type–based diet suggests a linkage between one's culture and genetics, and one's dietary traditions. Dr. Price showed that even though each of the different groups had a different type of cultural and genetically

adapted diet, each was able to prevent many of the diseases now associated with our modern diet. Of course, it would be difficult to go back and trace one's specific cultural diets. However, now through blood type, we are able to provide at least some type of basic blueprint for each individual to follow in order to achieve some level of their past genetic dietary format.

Point Two: Fat is an important part of any sound diet, including animal and butter fats, as well as organ meats, marine oils, fish, and eggs. Most nutritionists of the modern age have condemned fat as a bad substance to be avoided, and have promoted low-fat diets as a way to improved health. However, as Dr. Price noted, fat was probably one of the key elements why these primitive peoples attained such superior health and fitness. In a low-fat diet, many of the fat-soluble vitamins, which are vital for the assimilation of other proteins, minerals, and other water-soluble nutrients, are eliminated. The problem with eating present-day animal source fat is the high level of toxins from chemical pollutants contained in the fatty tissues.

Point Three: A diet high in refined sugars and processed products contributes to serious nutritional deficiencies as well as damaging the internal organs and glands. We must exclude these kinds of foods from our diet.

It is evident from Dr. Price's work that our modern culture has lost touch with its traditional dietary roots. Is there any doubt why we see an ever-increasing rise in chronic diseases such as cancer, heart disease, migraine headaches, dental caries, and numerous other conditions? If modern society is to survive and overcome these threats to health and life we must begin reincorporating the fundamentals of ancient nutritional wisdom back into our lifestyle.

Much of the nutritional knowledge primitive man possessed was passed down from one generation to the next. This ensured that each subsequent generation would have the maximum potential for survival as well as the opportunity to enjoy their full genetic health potential. Therefore, sound nutritional advice must be taught in schools from kindergarten through college in order to reeducate our young people in the ancient wisdom of basic dietary truths.

Primitive peoples usually required that newly married couples, and especially the women prior to conception, undergo an intensive nutritional fortification program. This was seen as nutritional insurance so that babies would be born optimally healthy. It is important that breast feeding be reinstituted in our society to reduce the chance of poor neurological, physiological, and dental development.

We must turn our backs on the "civilized" foods that line the shelves of our food markets. We need to take the time to prepare nutritional meals, instead of a 10-minute quick fix with hamburger and some processed side dish. Many refined fats used in the preparation of potato chips, French fries, crackers, pastries, commercial cereals, and breads must be avoided because these fats are associated with heart disease and aging.

Refined sugar in all forms must be eliminated. It is one of the key elements in the deterioration of our health and our teeth. Many of the refined breads and flours need to be substituted with sprouted wheat breads and whole grain flours, free of chemical preservatives.

You are what you eat. A nutrient-poor diet full of chemicals cannot create the good level of health you seek. It takes a diet of wholesome food to create good skin and appearance, optimum brain and glandular function, a healthy liver and a healthy heart, and a solid structure of bones and muscles. Therefore, organically grown fruits and vegetables free of chemicals should be incorporated into our diet as much as possible. In addition, the use of organic meats and free range poultry which have significantly fewer pollutants than their commercial counterparts should be used when meat is part of your blood type–specific diet.

We must also return to sustainable farming techniques that avoid the use of chemical pesticides and fertilizers. Current methods have broken the cycle of regeneration that accounted for the high nutrient levels found in the foods of most primitive diets. Moreover, such methods pollute groundwater and deplete the nutrient level in soils. Vegetables and fruits now have little taste — and less nutrient content — because commercial farming production emphasizes quantity over quality. The level of nutrient intake has declined steadily over the last 100 years and today surveys continually indicate widespread nutritional deficiencies among the U.S. population.

We must also begin to understand that this era of synthetic chemicals and drugs has sharply increased our exposure to substances that are toxic to the body. We are bombarded with thousands of indoor and outdoor chemicals. Perfumes, hair sprays, synthetic carpets and car exhausts, just to name a few of a countless number of typical sources, which expose us to an avalanche of chemical compounds. This significantly prevents the development of our full genetic potential which we all inherently possess and should enjoy.

The majority of these chemicals are derived from cold tar and petroleum-based compounds, which are completely foreign to man's cellular machinery. Residues of chemicals are now found in most living species from the Arctic to the Antarctic. Phytoplankton, organisms found at the bottom of the food chain and which are mandatory for the production of oxygen needed for our survival, are tainted with petroleum by-products.

These chemicals move up through the food chain. Eventually they end up in human beings. They have been shown to affect the sex hormones and various other reproductive functions of numerous species. Many frog species throughout the United States are appearing with birth defects, such as missing or duplicated legs. This is confirmation that many of our streams, rivers, and lakes are being contaminated by chemicals, possibly altering certain biochemical processes, making the frog more susceptible to infections from bacteria or parasites. Even polar bear offspring are now being found with both male and female sex organs. Scientists believe this is being caused by exposure to PCBs, DDT and other chemical pollutants in the environment.

Modern man has lost the tribal wisdom which kept him emotionally and physically sound from one generation to the next. As Dr. Price stated, "Life in all its fullness is Mother Nature obeyed." The laws of God and nature are immutable, and they cannot be broken without retribution. The New Millennium Diet provides the systematic approach for reconnecting us to traditional wisdom and our dietary roots. In the process, it gives us a practical road map for achieving superior health.

My deep appreciation goes to Dr. Price for his great insights and to the Price-Pottenger Foundation which today continues to promote these *back to basics concepts* to prevent the further decline of health in our society. I hope you can join me in reeducating yourself and your family in a way of eating and thinking that can change your health, the health of your family and ultimately the health of the planet which sustains our future generations. ■

Keith DeOrio, M.D., D.(Hom.)Med.
January 2000, Santa Monica, CA

Part One

"READY"

Understanding the Roots of the Diet

CHAPTER 1

Dietary Evolution

During the past twenty years there has been an explosion of diet plans promoted in the United States. Unfortunately, most of them have failed to produce the desired level of weight loss and control for practically all those people who have tried them. These plans, mostly restrictive in nature, have attempted to accomplish their proclaimed goals by reducing the consumption of either proteins, carbohydrates, fats or meats. The originators of these plans promoted the idea that by skewing such foods, either up or down, people would be able to lose weight. They could not have been more wrong! Despite the inundation of weight loss plans, obesity has increased by 30% in the last 10 years.

Only recently has there been a movement towards a more balanced and individualized approach to weight control. In 1995, Barry Sears, Ph.D., authored *The Zone*, which promoted the so-called 40-30-30 balance concept of food management. His book prescribes a daily calorie intake derived from 30% protein, 40% carbohydrates and 30% fats. In 1996, Peter D'Adamo, N.D., authored *Eat Right 4 Your Type*. His book prescribes the management of food based upon an individual's blood type and genetic heritage. Both books were on the *New York Times* bestsellers list for months and enjoyed phenomenal success. The popularity of these new approaches only confirms that millions of Americans are still looking for the right dietary program.

Even though these approaches have made great headway, they are not foolproof. Diet and health research continues and every day we are learning more and more about how the body processes foods. My diet program uses both Dr. Sears and Dr. D'Adamo's approaches as a springboard to move into the next level of dietary success.

To really understand where we're going, we must understand where we've been. So, in the following pages, let's review some of the dietary concepts popularized in the last two decades. It's important to understand the evolution of these diets, their benefits, and their pitfalls, to appreciate the next generation of nutrition…**The New Millennium Diet**!

The Restrictive Diets:
Feast or Famine

These dietary plans promote a reduction in the amount and consumption of either proteins, carbohydrates, or fats to achieve *weight* loss. People who try these kinds of diets are usually unsuccessful in achieving their desired goals. They feel hungry during the diet and after dieting put weight back on as quickly as they took it off.

In most cases, the dieter enters into what is known as *starvation mode*. This happens because of the body's prehistoric and ancestral tendencies towards "feast or famine." In other words, the sudden reduction in food intake causes the body to think that it won't be receiving food for a long period of time. Consequently, the body begins to conserve and store fat, in preparation for "famine." So, the dieter's fat loss reaches a plateau and you stop losing weight.

The sad thing is, when dieters are in the throes of the restrictive diet, they lose a significant amount of lean muscle mass. Even worse, they ultimately regain their original weight plus extra pounds ... only to have it all come back as fat! Muscle mass is not restored. This unfortunate situation leads to feelings of remorse and despondency, and reinforces the belief that the dieters are unable to control their eating habits.

Let's review some of these plans a bit more in detail.

High-Carbohydrate — Low-Protein — Low-Fat Diets

For many years, traditionally trained dietitians and nutritionists have recommended that the majority of calories come from approximately 65% carbohydrates, 20% proteins, and 15% fats. There are many different diet plans that preach this high-carb/low-protein/low-fat approach. Frequently, this skewed balance of foods causes disturbances in the body. The typical meal usually gives the person the short-lived effect of feeling good, but for most people it leads to significant blood sugar and hormonal imbalance. It generally produces hormonal irregularities with high levels of insulin and low levels of glucagon. As a result, within a few hours after the meal, you bottom out.

Here's what happens in your body: You lose energy and your brain doesn't seem to function at peak performance. Many people who work in offices complain of the "after-lunch snooze period." They come back from lunch and they can hardly keep their eyes open. Almost always, they've gone out and had a high-carb lunch and then come back to fight the hormonal imbalance at their desk. When this happens a message is sent by the brain to the body for some immediate fast-acting fuel. Typically, the person craves high-carbohydrate food containing large amounts of sugar ... from candy bars to soft drinks or other sugary snacks. This is why people find themselves at the candy machine for the "afternoon snack break."

With a low glucagon level, it is very difficult for the body to access carbohydrate reserves in the liver ... even though the energy equivalent of two to three candy bars of fuel is stored there at any one time. This condition begins continual cycles of increased insulin and reduced glucagon. It creates for the dieter insatiable cravings and a desire for sugary snacks occurring on a frequency of every two to three hours. It's a vicious cycle!

Endurance athletes will often undertake what is known as *carbo loading*. They will derive 75% of their calories from carbohydrates, 15% from protein and the other 10% from fat. This initially results in an increased boost in their energy level, but frequently is followed by a slump in both their physical and mental performance. This is commonly known as *hitting the wall* in marathon running, the *bonk* in cycling, and the *loss of focus* in tennis. Nowhere was this dietary regime seen more dramatically than in the early days of triathlons, when contestants used to *load up* in the ritualistic prerace pasta feasts. Many of them hit "the wall," painfully learning the lesson of relying on carbohydrates for sustained energy under extreme physical exertion.

Nearly all people who consume large amounts of high-carbohydrate meals complain of mid-morning or mid-afternoon drops in energy. This is particularly true in the afternoon when drowsiness overtakes them within a hour or so after eating lunch. The carbohydrates in the meal have caused an increased release of insulin, which then lowers their blood sugar. This condition, in its chronic phase, is medically known as hypoglycemia. Low blood sugar level is a frequent cause of fatigue, depression, irritability, severe sugar cravings, water retention, gas, bloating, poor exercise tolerance, and reduced mental concentration.

In general, the majority of people who follow high-carbohydrate diets develop significant food cravings and hormonal swings. This situation over time may precede the onset of adult diabetes and other more serious problems such as a greater propensity for arterial and heart disease.

High-Protein — Low-Carbohydrate — Low-Fat or High Fat Diets

This type of diet regime is similar to the one just discussed. The basic difference is that it favors a diet high in protein rather than carbohydrates. But there's a problem. The body, in its attempt to replace missing carbohydrates needed for fuel, breaks down muscle tissue and converts it to carbohydrates. Reduced muscle mass leads to a reduced metabolic rate. This is because muscle is a very metabolically active tissue. Muscle cells burn fat efficiently. Moreover, these diets cause increased insulin release, which leads to greater fat storage. When high fat is consumed along with high protein such as occurs in the Atkins diet, much less insulin is released. However high acidity is acheived (ketosis) as is the desired goal but as any holistic physician or practitioner knows, acidifying the blood leads to ill health in the long run. More will be discussed on this topic later, but if you value your health avoid this approach.

It is estimated that more than 90% of the people who go on high-protein/low-carbohydrate diets gain back the weight they lost within the first three to six months after completing the program. Often they put on an extra 5 to 10% of their body weight after the diet because of the internal organ and glandular trauma caused by such a diet.

Vegetarianism

Vegetarianism has been commonly viewed as the dietary poster child of the alternative medicine movement. It has been promoted by many nutritional gurus over the course of the last century, such as Misho Kushi, Dr. Michael Klapper, John Robbins and Dr. Dean Ornish. They have promoted vegetarianism based on economic, environmental, nutritional, and philosophical grounds. Many people who choose a vegetarian diet do so because of their religious and/or moral beliefs. Killing animals for food or any other purpose carries either a *karmic burden* or goes against the *laws of nature.*

Vegetarians eat vegetables, fruits, and grains. Some eat eggs or dairy products. A true vegetarian — a vegan — does not eat any kind of meat or animal protein. This represents a high-carbohydrate, low-protein, low-fat diet that works well for some people. It does not work well, however, for the majority of people, as the proponents of this eating style would have you believe. As you will see, the vegan approach should really be followed *only* by certain blood types and not others. The next chapter will explain the reason why.

Low-Fat Diets

According to most modern day diet plans, fat is considered the worst thing a dieter can eat. For this reason, low fat has become the anthem of many dieters. Some plans recommend a maximum of 10–15% fat, with lowered proteins and unlimited amounts of carbohydrates. The fear of fat promoted by such diets has led to an excess of carbohydrate consumption and contributed to erroneous eating habits. Americans have, in fact, gained 30% *more* weight over the last decade compared to the previous decade.

The media have promoted the dangers of high-cholesterol and high-fat diets because of their connection to heart disease, obesity, and cancer. Now, millions of individuals are consuming fat-free cookies, breads, crackers, muffins, and bagels. They do so in the belief that this particular dietary plan is the answer to their weight concerns and health-related problems. However, in my clinic, I have seen disturbing effects from these low-fat, high-carbohydrate diets. In most cases, the results of these diets tend to be devastating, especially for individuals who are *slow burners*. This is a term used to describe individuals who have a very low metabolic rate. Their increased consumption of carbohydrates leads to increased insulin production and greater fat storage.

Low-fat diets can also result in essential fatty acid deficiencies. Essential fatty acids are fats required for proper body function. They can be found in seeds, nuts, or cold-water fish. Symptoms associated with low fatty acid consumption include dry skin, poor hair and nail growth, mood swings, allergies, fatigue, and immune-related disturbances. In reality, *the less fat you consume, the fatter you become, and the more your health is compromised.*

The Next Step Closer ... Dietary Balance and Individuality

The concepts promoted by Barry Sears and Peter D'Adamo were major turning points in dietary planning. Their concepts basically turned the dietary world upside-down. This balanced approach to diet planning went against all traditional methods. The thought of using one's blood type as the key to weight control and good health was unthinkable. Of course, at one time, people also thought the world was flat. Let's review these plans.

Enter the Zone ... Balance

The Zone diet was introduced in 1995 by Barry Sears, Ph.D. The 40-30-30 concept of eating (40% carbohydrate, 30% protein, and 30% fat) in each meal was a phenomenon that spread rapidly across the United States and the world.

The Zone has been embraced by many people, including world-class athletes, movie stars, fitness buffs, diabetics, and people just looking to lose weight and improve their overall health. The Zone concept, however was not appreciated by everyone. It generated a tremendous amount of controversy within the traditional nutritional and dietary fields. Its emphasis on an increase in protein and fat and a reduction in carbohydrates contradicted the high-carbohydrate, low-protein, and low-fat consumption that had been long recommended.

The ratio of proteins, carbohydrates and fats in the Zone achieves appropriate hormonal balance, a metabolic state in which the body can work at optimum efficiency. If an individual is not in hormonal balance, significant disturbances occur in the body, such as hunger, mood swings, decreased mental focus, reduced productivity, and generalized fatigue and listlessness.

One of the benefits that a Zone-balanced meal can provide, for both athletes as well as the average individual, is that foods can be used for their "drug-like" effects. Today the concept of using foods as drugs is rapidly becoming more widely accepted. Before, people used food merely as fuel for the body, and to get them through the day. However, new research indicates that foods have powerful physiological effects on our mood, mental performance, and physiological functions.

Maintaining the Zone balance of 40-30-30 helped many people achieve their desired weight better than any other previous diet plan. The decrease in carbohydrates with the increase in protein and fat consumption will definitely lead to improvements in overall health. Better health lessens the chances of catching colds, the flu or serious infections. More importantly, you minimize the probability of acquiring chronic conditions, such as allergies, cancer, diabetes, and heart disease.

Where the Zone Leaves Off

For the most part, I like the plan and consider it to be one of the best available today. My main concern with this diet regimen is that it fails to take several important points into consideration: (1) the inherent genetic and cultural aspects of the individual, (2) the energetic properties of the body and food, and (3) the toxicity of food. These are essential considerations for achieving a complete dietary plan.

Your Blood Type Is the Key...
Individuality

In 1996, Dr. Peter D'Adamo authored *Eat Right 4 Your Type,* which became very popular among diet devotees. His book prescribes the use of certain foods based on individual blood type and genetic heritage. Dr. D'Adamo contends that foods contain certain immunological factors specific for each blood type. Therefore, knowing what *food to eat or not eat,* based on your specific blood type, can prevent illness, improve health and maximize fat loss.

He also asserts that your blood type has the power to affect many different aspects of your life, such as physical performance, sexual vigor, emotional and mental well-being, risk factors for various diseases, life span, and even personality characteristics.

I am in complete agreement with his concept. Based on my research and clinical experience, I have found utilizing one's specific blood type can play a vital role in determining a person's health and dietary protocols. Every single cell in the body contains the human DNA code — the blueprint for our entire body. As incredible as it may seem, an entire human being could be made from one single drop of blood, once the technology is available to unlock the code. This fact supports the concept that using the four blood type antigens, known as O, A, B and AB, could be the key to finding a proper diet in order to achieve the highest level of health.

In his book, Dr. D'Adamo explains how blood type is based on one's race, culture, and geographical ancestry. Type O is the oldest blood type. Type A evolved as the result of the agricultural revolution. Type B has been reportedly associated with migration into harsher and colder climates. Type AB is the newest blood type, which came about from the intermingling of A and B groups. His theory considers the probability that the different blood types evolved because of the environmental challenges confronting early man. More likely than not, our blood types are continuing to evolve due to social, economic and environmental conditions that we face in our daily life. We just won't be around to see the final outcome.

It is very conceivable, then, that your blood type does indeed contain the powerful genetic outline of your body's constitutional makeup and dietary requirements. By utilizing the foods specific for your blood type and avoiding those that are not, you could very well maximize your genetic potential. In addition, one could improve resistance to disease, slow and reverse the aging process, and enhance the body's natural tendency for achieving one's ideal height and weight.

Man Cannot Eat by
Blood Type Alone

As stated earlier, I have found that my patients' blood type is a critical component in the development of a successful diet plan. However, the problem with following a strictly blood type–based diet regimen, as prescribed by Dr. D'Adamo, is its lack of direction in the areas of: (1) achieving the proper balance of protein, carbohydrate and fat, (2) incorporating the energetic properties of Yin and Yang in relation to food, and (3) failing to fully acknowledge the issue of toxins in our food supply; again, some of the essential factors which were lacking in the Zone approach.

Man Cannot Eat by
the Zone Alone

Moreover, I have found that the 40-30-30 dietary approach, most commonly associated with the Zone, does not apply to every blood type. My research indicates that the balance of 30% protein, 40% carbohydrates, and 30% fat only applies to Types O and B. Types A and AB must follow a 25-50-25 percent dietary plan, i.e., 25% protein, 50% carbohydrate, and 25% fat. Consideration of these differences in the dietary balance of each blood type, plus the additional factors promoted in the New Millennium Diet, are *mandatory*, in my opinion, for achieving an optimum dietary plan paradigm.

The Final Step ... The New
Millennium Diet Program

The **New Millennium Diet** is a program for a lifetime of healthy eating, not just for quick weight loss. It has been designed to incorporate the best of past and present dietary technology for maximum synergistic effect. It will consider you as a unique individual with special needs. You will see that you are following a systematic and scientific path toward total health, hormonal balance, fat loss, and longevity. Applying the concepts outlined in the New Millennium Diet will allow you to accomplish the following:

- Achieve your desired body weight by decreasing your body fat percentage while increasing your lean muscle mass.

- Enhance your immune system and protect you from many of the new, resistant strains of bacteria, viruses, and exotic infections now on the increase throughout the world.

- Reduce the risk of developing serious diseases such as cancer, diabetes, and cardiovascular illness.

- Slow down the aging process by reducing the rate at which cell degeneration occurs while facilitating the repair of damaged tissues caused by poor dietary habits.

- Reduce your level of stress by eating good foods that calm rather than agitate the body.

- Achieve maximum sexual potency for a lifetime.

By following this new dietary approach, you can enter the new millennium with a body slim, fit, vital, and worthy of admiration ... a strong immune system ... a mental perspective that will give you a cutting edge advantage in all aspects of your life. ■

CHAPTER 2

Your Blood Type Is the Key… Individuality

The First Piece of the Puzzle

Elixir of Life

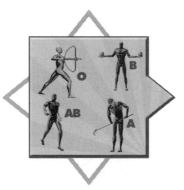

For ancient cultures, blood was regarded as a sacred symbol of life. Today, we know that it is the essence of life itself. Countless scientific investigators have reaped great discoveries about the nature of life by studying the composition and function of blood. The average adult has about five liters of blood coursing through his or her network of veins, arteries, glands and organs. Like a great delivery system, blood transports life-sustaining elements, moving essential nutrients from food and hormones from glands throughout the body. It delivers bacterial- and viral-destroying substances to tissues and removes harmful wastes and toxins. We are alive because blood carries oxygen from the lungs to the tissues, and carbon dioxide as waste from the tissues to the lungs. Blood is indeed the ultimate elixir of life.

Four Blood Type Antigens

The typing of blood plays a major role in understanding the mysteries of the human body, even helping us optimize our health and diet. To learn more about this, we first need to consider a few facts about antigens, which are specialized sugar or protein molecules. Antigens are found in all living things ranging from humans to amoebas. Antigens enable an organism's cells to identify and "mark" themselves as different or "nonself" substances that have entered the body.

Among the most significant antigens in the human body are the blood type antigens, present in the membranes of red blood cells. They are four in number, each with a unique chemical structure, and are known as A, B, AB, and O. These molecules, in fact, determine a person's specific blood type. If your blood type is A that means your blood contains antigen A. Type B's have antigen B. AB's have antigen A and B. People with O type blood, however, have technically no antigens associated with their red blood cells, except a sugar molecule known as fucose.

Blood type antigens represent a critical arm of the immune system. The body uses them to distinguish its own tissue from foreign antigens commonly found on bacteria, viruses, parasites, or food.

Most antigens are sugar molecules that combine to form distinctive antigen structures. The simplest of these sugars is known as fucose. It is found alone in Type O blood without any of the other biochemical substances that are combined into antigen complexes in other blood types. In A, B and AB types, fucose is used as a building block upon which other molecules are added to form more complex antigens. Blood Type A antigen is formed when the fucose is partnered with a sugar substance called N-acetyl-galactosamine. Type B is formed when fucose binds with another sugar called D-galactosamine. Type AB antigen results from fucose combining with N-acetyl-galactosamine and D-galactosamine. Illustration 2-1 shows the various blood type molecular configurations.

Illustration 2-1
Blood Type / Antigen Diagram

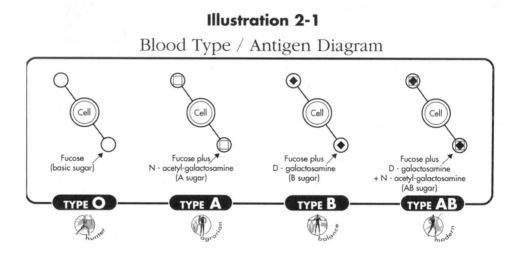

Within individual blood types there is an additional identifying element called the Rh factor. This relates to whether your red blood cells have certain special antigens. If they do, you are considered positive. If not, you are considered negative. For instance, you may be a blood Type A positive. There are some differences in acceptable foods between positive and negative persons who have the same blood type. We will cover those differences later in the book.

Evolution of Man's Four Blood Types

Blood type is critical in understanding how we have evolved, how we have adapted to changing environmental situations, and how food can impact our physical bodies, especially our organs, glands, and cells.

The human species evolved over a million years ago and is believed to have first appeared in Africa. The first real humanlike creatures, known as Neanderthals, emerged about 500,000 years ago. Prehistoric man's crude diet basically consisted of fruits, nuts, seeds, vegetables, and scavenged animals. Current ethnographic data suggests that primitive man's diet was made up of 35% plant material and 65% animal proteins.

Many of these foods contained a wide assortment of parasites, bacteria, and viral organisms which posed a threat to survival. Over time and continued exposure to these organisms, a process of survival of the fittest endowed the blood type with certain adaptation properties that essentially rendered individuals highly resistant to these threats. Adaptation to the environment can thus be slowly passed over many thousands of years to ensure the long-term survival of the species.

The development of human blood types is seen as correlating with the movement of the original humans from one climatic zone to another. As man's food supply and environment changed, the immune system and dietary functions had to adapt in order to survive this evolutionary process. The migration of people over time led to changes not only in blood type, but also in bone structure, skin color, eating habits, and other characteristics.

Blood Type "O" — The Hunter

 Blood Type O is considered to be the oldest type on the planet. Development of conscious thought and organized hunting moved the human species to the top of the food chain. Early man's use of tools and weapons, and the pursuit of game, furthered his expansion into new territories. Cro-Magnon man, appearing around 40,000 B.C., was an especially effective hunter.

Inadequate food supplies and poor weather conditions forced early man to continually migrate. The migration pattern is believed to have led out of Africa into Europe and Asia around 30,000 B.C. This allowed blood Type O to become well ingrained in the population, and is the reason why this is the most common blood type of modern civilization.

At the present time, it is estimated that Type O individuals make up 40–45% of the world population. The modern day blood Type O individual is genetically programmed to eat a higher protein–moderate carbohydrate diet. In addition, the digestive tract of such persons reacts poorly to dairy products and to wheat- and grain-based foods. If a Type O fails to eat in this manner, physical and mental health can be seriously compromised. This is why I recommend O blood types consume 30% of their calories in the form of protein, 40% in carbohydrates and 30% in fat.

Blood Type "A" — Agrarian

 It is theorized that blood Type A appeared somewhere in the Middle East or Asia sometime between 25,000 and 15,000 B.C., around the time of the Neolithic Period or New Stone Age. Some of the Type O hunters and gatherers evolved into Type A agriculturists because of unreliable food sources in the new areas to which they had migrated. The domestication of animals and the improvement in agricultural technique led to the cultivation of sustainable edibles such as grains, corn, and root foods. Man's digestive tract and immune system gradually adapted to these changes. While Type O was a meat eater, Type A thrived on a lower protein, near vegetarian diet. The only thing these blood types had in common was a poor tolerance to dairy products. Since Type A individuals require less protein than Type O's, my recommendation is 25% of their calories come from protein, 50% from carbohydrate and 25% from fat.

The changes in the style of living necessitated a new psychological and intellectual approach to survival. Realizing that certain foods grew better during certain climactic periods allowed Type A people to anticipate and plan their harvest times. The emergence of Type A occurred rapidly because of the need for adaptation and survival in a growing communal setting that produced greater infection and pollution than what was normally experienced by the roving Type O Cro-Magnon man. This adaptation to Type A appears to have endowed people with a higher resistance than Type O to diseases such as the bubonic plague, smallpox, dysentery, and typhoid fever.

Today, the Type A blood line is widely found among Europeans. Many Type A individuals are concentrated along the Mediterranean, Adriatic and Aegean Seas, particularly Spain, Sardinia, Corsica, Turkey and the Balkans. The Japanese population also has a high concentration of Type A individuals. At the present time, it is estimated that this blood type makes up 35–40% of the world population, making it the second most common blood type.

Blood Type "B" — Balance

 It is believed that the B blood type developed between 15,000 and 10,000 B.C., in the Himalayan Highlands, the area now known as India and Pakistan. The migration and intermingling of blood Types O and A led to the evolution of Type B. It is thought that Type B evolved as a result of harsh climactic influences. The mountainous regions of Pakistan and India are much colder compared to the unbearable heat of eastern Africa.

As Mongolian migration occurred throughout Asia, Type B was spread throughout the region. Domestication of herding animals was a characteristic trait of the Type B individual. The B in Type B stands for balance — the balance that exists between nature and civilization. People with this blood type are usually tolerant of a wide variety of foods. Type B individuals are found throughout China, India, Mongolia, Japan, and the Ural Mountains of Russia. Germans and Austrians also have high concentrations of Type B relative to their Western counterparts. At the present time, it is estimated that Type B accounts for 10–15% of the world population, the third most common blood type. Type B individuals require the same ratio of macronutrients as blood Type O individuals. Type B's should eat a diet consisting of 30% protein, 40% carbohydrate and 30% fat.

Blood Type "AB" — Modern

Blood Type AB is a more recent development. Essentially, it is the combination of blood from both blood Types A and B. This is believed to have occurred about 1,000 to 2,000 years ago, during the time the Mongol hordes were attempting to conqueror the Roman Empire and European civilizations. This is an uncommon blood type, which anthropologists have not found evidence of prior to 900 A.D. It is estimated that this type currently accounts for the remaining 5% of the world population.

It appears that Type AB's tend to have a greater ability to fight bacterial infections because of the mixing of both Type A and B immunological systems. Possessing this blood type possibly reduces the chances of developing allergies and autoimmune conditions such as rheumatoid arthritis, lupus and scleroderma. On the other hand, Type AB's have a greater chance of developing cancer because of the lack of specific antibodies required in the fight against this disease.

In terms of diet, Type AB resembles Type A, except that there is better tolerance to dairy products. Type AB's should consume 25% of their calories in the form of protein, 50% in carbohydrate and 25% in fat.

The concepts of migration and development of Type A from Type O and beyond are only hypotheses. They are not absolute explanations for the differences seen in the dietary characteristics of individuals with these blood types. However, we do know that blood Types O, A and B date back to very ancient times. The information encoded in each blood type, if it were possible to transcribe, would provide the correct genetic blueprint of the foods required to maintain our bodies in peak vitality and health.

The Immune System: Reaction to Foreign Antigens

Blood type is the critical aspect of our immune system function that allows our body to make determinations about whether or not we are being invaded by various microorganisms. If a foreign substance or antigen has entered our body, the immune system will attack it and remove it from the system. In certain situations when the system goes haywire, it can even attack itself. This is what commonly happens in autoimmune conditions.

Antibodies

The immune system appears to have an *intelligence* separate from the mind. It has the ability to determine subtle differences that exist within one substance that may be *foreign* to the body, versus a substance that is recognized as *self*. When foreign antigens enter our body, the first thing that the immune system does is produce specialized cells known as antibodies, which attack, destroy, and remove these foreign intruders from the body. The system has a capability to produce an enormous number of different antibodies, even if the alien substance has never before been detected in the body.

Tests using unknown materials from an asteroid, believed never to have been present on Earth, have proven this ability. When these substances were introduced into a human body, the immune system was able to identify these galactic foreign bodies and create an antibody specific to that substance. This suggests that the immune system can create countless combinations for the identification and destruction of any type of foreign invader.

Agglutination

The immune system not only has the ability to attack foreign substances that are non-living or unknown, it can also attack living foreign substances. This is the area where it performs the majority of its work: attacking microbes such as viruses and bacteria. When an antibody attaches to an antigen on any one of these microbes, it causes a clumping reaction known as agglutination to occur. Once this agglutination takes place, the body is then able to eliminate the microbe. Most microbes attempt to evade this type of attack by creating defenses against the antibodies or hiding within the immune system cells. The HIV virus is one of the best known for pulling off this masquerade.

Besides attacking microbes, antibodies can cause an agglutination reaction against certain types of foods. This agglutination can be seen in a microscope as a gluing together of red blood cells. When this happens, improper digestion has occurred, preventing the normal breakdown and assimilation of the food. In many cases, this reaction triggers an allergic response and eventually leads to other medical problems. Understanding how blood type antibodies react to various foods is vital for optimum health and well-being. This knowledge gives us a specific range of foods that offer good compatibility with our bodies.

Blood Donation

Blood type antibodies also explain why people require a specific type of blood when blood is exchanged between humans. This discovery was made by Dr. Carl Landsteiner, an Austrian physician, more than 100 years ago. He found that there were unique distinctions between people's blood. These differences had to be identified if blood transfusion were to provide life-saving benefit.

Subsequent medical research determined the specific facts concerning the exchange of blood. It was found that Type A blood carries anti-B antibodies, therefore Type A individuals reject blood Type B. Type B blood carries anti-A antibodies, therefore Type B individuals reject blood Type A. Consequently, Types A and B are unable to exchange blood.

Type AB blood does not have any A or B antibodies, therefore AB individuals can accept any other type blood without harm, since they carry both A and B antigens. However, Type AB blood would be rejected by all other blood types.

Type O blood carries anti-A and anti-B antibodies, therefore blood from a Type A, B, or AB individual would be rejected. A Type O person cannot receive blood from anyone else except another Type O. Type O individuals can give blood to all people, and are therefore considered to be universal donors. Table 2-1 shows these properties.

Table 2-1 Exchange of Blood Type

Blood Type	Antigens	Antibodies	Reject Type
O	No Antigens	Anti-A & Anti-B	A & B
A	A	Anti-B	B
B	B	Anti-A	A
AB	A & B	No Antibodies	None

The reactions that take place between different blood antigens are very powerful. In fact, they are so powerful they can be seen by the naked eye. *Foods contain antigens* that are similar to Type A or B antigens. Therefore, they have the same potential to cause severe reactions in certain blood type individuals. This explanation helps in the understanding of why certain foods are harmful to certain blood types, while being perfectly tolerated by another. One man's food is another man's poison. This old saying can now be scientifically understood.

Lectins: Key to Food Selection

Special Proteins

There exists in nature and in the foods we eat special proteins known as lectins. *The unique thing about food lectins is that they are very similar to the antigens that are associated with blood type.* Lectins can cause a tremendous amount of disturbance when exposed to the wrong person's blood. These proteins have powerful agglutinating characteristics, which can cause immune system dysfunction. They can also damage the delicate function of organ and glandular tissue.

Lectin disturbances are blood type specific. Scientists can determine which foods react with which blood type. This makes lectins an enemy within a person of an opposing blood type. For example, we know that dairy products tend to have Type B qualities. Therefore, if a person with either Type O or A blood drinks milk, the process of agglutination occurs. The agglutinated complexes could then develop in the intestinal tract causing damage to the intestinal lining. In addition, the complexes could be absorbed into the bloodstream where they can cause problems to organ or gland function.

Over a long period of time, this can lead to serious illnesses such as Crohn's disease, diabetes, kidney failure and cancer.

The interaction between food and blood dates back thousands of years into man's distant past. Unlocking these dietary truths can provide a key to the understanding of our ancestors' eating habits. This knowledge reveals the types of foods that can harm your body and the types of foods that can heal.

Common Diseases Associated with Incompatible Blood Type Food Choices

- **Allergies**

I believe lectins are one of the primary reasons why many people develop food allergies or intolerances. When "bad" lectins enter the body through foods, reactions usually occur if the liver, kidneys or immune system fail to remove these substances. We call the reaction an *allergy attack*. Repeated exposure undermines the body's ability to offset these toxins. Reducing the amounts of incompatible food lectins in the diet can reduce the number of allergens floating around in your blood. Allergens are substances that cause reactions, such as pollen and food that may be offensive to us. Reducing the lectins in turn reduces the release of histamines, and minimizes common allergic symptoms such as itching eyes, running nose, asthma and/or eczema. You must realize that the lectins, in and of themselves, are not necessarily bad. Rather, *it is the body's reaction to lectins that is the essence of the blood type–diet connection.*

- **Nervous System**

The nervous system is very sensitive to agglutinating lectins. I have seen people with Alzheimer's or Parkinson's disease make tremendous strides when certain lectins were removed from their diet. Significant improvement in mental functioning and nervous system control typically occurs within 3 to 6 months after starting the New Millennium Diet. Even hyperactivity disorders can be improved by removing agglutinating lectins.

- **Arthritis**

Studies have shown that rheumatoid arthritis can be induced by injection of certain toxic lectins into the knee joint of rabbits. Food allergies play a significant role in arthritic diseases. The nightshade plants, such as eggplant, tomatoes, potatoes, and bell peppers, have high levels of lectins. Their agglutinating effect on sensitive people can be very powerful. Readers with arthritis should immediately remove these kinds of foods from their diet and follow a strict blood type–compatible diet for maximum joint health.

Frequently, I have patients following the blood type–based diets who are still continuing to have symptoms. Such individuals may have unusual lectin–blood type incompatibilities that require further assessment. For these patients, I recommend a specialized blood typing panel test provided by Rockwood Natural Medicine Clinic in Portland, Oregon (Phone: 503-667-1961). This test can more accurately determine a person's blood type–food interactions.

Another procedure known as the Indican Test is one of the best ways to identify whether you may still have lectin incompatibilities, even though you have been strictly following an individual blood type diet. The test reveals toxic metabolites in the urine that occur as by-products of undigested and improperly metabolized proteins. These by-products build up in a person's body and then are excreted in the urine. If the person consumes too many toxic lectins, a level of toxic metabolites is registered. Based on the results of the Indican score, the appropriate dietary adjustments can be made to correct the problem. It could take several adjustments in order to optimize the diet for an individual.

Cultural Aspects of Blood

In 1980, Toshitaka Nomi wrote the book *You Are Your Blood Type,* which sold 6 million copies. The book profiled various blood type personalities. Even in different cultures, blood type has emerged as a factor to help in understanding how people think, how they feel, and how they act in certain situations. In Japan, for instance, an individual's blood type is given considerable importance. The Japanese term *ketsu-eki-gata* is used to define the type of analytic process conducted by corporations and businesses for determining the personality characteristics of their employees based on blood type. *Ketsu-eki-gata* is also used in market research to determine the buying habits of certain blood types.

Conclusion

Understanding our ancestral linkages to diet provides a partial explanation as to why lectins are important and why certain blood types have evolved. However, I do not believe that this gives us the complete answer. Anthropologically, a limited amount of information is available to document the lectin–blood type theory. However, more recent scientific studies involving the role of lectins in foods have clearly substantiated the fact that lectins can cause internal organ damage and eventually lead to disease.

My intention here is not to scare you from eating, but rather to drive home the point that certain foods can lead to disease, depending on your blood type. You need to avoid incompatible blood type foods, or at least reduce consumption of them, to maintain and improve your health.

Further, by understanding the interactions of lectins in foods and blood type, you can now begin to see how a synergism of many concepts is required to create an optimum dietary plan ... a giant puzzle of individual dietary pieces that must be identified and put into place before the whole picture is revealed. ■

Chapter 3: The Next Piece of the Puzzle ...

Macronutrient Balance — Enter the Zone!

CHAPTER 3

Zone and Macro-Nutrient Balance

The Second Piece of the Puzzle

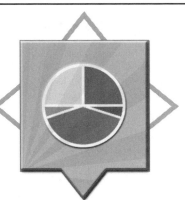

What Is the Zone Diet?

The idea of balancing dietary macronutrients — proteins, carbohydrates and fats — in a 40%, 30%, 30% ratio at each meal was popularized in 1995 by Barry Sears, Ph.D., in his national bestseller, *The Zone*. The plan allowed more protein and fat to be put back into our diets. This allowed us to reexperience the health benefits of eating the correct fats without causing heart disease or other fat-related problems. Sears's diet also pointed out that refined carbohydrates, such as white flour products, should be avoided, and that pastas, potatoes and cereals be consumed in moderation. Further, it revealed that these carbohydrates, which rapidly release their sugar contents in the body, cause increased insulin production and an excess accumulation of fat. These new ideas were revolutionary, going against the traditional dietary plans of the past.

The Zone concept received wide acclaim because it was fairly easy to use and worked for many people. One could easily determine daily protein requirements based upon lean body mass and an activity level factor, and use a unique conversion factor termed a *block* to help balance out the macronutrients in the recommended 40-30-30 ratio at each meal.

The 40-30-30 *balanced* approach prevented the development of cravings for sugar-containing foods because the ratio creates hormonal stability. Hormonal stability is extremely important for physical and mental well-being. However, the problem with the 40-30-30 ratio, as explained in Chapter 2, is that it works well for blood Types O and B, but not for Types A and AB. As a result of this difference, I have given the name *Macrobalance*™ to my newer approach which addresses the needs of all blood types.

Understanding Macrobalance™: The Basic Physiology of Hormonal Systems

It is important to understand the different hormonal systems in order to appreciate how diet has the potential to affect our bodies and why Macrobalance™ is essential for good health. These systems literally produce hundreds of different types of hormones which perform thousands of functions within our bodies each day. When the systems are in balance you feel well. When they are out of balance, medical problems often develop. Fundamental to the understanding of Macrobalance™ is the relationship of hormones within our body.

There are three main hormonal systems: the endocrine, paracrine, and autocrine systems. They provide the major chemical messengers which control almost every type of known body function. These hormones carry messages which usually evoke some type of action within a target cell or organ.

Endocrine Hormones

The endocrine system is a "long distance network" within the body. It allows for the relay of certain messages either from the brain or other glandular systems to distant cells and organs. The types of hormones that are secreted by the endocrine system remain for long periods of time within the bloodstream. This fact has made it relatively easy for scientists or physicians to measure and evaluate their function. As a result, there is a tremendous amount of data available on how these particular hormone systems operate.

Paracrine and Autocrine Hormones

Like the endocrine hormones, the paracrine hormones travel between the cells that secrete them and the cells they target for action. However, the paracrine hormones travel a shorter distance than endocrine hormones. In contrast to both endocrine and paracrine hormones, the autocrine hormones work directly on the cells that secrete them. These hormones feed back onto the cell that secretes them, thereby directly regulating their own action.

Scientists have very little time to obtain samples of the autocrine and paracrine hormones due to the shorter distances between the releasing cell and target cell. Therefore a limited amount of data is available on paracrine and autocrine hormones compared to the endocrine hormones. We do know that the short distances between the releasing and the target cell results in these hormones having a much greater physiological impact at much lower physiological concentrations.

Maintaining a balance of these three hormonal systems is important for good health. Volumes could be written on them. However, we will limit our discussion to the endocrine system hormones because of the key roles they play in dietary planning.

Endocrine Hormones: Insulin and Glucagon

Insulin and Glucagon Axis

Each of these systems has paired sets of hormones referred to as an axis. This means that certain hormones operate in pairs to produce opposite functions. In the endocrine system, for instance, a pivotal axis exists that involves the hormones insulin and glucagon. Knowing how these substances work is key to understanding how one enters a Macrobalance™ state. Insulin and glucagon play a vital role in controlling blood sugar levels, which is essential for optimum body and brain function. These hormones are also the key to unlocking your excess fat reserves and maintaining ideal body weight.

Insulin

Insulin is produced by the pancreas in response to elevated sugar (glucose) levels in the blood. It stimulates the liver and the muscle cells to store the excess sugar or use it for fuel. If glucose is not used as fuel, then insulin acts as a storage hormone converting the sugar from surplus dietary carbohydrates in order to be stored as fat in the body.

High insulin levels support increased fat storage, whereas low insulin levels reduce the amount of calories that are being stored as fat. This means that if you want to lose weight, you must reduce the amount of insulin released at each meal. You need just enough insulin to support the metabolism of glucose as fuel to meet bodily demands. Proper insulin levels also allow other hormones to function more efficiently, especially the female hormones that control PMS and fertility. However, when insulin levels are incorrect, numerous hormone imbalances can occur that cause excess weight, cancer, diabetes and other dangerous conditions.

Insulin resistance, a fairly common condition, occurs because of too much insulin in the body. This condition is known as hyperinsulinemia. In the face of constant excess insulin, the cells of the body simply don't respond to the hormone as they normally would. They lose their sensitivity to insulin and thus the hormone is no longer able to properly regulate blood sugar. In most cases, this situation causes a significant accumulation of excess body fat in addition to other types of hormonal disturbances.

Glucagon

Glucagon is the biological opposite of insulin. Instead of storing sugars it is considered a sugar mobilizing hormone. Glucagon initiates the release of stored glucose in the liver. Once glucose is released from the liver it enters the bloodstream where it helps to balance energy levels.

Hypoglycemia or Low Blood Sugar

Many Americans are affected by hypoglycemia, also known as low blood sugar. This condition frequently occurs after eating a meal high in carbohydrates or sugar. The flood of sugar in the body causes excess insulin to be produced by the pancreas. This rapidly drops the level of glucose, or blood sugar. The brain, which functions predominantly on glucose, now begins to lose its fuel source. The high level of insulin causes the sugar to be stored and used by the rest of the body instead of the brain. Consequently, the brain enters a dull, sleeplike state. This state of hypoglycemia or low blood sugar usually occurs within 15–30 minutes after eating a heavy sugar or carbohydrate-rich meal. The brain is not the only organ to be affected by these abrupt swings in blood sugar. Common problems associated with hypoglycemia include lack of energy, weakened immune system, glandular imbalances and weight gain.

When this hypoglycemic scenario occurs, and the blood sugar level of the body is low, the brain signals the body to consume more food in an attempt to restore the blood sugar to a normal level. Most people experience this as a craving for sugar or sweets. If the cravings are fulfilled, as they often are, people eat more sugar. This starts the cycle all over again. If the pancreas is thus stimulated to release insulin continually, insulin resistance or hyperinsulinemia can develop. It is evident that when this hypoglycemia cycle occurs, individuals consume a great deal of food in an effort to pacify their cravings. Consuming additional calories in conjunction with high levels of insulin results in excessive weight gain and, many times, in obesity.

Balance of Glucagon and Insulin

The body stores glucose as glycogen. Glycogen is a reserve energy source which is directly controlled by the hormone glucagon. When the body's demands for energy peaks, glucagon converts glycogen to an energy source usable by the body. The proper balance of glucagon and insulin is critical for overall hormonal balance and health.

The release of insulin is stimulated by glycemic foods, that is, predominately sugar-containing foods such as carbohydrates, bread, and pastas. Insulin, as we have noted, regulates the storage of excess sugars. Glucagon, stimulated by dietary proteins and physical exertion, causes a release of stored sugars, making them available for energy use by the body. The critical balance between glucagon and insulin depends on three things:

1.   The amount of calories consumed at the meal.
2.   The ratio of protein to carbohydrates.
3.   Whether or not the appropriate blood type–based foods are consumed.

To prevent the harmful hypoglycemic cycle previously described and to maintain the proper balance of glucagon and insulin, we must eat within the correct Macrobalance™. Utilizing the appropriate ratios of proteins, carbohydrates and fats, and ensuring they are blood type specific, allows us to appropriately regulate blood sugar levels, maintain proper insulin to glucagon balance, and eliminate cravings and abnormal hunger.

It is worth emphasizing that eating the wrong blood type–based foods can upset the delicate balance between insulin and glucagon. As we have seen in Chapter 2, this is due to the negative influence of lectins on the internal organs necessary for proper digestion.

Eicosanoids—Microscopic Hormone Regulators

The insulin-glucagon balance is critical for yet another reason. In 1982, the Nobel Prize for medicine was based on the early research into what are now known as eicosanoids (pronounced eye-kah-sah-noids). These little-known hormones, produced by the paracrine and autocrine axes, regulate either directly or indirectly every single significant body function. Until recently their short lifetime in the bloodstream prevented in-depth study. It was not until the early 1970s that researchers were able to begin looking closely at this class of hormones. This recent research has concluded that these hormones are made by every cell in the body and are extremely important when considering the effects of food on hormonal regulation.

Eicosanoids influence almost every system in the body, including the immune system, the central nervous system, the cardiovascular system, the reproductive system and the neuromuscular system. All these systems, in some fashion, are dependent upon eicosanoids for their intimate minute by minute cell processes. Some more common eicosanoids include prostaglandins, leukotrienes, lipoxins, thromboxanes, and hydroxylated fatty acids.

Eicosanoids: Check and Balance

There are two specific classes of eicosanoids, which act as a check and balance system among this group of hormones. This arrangement is similar to the check and balance effects found in the insulin-glucagon axis. However, unlike insulin and glucagon, minute disturbances in the eicosanoid balances are enough to lead to ill health.

Equilibrium in the functioning of bodily systems is the goal of the eicosanoid check and balance arrangement. For example, if too many platelets clump in the bloodstream, there is an increased risk of clots. If not enough platelets clump a person could bleed to death. "Good" eicosanoids prevent platelet aggregation. "Bad" eicosanoids promote their clumping. An imbalance in either of these two types of eicosanoids could result in a dangerous situation. This analogy between good and bad eicosanoids is also reflected in the concepts of yin and yang, discussed in Chapter 4.

Let's look now at how the balance between "good" and "bad" eicosanoids affects the immune system. Too many "good" eicosanoids can lead to a hyperstimulated immune system response, such as occurs in chronic fatigue immune system dysfunction. Too many "bad" eicosanoids can lead to a depressed immune response. Most diseases manifest because of an imbalance in eicosanoid harmony, including pain syndromes, inflammation, and high blood pressure.

Here, at a glance, are some of the characteristics of eicosanoids and how they are classified:

Good Eicosanoids	Bad Eicosanoids
• Inhibits platelet aggregation	• Increases platelet aggregation
• Enhances immune response	• Decreases immune response
• Prevents cell proliferation	• Increases cell proliferation
• Induces vasodilatation	• Promotes vasoconstriction

Food as a Hormonal Regulator

Understanding the effects of food on insulin, glucagon and eicosanoid activity within the body enables you to look at food as not just a source of fuel but also as a major factor in hormone regulation. Each and every meal we eat must be properly balanced so that the following four to six hours of physiological function will be optimally regulated.

Wellness is the optimum functioning of all bodily systems, and this functioning leads to a balanced mind, body and spirit. Most Americans today know little about wellness, and a lot about disease. They know little about the hormone systems and how food impacts these systems, creating either good or bad health. The New Millennium Diet is specifically designed to support these essential life-bearing systems. This systematic simplified dietary plan will help those individuals interested in obtaining peak performance and ideal health achieve their goal. Consequently, in order to have a thorough understanding of this plan so that it can be incorporated into our daily lives we must review the building blocks of our diet, the macronutrients.

The Macronutrients

Carbohydrates: The Unknown Fat Connection

What Are Carbohydrates?

Carbohydrates, the primary source of energy for all body functions, especially muscular contraction, are composed of carbon, hydrogen and oxygen. Immediate energy is provided by carbohydrates when carbon is combined with the oxygen in the bloodstream. Our main sources of dietary carbohydrates are vegetables, fruits, grains, and sugars.

Glycemic Index: Simple and Complex Carbohydrates

Carbohydrates are grouped into two basic categories, simple and complex. Such designations are primarily a function of the glycemic index of the particular carbohydrate molecule. The index allows us to determine precisely the rate that carbohydrates enter the bloodstream.

Complex carbohydrates enter the bloodstream at a slower rate and therefore have a lower score on the glycemic index. Simple carbohydrates and sugars enter rapidly and have a higher glycemic score. Many of the processed or refined carbohydrates are simple carbohydrates and have a high glycemic index. Refined carbohydrates such as white flour, pastas, white rice, white flour bagels and breads, and cereals have a very negative effect on our hormonal systems. These high glycemic foods work against the body's natural homeostatic patterns. In truth, they are harmful to the body if they form a regular part of the diet.

Complex carbohydrates are more complicated structures. They are slowly digested and break down into three simple sugars. These sugars are glucose, fructose and galactose. Glucose is found in cereals, breads, starches, pastas, grains and vegetables. Galactose is found in dairy products. Fructose is the sugar found in fruit. Fructose has the slowest rate of entry relative to glucose and galactose. Many fructose-containing foods contain fiber, a nondigestible form of carbohydrate.

Fiber, or roughage, makes up most of the material substance of carbohydrates and gives bulk to food. Fiber has no effect on insulin release. However, it does slow down the rate of carbohydrate entry into the bloodstream. In general, the more fiber present in a particular carbohydrate food, the lower its glycemic index, and the slower the rate of entry of its sugar components into the bloodstream. If there is no fiber in the carbohydrate food, then the glycemic index increases significantly.

Low-glycemic foods like proteins and fats are not rapidly converted into sugar and consequently do not cause rapid swings in blood sugar levels. Proteins and fats actually act as a buffer, shielding the potentially negative effects of certain carbohydrates. Fat is one of the best regulators of blood sugar levels, whereas proteins have more of a neutral effect. That is why it is imperative to eat some type of good fat along with every meal. This slows the entry of sugar into the bloodstream.

Foods, even if they score high on the glycemic food index, can be balanced in terms of their insulin-stimulating tendencies when placed in the proper ratio of proteins, carbohydrates and fats. If one were to eat a chocolate candy bar and add an adequate amount of protein and fat, the negative insulin-stimulating effects on the body would be significantly reduced. However, I do not recommend eating this type of food.

Glucose: Fuel for the Brain and the Body

When food is broken down in the digestive tract, glucose is the main sugar released into the bloodstream. High-glucose carbohydrates, such as refined flour, breads and pastas, are broken down rapidly, whereas the other two sugars — galactose and fructose — must first be converted into glucose prior to entering the blood. This conversion process takes longer.

Glucose is the main carbohydrate used by the brain for fuel. It is estimated that the brain, when at rest, uses approximately two-thirds of the carbohydrates circulating in the bloodstream. Stored glycogen is not available for use by the brain. The glycogen stored in the liver must be converted to glucose before it becomes available for use by the brain. However, the liver has a very small capacity to store carbohydrates as glycogen. After 10 to 12 hours, these reserves must be replenished; otherwise, a hypoglycemic or low blood sugar state will occur. Because of this potential, it is important to maintain a certain level of carbohydrates, not, however, the 60 to 65% of total calories as recommended by the American Diabetes Association. This amount is way in excess of bodily needs and much of it is put away by the body as fatty tissue. Even though carbohydrates are essentially **fat free**, they end up as excess fat in the body.

Table 3-1, the Glycemic Index chart, provides a number of common foods and their respective glycemic index. High glycemia is considered greater than or equal to 70%, moderate glycemia is equal to 40 to 69%, and low glycemia is 39% or less.

Table 3-1 Glycemic Index of Selected Foods

High Insulin Stimulators	Moderate Insulin Stimulators	Minimum Insulin Stimulators
> 100% Glycemic Foods Cold Cereals French Baguette Instant White Rice Maltose Millet	**60–69% Glycemic Foods** Apple Juice Apple Sauce Beet Bulgar Wheat Couscous Macaroni Pinto Beans Pumpernickel Rye Raisins Snickers Candy Bar Spaghetti Wheat Kernels	**30–39% Glycemic Foods** Apples Black-eyed Peas Breaded Fish Sticks Chick Peas Ice Cream Pears Skim Milk Tomato Soup Whole Milk Yogurt
100% Glycemic Foods Glucose White Bread Whole Wheat Bread		
90–99% Glycemic Foods Apricots Carrots Corn Chips Grape Nuts Parsnips Shredded Wheat Whole Meal Barley		**20–29% Glycemic Foods** Cherries Fructose Grapefruit Lentils Peaches Plums
	50–59% Glycemic Foods Barley Custard Dry White Beans Green Bananas Lactose Peas Potato Chips Sucrose Yams	
80–89% Glycemic Foods Bananas Brown Rice Corn Honey Mangoes Papayas Rolled Oats Rye Shortbread White Rice	**40–49% Glycemic Foods** Bran Butter Beans Grapes Lima Beans Navy Beans Oatmeal Orange Juice Oranges Peas Sponge Cake Sweet Potatoes Whole Grain Rye	**10–19% Glycemic Foods** Peanuts Soy Beans
70–79% Glycemic Foods Buckwheat Kidney Beans Oatmeal Cookies Wheat		

Fats: The Real Story

What Is Fat?

The fats we eat and the fat in our body are made up of three fatty acids and an alcohol molecule called glycerol. Depending on the number of fatty acids added to the glycerol molecule, fats are classified as monoglycerides, diglycerides or triglycerides.

There are a number of essential fatty acids, also known as EFAs for short. The most common belong to the omega family of fats. They consist of omega 3, omega 6 and omega 9 fatty acids, and include alpha-linolenic acid, linoleic acid and arachidonic acid. EFAs cannot be made by the body. They must be obtained from our food. Therefore it is imperative that we consume enough on a regular basis to meet our body's needs. The typical American diet is extremely low in valuable EFAs. Many of the low-fat diets hyped today are equivalent to nutritional suicide.

Essential Fatty Acids: Important for Health

Fat has gotten a very bad rap. Fats are essential for good health, necessary for the production of numerous hormones, membrane structures and blood vessels. They are extremely important for proper nerve conduction. They make up the myelin sheaths surrounding the brain and other nerve systems within the body. They are vital for the production of eicosanoids, the important hormones we just discussed. Fats also provide a large amount of stored energy, yielding approximately 9 calories per gram. Fats stimulate the release of cholecystokinin from the stomach, a substance that indicates to the brain that satiety has been achieved. Fats are also important in oxygen transportation, calcium absorption, and in the absorption of certain fat-soluble nutrients such as vitamins E, D, A, and K. Fats have a very positive effect on cellular structure, and specifically help to maintain cell membrane strength, integrity and resilience.

Good Fats vs. Bad Fats

Fats can be considered either good or bad. "Good fats" include olive oil, canola oil, flaxseed oil, hemp seed oil, fresh cold water fish oils, certain nut fats, seeds and avocados. These "good fats" generally tend to be mono or polyunsaturated fats.

Generally speaking, "bad fats" are those fats that are fried, oxidized, heat processed, or hydrogenated. Hydrogenation involves taking a "good" poly-unsaturated oil and bubbling hydrogen gas through it. This causes a restructuring of the oil's chemical bonds. Food manufacturers hydrogenate fats to delay rancidity (oxidation) and increase the shelf life of the product. Both heating and hydrogenation, however, create an unhealthy and dangerous oil known as a trans-fatty acid. Many foods now are made with these "bad fats." You see them as processed vegetable oils, margarine and vegetable shortenings. The major concern is that these unnatural trans-hydrogenated fats, derived from both partially hydrogenated oils and fully hydrogenated oils, are the main culprits in our concerns about fat. Not only do these trans-hydrogenated fats lead to both cancer and heart disease, but they have also been associated with accelerated aging, suppressed immune system function, and a reduced ability to absorb vital essential fatty acids.

Many potent chemicals and pesticides are stored in the fat of animals. The New Millennium Diet promotes the use of meat products for select blood types, but these meats should be lean and organically grown. Organically grown meats have the lowest exposure to environmental poisons and chemicals. Chapter 5 discusses the many poisons in our food supply and environment and gives specific recommendations on how to avoid them.

Saturated Fats Are Not Always Bad Fats

Saturation of a fat does not necessarily mean the fat is bad. Generally speaking, saturated fats have been believed to be "bad fats" because they reportedly cause hardening of the arteries and elevated cholesterol. But, according to Dr. Mary Enig, an expert on fatty acids, saturated fats do not actually cause heart disease. In her opinion, a great deal of propaganda has been circulated because of political and economic factors implicating saturated fats as one of the main factors in cardiovascular disease. Dr. Enig points out that in certain island societies where large amounts of fat are consumed, either in the form of coconut oil or palm oil, there is no significant increase in heart disease or other cardiovascular-related conditions.

Fat Does Not Make You FAT!

A misconception perpetuated by many modern weight loss programs is that fat makes you fat. This is far from the truth. Weight loss diets that are low in fat or fat free are harmful. These programs do not supply the body with the necessary essential fatty acids and over time can cause serious health problems.

A study in the 1950s, conducted by Kekwick and Pawan at the University of London, showed that fat is not the culprit in weight gain. Study participants were placed on a 1000-calorie a day diet which was extremely high in fat. Approximately 90% of the total calories came from fat. The participants on this high-fat diet lost considerable weight. A second group of participants were placed on a high-carbohydrate diet. Here, approximately 90% of their food was in the form of carbohydrates. This second group had no weight loss over the same period of time.

Permanent weight loss requires a diet which balances the macronutrients properly. Sufficient carbohydrate levels are vital for maintaining even blood sugar levels. A sufficient amount of dietary fat is also needed so that the body can maintain the overall health of the nerves, hormones and cell membranes.

Protein: The Amount Is the Key

Complete protein is necessary for sustenance of life. Protein provides the basic structural material for all living things. It is the main constituent in our body, second only to water. It is the principal ingredient in muscles, skin, hair, cells and enzymes. Proteins are composed of 22 amino acids, nine of which are considered essential, that is, they are not produced by our body and must be obtained from our food supply on a regular basis. If the body does not receive these necessary amino acids, the basic process of protein synthesis in the body is put in jeopardy and can cause a variety of serious health problems.

It is essential to eat the correct amount of proteins. A number of diets today call for high amounts of protein, thereby reducing the amount of carbohydrates. After considering carbohydrates and their ability to generate fat in our bodies, a high-protein diet may seem logical. When one undertakes a high-protein diet, initial positive results are indeed seen, but if maintained for an extended period of time the dieter can have serious consequences, including kidney damage and bone calcium depletion. In addition, high-protein dieters routinely regain the weight they lost and put on as much as 15% more weight than when they started the diet.

High-protein dieting leads to a metabolic state known as ketosis. It occurs when insufficient amounts of carbohydrates are eaten and the body attempts to inefficiently utilize fats for energy. Initially body water is lost. Here is the weight loss that people see. But then the body produces abnormal by-products known as ketone bodies, substances that cause a shift from a neutral pH to an acidic pH inside the body. Normally we function within a neutral pH range. Ketosis means the body is in an undesirable acidic state. This acidic state accelerates aging and disease.

A second problem that occurs from a high-protein diet is the creation of a large number of free-floating amino acids in the blood. Amino acids are the building blocks of protein. This development causes the body to produce insulin, which acts as an agent to convert the amino acids into fat. The process occurs in a similar fashion to the body's response to excess carbohydrates.

The third and most shocking problem of high-protein diets is the actual changes to fat cells exposed to excess protein conditions. Research is showing that fat cells are actually changed, that is, they have a greater tendency to accumulate fat. Fat cells thus get fatter, so to speak. This increased fat cell activity could be one of the reasons why individuals placed on high-protein diets eventually gain back more weight than when they first started the diet.

Extremism or excess is not a natural state for our bodies. Continuing on these types of programs can create great frustration and health problems. The body is designed to work within certain balanced parameters. The New Millennium Diet uses the Macrobalance™ approach to incorporate the correct ratio of carbohydrates, fats and proteins.

Balance is the key to diet, health, career and lifestyle. Macronutrient balancing supports the body's desired tendency to function in a neutral pH (healthful) zone. A strong immune system and cardiovascular systems are all dependent on having neutral pH blood. The New Millennium Diet is the way to get you there and keep you balanced for a lifetime. ■

Chapter 4: The Third Piece of the Puzzle ...

Age-Old Traditions: Yin and Yang, the Energy Concepts

Yin and Yang— The Energy Concepts

The Third Piece of the Puzzle

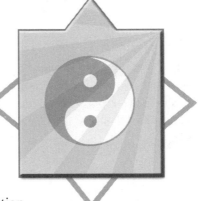

All movement, change, and interaction in creation are explained by the ancient Chinese concepts of Yin and Yang. Yang is the name given to energy that has an external, centrifugal, outward movement or expansion. Yin is the name given to the energy that reflects centripetal, inward, and contracting movements. The forces of Yin and Yang are basic primal substructures of all creation.

Everything in the universe is in unceasing motion. Life turns into death. Death into rebirth. Night changes into day. Activity changes into rest. Youth turns into age. Yin and Yang are the balancing of these universal forces as they appear on earth and in the biological world. Understanding them helps us achieve harmony with our immediate environment and with the universe as a whole. Psychologically, this condition of balance and harmony is called *happiness*. Biologically, we refer to it as *health*.

Yin and Yang are also known as unifying principals because they exemplify the relationship between what appear to be opposite forces, yet at the same time are complementary and unifying. One example of this is man and woman. Although they are opposite in many ways, they also have complementary needs including primordial needs that result in the perpetuation of the species.

In China, the universal process of change is known as Tao. Taoists base their teachings on the underlying principles of Yin and Yang. In Judaism, the principle of complementary forces is expressed by the symbols of the six-pointed star of David with its balances and intersections of descending and ascending triangles. The ancient Greek philosopher Empedocles envisioned the universe as an infinite playground of two opposite yet complementary forces he called *love* and *strife*.

In Western cultures, these similar thoughts and ideas have been expressed by many well-known philosophers. Ralph Waldo Emerson, one of America's greatest thinkers and writers, expressed the principle of Yin and Yang in his essay titled "Compensation." He wrote:

> Polarity, or action and reaction, we meet in every part of nature; in darkness and light; in heat and cold; in the ebb and flow of water; in male and female; in the inspiration and expiration of plants and animals; in the equation of quantity and quality in the fluids of the animal body; in the systole and diastole of the heart; in the centrifugal and centripetal gravity; in electricity, galvanism and chemical affinity.

The principles of Yin and Yang are now finding their way from ancient esoteric texts into our modern Western culture because the teachings are as true today as they were 4,000 years ago. Understanding the changes that govern our lives and our natural world, and recognizing the interconnectedness between these complementary and opposite forces, help us achieve a better balance of mind, body, and spirit … and ultimately our health and well-being. The principles of Yin and Yang, as they relate to the energy in food and one's health, are key components of the New Millennium Diet.

Yin and Yang — 4,000-Year-Old Ideas

The principles of Yin and Yang have been studied and practiced for more than 4,000 years by Chinese healers. In the last 30 years they have been applied in the United States and other countries of the Western world. A major aspect of these ancient teachings is the *Macrobiotic Diet,* which recognizes that certain inherent energetic qualities of food can generate beneficial or harmful changes to health and well-being. This system has enjoyed great success worldwide because of its emphasis on a balanced approach to diet and lifestyle. For some people, it has worked very well. For others, it is too demanding, with limitations that prevent wider acceptance. I believe that by including the concept of energetic qualities of food, a more comprehensive dietary program can be developed that will lead to optimum health. For this reason, I have added the principles of Yin and Yang to the concepts of blood type and Macrobalance™ in order to create the total synergistic foundation of the New Millennium Diet.

Divergent Concepts of Food and Medicine

Western vs. Chinese Food Selection

In Western culture, the selection of food is determined by the presence of proteins, carbohydrates, fats, vitamins, minerals and calories. Foods that contain similar amounts and portions of these macro and micro nutrients are considered equivalent in biological value. Considering only these nutrients, a bowl of fruit and nuts is the equivalent to a peanut butter and jelly sandwich. The same amounts of proteins, carbohydrates, and fats exist in both types of foods. We know, of course, that the first example — fruit and nuts — consists of natural food, while the second example is processed food. They will have different physiological effects in the body, but on a macronutrient level their contents are considered equal.

In contrast to selection of food based upon macronutrient levels, the Chinese tradition-based food selection rests upon Yin-Yang principles and specific characteristics of an individual. These considerations are further influenced by climate, season, disease condition, and genetics. Yin tendencies include the night, moon, cold and winter. Yang tendencies include the sun, daytime, heat and summer. All foods are classified into either Yin or Yang categories, with the understanding that these are relative classifications. All substances vary from a greater or lesser spectrum of Yin or Yang tendencies. In other words, no food, animal, or object can be totally Yin or totally Yang.

One example of Yin and Yang in nature are cooling Yin plants — which tend to grow in more hot, Yang climates, while denser, heartier, more Yang plants tend to grow in more temperate, Yin climates. This change within climatic zones helps us to understand the importance of balancing the Yin and Yang within our bodies. This balancing enhances our ability to adapt to local climates and conditions.

When it's cold, we turn the heat on. When it's hot, we turn the air conditioning on. These actions are based on an instinctual desire to maintain homeostatic order — a healthy comfort zone, so to speak — within our systems. Yin and Yang, as it relates to food, is another way we can achieve homeostatic balance internally. When one gets out of balance, that is, either becoming too Yang or too Yin, disease begins to occur.

Western vs. Chinese Medicine

In the West, we view the body like an automobile. The brain is our on-board computer… the heart is our engine…the veins and arteries the gas line … the legs the wheels … all wearing down with age. Our doctors are trained like mechanics to repair this machine. They wait for a problem to happen and then try to fix it. Their thinking is reactive rather than proactive. Disease is considered as a foreign invader that must be attacked and destroyed. We use a potent antibiotic to kill the germ or surgically remove the worn-out part. As a result, we are always looking for that *silver bullet* to cure every problem and restore the body to good working order.

In contrast, Chinese medicine looks at sickness from a different point of view. The Chinese ask the question: "Why was your immune system so feeble as to get sick to begin with?" If you keep your immune system healthy by eating the proper foods in relation to your personal characteristics then you should not get sick. Sickness is the sign that your system is out of balance. Only by bringing your system back into balance can you expect to get well. In Chinese culture and medicine, foods and herbs are considered to have a very significant influence on the body. They have the potential not only to affect deep internal change, but also the power to maintain good health and heal certain conditions.

Depending on the Yin or Yang nature of the food consumed, we can influence the tendencies of our organs toward health or ill health. If we eat too many Yang-containing foods, such as meats, eggs, and hard, salty cheeses, this creates an imbalance. The imbalance will cause cravings for sugary, stimulating or cooling foods, such as coffee, alcohol, ice cream, soft drinks and fruits, all which tend to be more Yin. This is the body's attempt to balance out the disturbed energetic state created by consumption of excess Yang foods. A swing from too much Yin to too much Yang over an extended period of time leads to disease and ill health.

An example of too much Yin food consumption would be a hangover following the consumption of too much alcohol. This leads to an expansion of the cells and swelling of the tissues within the brain. The resultant pressure within the head creates the headache. A headache from too much Yang could arise if one were to eat an excess of meat that the body did not properly digest. From these examples you can begin to understand why aspirin, a very Yin medication, doesn't work for every type of headache. It doesn't help certain headaches that are a result of too much Yin because it increases the Yin state.

The concepts of Yin and Yang food can also be understood in terms of hot or cold or, more accurately, warm or cool. Yin is the cool element, and Yang is the warm element. If a person consumes excess amount of foods that are warming and heating, he or she will have a warmer, more Yang body. Unfortunately, this can lead to disease. The same applies if a person has a colder body. If he or she eats a lot of cooling foods, then the body will continue to get colder. This, too, leads to disease. The hot or cold concept is not necessarily the actual feelings of heat or cold, but more just a general state within the body. Within the spectrum of food we eat is a whole range of food with values that are heating, cooling or neutral. The goal is to attempt to eat foods that are not at the extremes, unless there is proper balancing.

There are a number of other types of states that foods can evoke in our bodies, depending upon whether they have certain characteristics such as damp, dry, strong, or weak. Food has a powerful effect on the human system, as we discussed in the section on foods and hormones, and through the understanding of these ancient Chinese concepts, we appreciate that the energy of foods can also have a dramatic impact on our bodily function. So, the old adage "you are what you eat" can now be appreciated for its full meaning.

Being too Yin is bad, just as being too Yang is bad. Maintaining a balance and harmony of the Yin and Yang energetic properties of food in relationship to one's individual characteristics is essential to happiness and good health.

The New Millennium Diet recognizes and understands the importance of the balance of Yin and Yang within food and within our own human bodies. This concept enables us to achieve a greater degree of true dietary balance.

The Body's Constitution in Relation to Yin or Yang Food

The constitution we inherited at birth contains tendencies toward being either more Yin or more Yang. While each person's constitution is unique and individual, there are many factors that can alter the general constitutional state during the course of a lifetime. They include eating the wrong foods, use of drugs, lifestyle, certain mental and emotional conditions, physical habits and attitudes. These factors create excessive Yin or Yang energies which then unbalance and interfere with one's God-given constitutional state.

In fact, the basis for disease, such as physical and mental imbalances, can be related in one form or another to either excessive Yin, excessive Yang, or a combination of both, in food choices, attitude, and lifestyle.

These principles also apply to herbs, nutrients, chemicals, and any other types of substances to which we are exposed. Exposures can be both endogenous or exogenous. Endogenous means that they occur inside the body. Exogenous means they occur outside the body. If a person has low energy and frequent colds, and has been given warming herbs and a balanced diet, yet fails to heal after weeks or months of taking the appropriate herbs and diet, one has to suspect this person might be consuming the wrong foods for his or her constitutional state. One of my patients, as an example, was consuming excess fruits and juices in the belief that they were healthy and good for him. Technically these foods are healthy, but they were too Yin for his constitutional state. They caused poor digestion, decreased immune function, fatigue, and excess mucous production. When these foods were eliminated, his health improved significantly. This shows how consuming the wrong energetic foods can be detrimental to your body's constitutional state.

Therefore, if we can determine a person's present constitution and state of health we can utilize the Yin and Yang qualities of food to balance out the natural and/or altered constitutional excesses or deficiencies.

Table 4-1 lists excess Yin symptoms and Table 4-2 presents excess Yang symptoms. Review these lists and determine which of these symptoms apply to you. Add up the total number of symptoms in each category to help you establish whether your constitution tends to be more Yin or more Yang.

Table 4-1 Excess Yin Symptoms

- Aversion to cold
- Clear discharges either in urine, stool, or nasal secretions
- Cold extremities
- Coldness
- Craving heat
- Diarrhea
- Excess need for sleep
- Frigid appearance
- Slowness, lethargy
- Very little sweating or no sweating
- White-tongue
- Any bloody discharge in stool or urine
- Aversion to heat
- Bloody noses
- Burning digestion
- Constipation
- Cravings for cold foods or drinks
- Dark and scanty urination
- Dryness internally or externally

Table 4-2 Excess Yang Symptoms

- Lack of circulation
- Loose stools
- Low blood pressure
- Moist tongue
- No thirst
- Pale
- Poor appetite
- Poor digestion
- Slow pulse
- Fast pulse
- Fever, increased thirst
- Infections
- Inflammations
- Irritability
- Red face or eyes
- Red tongue
- Strong appetite
- Sweating easily
- Thick and hot feeling of excretions
- Yellow coated tongue
- Yellow mucus in the stool or urine

Neutral/Balanced Constitution

If none or just a few of these symptoms applied to you, then you have a neutral or balanced constitution. This is the optimum level you want to achieve. People with this constitution usually experience less disease and maintain a higher degree of health through their life than those who are at either one of the extremes.

Yin Constitution

If the greater number of the Yin symptoms applied to you, then your constitution tends to be more Yin. You want to place an emphasis on consuming more Yang food to balance out the Yin excess. An extreme of these symptoms signifies poor health. It is associated with coldness and tends to cause sedation and a reduction of body movement because there is lack of internal heat, usually associated with fatigue and weakness.

Yang Constitution

If the greater number of the Yang symptoms applied to you, then your constitution tends to be more Yang. You should emphasize eating more Yin food to balance out the Yang excess. An extreme of these symptoms also signifies poor health. It is associated with heat and extreme activity in the body, with a tendency towards restlessness.

In many cases, you can minimize or even eliminate the symptoms described above by bringing balance back into your food, according to the Eastern tradition. That means eat more Yin foods if you have an excess of Yang, or eat more Yang foods if you have excess of Yin. If you are suffering with more serious conditions, I would recommend that your Yin/Yang food prescriptions be determined under the advice of an astute practitioner who understands the art of Chinese medicine.

By knowing your specific constitution you can make the proper adjustments in the foods you consume, the herbs you take, and the nutrients that you utilize. This will help you to rectify your inherited and/or altered imbalances, and bring them into a healthy balanced range. I consider this energy balance to be part of the overall *Macrobalance™ concept*.

Thus, *Macrobalance™* in my opinion is not simply a matter of understanding the ratio of protein, carbohydrates, and fats. It also requires an understanding of Yin and Yang, and how blood type–compatible foods either hinder or enhance the pursuit of balance. If you are too Yin or too Yang, you are outside of the *balance*, and need to consume the proper foods to help bring you back into the correct energetic state.

New Millennium Diet Use of Yin and Yang Food Groups

You now have an idea of how the energy in food can influence our internal organ function, constitutional states or disease states. If one desires to be appropriately fit and have a low body fat percent and a high lean muscle mass percent for one's gender, age, or fitness level, it is vital to incorporate the energetic qualities of foods, as well as the appropriate macronutrient ratios.

I'm now going to discuss in some detail how we use the energy of food in the New Millennium Diet. Graph 4-1 shows the Yin and Yang food groups we will apply in our plan. You will note that most Yang foods tend to be protein-based foods, whereas most

Yin foods tend to be more carbohydrate and fat based. The protein-based foods are more Yang than carbohydrate-based foods because plants tend to be eaten by animals, which concentrate the energy. We have categorized and assigned a numerical rating (score) to these food groups.

At this point of the discussion, I am assuming that you have read Chapter 2 and know your blood type, and that you know your constitutional state, that is, whether you tend to be more Yin or Yang. Knowing these factors about yourself will enable you to more fully relate to the last part of this chapter. Let's review the Yin and Yang food groups in more detail.

Graph 4-1 Yin and Yang Food Groups

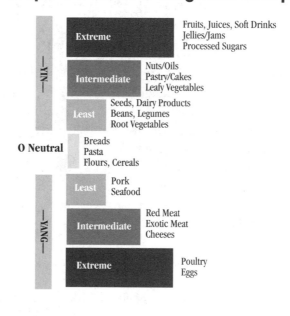

YIN

Extreme	Fruits, Juices, Soft Drinks / Jellies/Jams / Processed Sugars
Intermediate	Nuts/Oils / Pastry/Cakes / Leafy Vegetables
Least	Seeds, Dairy Products / Beans, Legumes / Root Vegetables

0 Neutral — Breads / Pasta / Flours, Cereals

YANG

Least	Pork / Seafood
Intermediate	Red Meat / Exotic Meat / Cheeses
Extreme	Poultry / Eggs

YIN FOOD GROUP	NEUTRAL FOOD GROUP	YANG FOOD GROUP
• Extreme Yin Food Score = -3	• Yin or Yang Score = 0	• Extreme Yang Food Score = +3
• Intermediate Yin Food Score = -2		• Intermediate Yang Food Score = +2
• Least Yin Food Score = -1		• Least Yang Food Score = +1

Extreme Yin Food Score = -3

All sugars, fruits, jams, juices and candies are in this category. The same rating has been given to sugar whether raw or processed.

If eaten in excess, these foods can do the following: lower body strength and resistance; cause loose stools and diarrhea; recurrent cold and flu; poor digestion; excess mucus; chronic asthma and other lung problems; low back pain and sciatica; impotence and infertility.

Eating too much fruit or fruit juices can cause excessive dampness in the body leading to an excessive Yin state. If you are suffering with systemic candidiasis, consuming excess amounts of fruit can be detrimental to your recuperation, since fruits can be rapidly converted into sugar, which feeds yeast. The excess Yin makes the yeast grow more rapidly because it affects the spleen, a vital organ that keeps candida in check.

All soft drinks, ice creams, pastries, cakes and related products should be avoided, not only because they contain a lot of sugar, but because they are also excessively Yin. Sweet-tasting diet drinks are just as bad for the body. Even if they have no calories, they have extreme Yin.

Intermediate Yin Food Score = -2

All leafy vegetables, as well as nuts, oils and other fats, are in this category. Leafy vegetables include lettuce, spinach, kale, and mustard leaf. Cooking these vegetables will make them less Yin. Eating them raw will allow one to fully access their Yin energies. Many people mention the importance of eating raw vegetables in order to benefit from their high enzyme content, but I've seen many sick people eating a predominately raw vegetarian diet who are just as sick as those who are strictly meat and potato eaters.

Too much raw and excessively Yin foods tends to thin the blood, cool the body down, and slow metabolism. This impedes digestive function and assimilation, and can lead to aches and pains, stiffness, anemia, arthritis, gas, bloating and lethargy. The most important thing to do is to try to individualize your eating habits and bring them into a balanced state for your particular genetic makeup, constitution, and blood type.

Oils and other fats include butter, canola, peanut, coconut, corn, hemp seed, cotton seed and olive oils, cream cheese, lard, and vegetable shortening. I consider olive oil the most desirable and peanut oil the least desirable of all the oils.

Least Yin Food Score = -1

The foods in this category include dairy products, seeds, beans and root vegetables. The term dairy products applies to all kinds of milk, yogurt and sour creams. It excludes hard, soft or salty cheese and egg products, which are in the Yang group. Milk can cause excess mucus production and poor digestion, especially in those blood types that are sensitive to milk, namely O and A. Many children are allergic to milk because of blood type incompatibility. B and AB types are better adapted to dairy products.

The seeds include flax, poppy, pumpkin, sesame, sunflower, and watermelon. The beans and legumes include all types from azuki to white. Beans contain protein; however, in our diet plan, we consider them to be carbohydrate-based foods. The root vegetables include beets, broccoli, carrots, eggplant, potatoes, peppers, sweet potatoes and many others.

Extreme Yang Food Score = +3

The foods in this category include poultry and eggs. These foods, like the -3 Yin foods, are considered extreme. They must be balanced with the opposing food; otherwise, if eaten too frequently without the appropriate balancing, the body will become ill.

Intermediate Yang Food Score = +2

The foods in this category include meat of both domestic and exotic types. The domestic meats include beef, internal organs, veal, lamb and mutton. The exotic meats include alligator, buffalo, ostrich, rabbit, rattlesnake and venison. I recommend that if you eat meat, you always use a little bit of raw ginger root. This helps to improve the digestion of meat and to facilitate the elimination of toxins that may come from this food.

I have seen many people who are vegetarians their entire life become significantly healthier and stronger when they begin to eat small amounts of meat. I have also seen other people who are consuming too much meat and who are blood Type A individuals become much healthier and stronger when they eliminate meat.

Excess meat consumption, especially in an A or AB blood type individual, can often lead to health problems. They include gout, rheumatism, constipation, hypertension, arthritis, stroke and cancer. That's why meat needs to be tempered by the appropriate amount of Yin foods, such as fruits, vegetables, and nuts, which are carbohydrate- and fat-based foods and which are required for proper Macrobalance™.

Least Yang Food Score = +1

The foods in this category include seafoods such as fish, abalone, clams, crayfish, eel, frog, lobster, oyster, shrimp, squid and pork.

Neutral Yin or Yang Food Group Score = 0

The foods in this category include grains, cereals, breads, pasta, and flours. They have no Yin or Yang tendencies in our context. However, it is important to note that grains were only introduced approximately 10,000 years ago during the agriculture revolution. People with Type A were the predominant blood type that emerged from that particular time period. Type A individuals do well on these foods. Others do not and have trouble with excess amounts of grains, especially wheat. Type O individuals, for instance, are extremely allergic to wheat.

Summary

The foods we eat slowly shift our body's constitution. If we eat too much of Yin food or too much of a Yang food, then that energy will push the body in a specific direction.

Hopefully, it's in the direction of balance; however, this is frequently not the case. If you eat a standard American diet, it's most definitely not the case.

What I ask of my patients, and what I'm asking of you in the New Millennium Diet, is if you're going to eat Yang or heating foods, then make the appropriate adjustments and eat a sufficient number of cooling or Yin foods to balance out any excess. This is especially true when you eat the extreme Yin or Yang foods. You cannot consume an excess of one type and hope to remain in balance. It is important to consume an adequate amount of low to intermediate Yin foods and similar Yang foods but, when one eats in the extreme, balance the effect with the opposing food.

If you eat too many Yang foods you will tend to develop congestion, a red neck and face, irritability, a loud voice, aggressive behavior, constipation, and toxicity in the blood and organs. These are warning signs of imbalance. If you eat too much of Yin food, you will tend toward poor digestion, gas, bloating, back pains, low immunity and resistance, poor mental acuity and focus, and excess body fat. For good health, your foods must be appropriately balanced. Frequent consumption of imbalanced foods is an invitation for disease. All factors must be accounted for, otherwise subtle imbalances will catch up with you over the course of a lifetime.

Our goal is not to make this complicated but to provide a simplified approach so that this plan can be easily incorporated into one's daily life. The systems that will be described when we bring the entire New Millennium Diet into focus will be simple enough for you to follow, yet comprehensive enough to achieve the desired results. In Chapter 7, I will show you how to use your Yin and Yang scores in planning a proper diet. In Chapters 8 to 11 you will find food charts for your specific blood type. They will designate the Yin or Yang score for each specific food. With them you will easily be able to balance each meal you eat.

Chapter 5: The Final Piece of the Puzzle ...

Toxins in Our Food

Hidden Food Toxins Identified

The Final Piece of the Puzzle

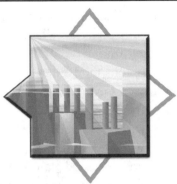

Chemicals are an important part of our modern age. They're used to produce plastics, paints, carpets, insecticides, pesticides, and today are used in the production of engineered foods. This huge introduction of chemicals over the course of the last 75 years has helped society in many ways but has also placed a huge burden on our physical and cellular systems. It is estimated that cancer has increased 1,500% since the time that America's first forefathers touched foot on this land. At the turn of the century, approximately 1 out of 33 deaths could be attributable to cancer. That's approximately 3% of all deaths. Presently, cancer strikes 1 out of every 4 American men and 1 out of 5 women.

There are a number of reasons why this large increase has occurred. High among them is the proliferation of chemicals in our food, air, water, and the environments in which we live and work.

Farmers today have some 60,000 to 70,000 different pesticide formulations available for use in order to eradicate insects, weeds, mold and fungi. These chemicals accumulate in the soil and over the course of decades accumulate to levels that can become toxic for both humans and animals. In addition, farmers use a wide variety of unique nitrogen-based fertilizing additives to enhance the growth and productivity of their crops.

Researchers investigating the health of prehistoric man have found only isolated evidence of cancer. The disease was statistically nonexistent 10,000 years ago and beyond. For one thing, the levels of toxic metals in prehistoric man compared to levels in modern man's tissues are significantly different. So-called toxic metals, such as lead, aluminum, cadmium and mercury are dangerous to the body of humans and animals at high levels. They have become much more prevalent in the environment in modern times due to their widespread use in industry. There is now, for instance, ten times the levels of lead in modern-day humans compared to our prehistoric ancestors.

Cancer has become a modern-day plague. Is there any greater indicator of that than among children today? Anthropologists have found no evidence of cancer among pre-historic children. Today it is widespread, indicative of our growing environmental contamination. The proliferation of chemicals and heavy metals is causing the body to break down at earlier ages. In addition, we see fetal cancers also increasing at a rapid pace. I believe that the consumption of toxic foods plays a major role in this startling development. There are literally hundreds of different chemical formulations found not only on the outer surface but also in the inner matter of food.

No dietary plan can call itself complete unless these issues are addressed. "The Zone," "Eat Right 4 Your Type," and "Macrobiotics" all fail to acknowledge the large numbers of truly poisonous foods that lie on our supermarket shelves. The New Millennium Diet goes one step further than these programs. It identifies the hidden toxins in foods and ranks them according to their severity.

This chapter will categorize foods according to the amount of toxicity they contain — low, intermediate or high. These differences are taken into account as I lay out the New Millennium Diet's food plan. Many foods that have in the past been considered acceptable because of a low glycemic index rating or for their blood type compatibility may actually be foods that have too large a toxic burden. Such foods are thus banished from consideration as a most beneficial or most favorable listing to an unfavorable listing.

Peanuts, for example have been considered to be highly compatible with A blood type individuals, but peanuts are probably one of the most toxic foods in the entire United States food supply. How can peanuts or peanut butter be included in a most beneficial listing if they contain over 180 different chemical formulations and residues? They cannot. That's why I have moved them down to the least beneficial listing. Organically grown peanuts merit a higher rating. I place them in a neutral position. Not higher than that, however, because peanuts are associated with serious mold infestations. One type of mold produces aflatoxin, a substance as toxic as the chemical dioxin, used in Agent Orange.

In my opinion it is crucial to take such chemical factors into consideration as we move into the New Millennium. Compared to our ancestors, we live in a completely different state of environmental conditions. This is why I believe it is necessary to purchase organic foods whenever possible. However, it can sometimes be difficult to obtain 100% organically grown foods.

If organic foods are unavailable, I highly recommend that food washes, available in many stores, be used to help remove as much toxic material as possible that is present on the surface of food. As I have stated, many times these toxins penetrate the skin of produce and are thus present in the meaty part of the food. This cannot be washed out, another reason why organically grown food is preferable to nonorganic.

Tap water is another source of contamination. Unless you have some sort of purification system in your home, simply washing food from the kitchen faucet may just add more chemicals to the food. I recommend that you obtain either a reverse osmosis system or some other type of effective home water purification unit to ensure that your family has clean, pure water. I would like to say that many of the inexpensive carbon filters on the market are truly inadequate for removing many chemical compounds. Carbon filters are fairly effective at removing chlorine, and help improve the taste of the water. But commonly found chemical compounds such as PCB, DDT, and dioxin can often pass through the carbon matrix. My choice is an advanced reverse osmosis system that can reduce the parts per million of toxins and other water constituents down to an extremely low level, somewhere around 10–15 parts per million. This is considered to be almost completely pure water. ProSana offers a multi-phase reverse osmosis system that provides this high degree of purification. Refer to the information at the end of the book.

It is up to each of us to take responsibility for our own health by striving to eat the highest quality and purity of food. The government has done little to reduce or control the levels of pesticides and other toxic chemicals in our foods, and has been much too lenient on the food industry. The Environmental Protection Agency, when it makes its evaluations of what are acceptable levels of toxins in foods, assesses each pesticide or chemical individually. However, each food contains more than a single toxin, and when we partake of a particular food we are likely ingesting a variety of substances that may have a different toxic nature when combined. Singling out individual chemicals, in my opinion, is a statistically inaccurate way of assessing the potential overall toxicity and carcinogenicity of an individual food. This system is in much need of improvement.

The foods you will find listed here in the most toxic category typically have 50 or more toxic residues or chemical substances, as determined by the FDA's Total Diet Study in 1986. Moderately toxic foods have anywhere from 20–50 toxic residues and the least toxic category usually has less than 10 such substances per food.

Cancer is one of many diseases that can be traced to toxins in our food supply. Others include degenerative brain disease, such as Parkinson's, Alzheimer's disease and dementia.

One widely publicized contaminant is aluminum, a metal known to interfere with nerve conduction in the brain, as well as in the peripheral nervous system. Growing health problems related to aluminum are thought to parallel its increased use during the last 100 years in the production of cookware, baking powders, antiperspirants, and even certain types of cheeses. High levels of this particular element are found in patients who have died of Alzheimer's disease. Using aluminum cookware, or even storing food in aluminum foil, especially if the food has a powerful acidic nature, can potentially leach aluminum into the food.

Dementia can also be traced to toxins that have built up in the brain tissue itself, leading to reduced brain cell activity. Mental retardation and low IQ scores in children could be associated with lead toxicity. A mother's exposure to lead or other chemicals before and during pregnancy, or afterward if she is breast feeding, could contribute to these conditions.

Coronary heart disease can be related to high levels of chlorine that get converted to chloramines when reacted upon by ultraviolet radiation. Elevated levels of PCBs and other toxins in the body have been connected in several studies to heart disease and hypertension. Chemicals place a huge burden on the liver, the organ that detoxifies and eliminates toxins and their by-products from the body. The liver becomes overstressed from excess exposure to toxic substances, leading to an increased production of cholesterol and other forms of fatty materials. The liver is also involved with regulating glycogen, insulin levels, and sugar levels in the body. A liver that is unable to store glycogen or regulate insulin levels effectively can contribute to the development of excess fat storage in the arteries as well as in the fatty tissues of the body.

Parkinson's disease may also have a connection to toxic chemicals, and specifically to the use of certain fungicides. These compounds are very fat soluble, and when they enter the body they can be deposited in the myelin sheaths, the fatty substance surrounding the nerve cells in the brain. Over the course of 20–30 years, this may lead to the tremors and limb rigidity seen in Parkinson patients.

There has been a huge increase in the number of patients suffering with chronic fatigue syndrome and environmental illnesses throughout the world over the last 25–30 years. I believe this is related to the large amount of chemicals not only found in our food supply but in our day-to-day environments — our homes, workplaces, automobiles, and even health clubs. People tend to spend most of their time inside some man-made structure. Many of these structures can be regarded as "sick buildings." They may have windows that do not open in order to improve the thermal efficiency and reduce heating and cooling costs, or they may have poorly maintained or inadequate ventilation systems.

Modern-day buildings contain hundreds of different chemical compounds that are used in the manufacturing of pressed plywood, carpets, draperies, roofing systems, and other cleaning agents. The polyvinyl flooring known as linoleum used throughout the world, for instance, is a major source of volatile compounds that are released into the air. Until the volatile gases have been sufficiently released from new linoleum, sensitive individuals may experience burning or itching sensations, and allergy-like symptoms. The closed environment of the home significantly reduces the escape of these noxious gases, literally causing months and potentially years of exposure. Many doctors have had a significant increase in the number of patients complaining of chemically induced conditions. Unfortunately, many have little knowledge about toxicology or industrial pollution so they are not able to offer much assistance to such patients.

The International Institute for Bau-Biologie and Ecology in Clearwater, Florida, is an organization dedicated to educating people about health hazards existing in the home and workplace. Ignorance of these hazards, the institute says, not only has an adverse effect on individual health but also on the health — and survival — of the planet. The Institute utilizes advanced knowledge developed in Europe over the last three decades to help people overcome such hazards when constructing or remodeling houses. For further information on Bau-Biologie and other ideas for maintaining a healthful living environment call (727) 461-4371.

Chemicals in our homes, buildings and food supply are not our only environmental problems. Electromagnetic fields bombard our immune system on a daily basis. EMF, as these fields are called for short, emanate from cellular phones, electrical appliances, computers, and even the electrical components in our cars. While numerous studies have been unable to fully implicate EMF as a potential health risk factor, many physicians throughout Europe have recognized this as a problem for decades.

The information you've just read should not depress you. It should alert you. I want to reinforce the fact that there are still plenty of healthy, nontoxic, and safe foods available in nonorganic markets. Combining these safe foods with the knowledge you are gaining now of blood type, Macrobalance™, and Yin and Yang energetics, will provide you with a new and protective dietary strategy not presently available elsewhere.

The remainder of Chapter 5 includes Chart 5-1, Commonly Found Chemical Pesticides, a "short list" of potentially toxic chemicals. These 42 chemicals are commonly found today in a variety of areas, but the most alarming is in our food supply. Following this chart, beginning with Table 5-1, I provide a listing of specific foods and their respective toxicity rating, low, intermediate or high. This rating is dependent upon the amount of chemical toxins found in the food. A great deal of the information in these tables was provided by the USDA Food Safety and Inspection Service.

As you review the toxicity ratings of these foods feel free to refer back to Chart 5-1, Commonly Found Chemical Pesticides, for a more detailed explanation of a particular chemical.

Chart 5-1 Commonly Found Chemical Pesticides

Pesticide	Use and Possible Hazard
Acephate	Insecticide used on citrus crops.
Aciflurofen	Herbicide used on rice, soybeans and peanuts. Dangerous carcinogen.
Alachlor	Herbicide. Human carcinogen.
Alar	Regulates growth, used on peanuts and apples from 1967–89. Carcinogen.
Aldicarb	Used on potatoes. Possible carcinogen.
Atrazine	Herbicide. Injures the adrenal glands.
Azinphos-methyl	Insecticide. Neurotoxin.
Baygon	Insecticide.
Benomyl	Fungicide. Carcinogen. Decreases sperm count.
Benzene	By-product of petroleum refining. Neurotoxin.
Bromacil	Herbicide.
Butylate	Herbicide. Possibly carcinogenic.
Butylated Hydroxyanisole (BHA)	Food preservative. Neurotoxin.
Butylated Hydroxytoluene (BHT)	Food preservative. Neurotoxin.
Captan	Fungicide. Serious contaminant of strawberries.
Carbaryl	Insecticide used on thousands of different crops. Carcinogenic.
Carbofuran	Pesticide. Accumulates in wildlife, especially birds.
Carbon Tetrachloride	Used in the production of chlorofluorocarbons which are refrigerants. Carcinogenic.
Carbophenothion	Used as an organophosphate pesticide.
Chlordane	Pesticide used in in-home fumigation. Can cause mutagenicity.
Chlorothalonil	Fungicide. Damages the thyroid and liver.
Dacthal	Herbicide. Possible dioxin contamination.
DDT	Insecticide. Banned but still shows up in our food supply and water supply.
Diazinon	Used on golf courses. Insecticide.
1,2-dichloroethane	Multiple uses. In particular, it is used to make vinyl chloride. Mutagenic and carcinogenic.
Dioxin	Insecticide 500,000 times more toxic than DDT. Carcinogen and mutagenic.
Fonofos	Insecticide.
Heptachlor	Insecticide
Lindane	Insecticide. Used in many shampoos, especially for lice, ticks and scabies. Possible carcinogen.
Malathion	Pesticide. Neurotoxin.

Methidathion	Pesticide. Associated with known birth defects.
Methylparathion	Insecticide.
Nitrate and Nitrite	Results from nitrogen-containing fertilizers and animal waste. Converts to nitrosamines in the stomach.
Parathion	Organophosphate pesticide.
Pentachlorophenol	Wood preservative. Fungicide and pesticide.
Phosmet	Pesticide. Carcinogen.
Styrene	Used to make styrene plastics. Neurotoxin.
Tetrachlorobenzenes	Industrial contaminant that affects our food supply.
Toluene	Used to produce benzenes, solvents, paints, resins and gasoline. Carcinogen.
Vinyl Chloride	Used to make plastics, rubbers, glasses and paper.
Volatile Organic Chemicals (VOC)	Toxic compounds found in drinking water.
Xylenes	Solvents, paints and adhesives. Carcinogen.

Food Toxicity Tables 5-1 through 5-7

Meat, Poultry and Exotics

Many people are aware of the large amounts of antibiotics being fed to our cattle, pigs, fowl, and now even to some buffalo and ostriches being raised for their meat. Sulfa drugs, as well as other chemicals and hormones, are also fed to livestock in order to compensate for poor management practices or bad environmental conditions. These are chemical measures taken to minimize bacterial infections and reduce the incidence of animals dying from disease before they are slaughtered. Such practices, however, lead to significant bacterial resistance that can be passed along to the human consumer.

Residues of various sulfa- and penicillin-based drugs are showing up in larger and larger levels in the animals evaluated by the FDA. It is estimated that 97% of all hog producers rely on feed medications to maintain their herds. This is only one of the reasons why eating pork can be a toxic experience. Outside of the fact that pork contains very bad lectins for all blood types, it also contains very high levels of antibiotics and other chemical residues which can seriously poison the human metabolic system.

It is estimated that between 40–95% of all chickens now raised in captivity are being fed antibiotics and other drugs to improve their appearance, increase their weight, and reduce the level of disease that occurs because of mass farming techniques. Somewhere in the range of 45–70% of all cattle that are now raised are given antibiotics and hormones in order to improve their size and appearance, and reduce the level of disease. It has also been noted that sulfamethazines as well as other antibiotics can have toxic effects on the human thyroid gland tissue. This could be one of the reasons why so many more thyroid cancers have developed since the beginning of the antibiotic era. Many people also suffer from sulfa allergies. Many individuals who experience reactions after eating pork or ham could be possibly reacting to the sulfa component of the residual antibiotic found in the meat. USDA meat inspectors are overwhelmed with the level of work that they are confronted with on a daily basis. Literally hundreds of millions of animals are slaughtered and taken to market yearly, and only a small fraction of them are actually examined and analyzed for bacteria, toxins, or chemical residues. This reality, therefore, places the burden on consumers to prevent or reduce their level of chemical exposure.

In addition to antibiotics, hormones are also being excessively used for livestock in order to reduce the fat percentage of the meat and to accelerate growth rate. Many of these hormones can pass into the milk of the farm animal and, in the case of bovine milk sources, this can be consumed by children who are very sensitive to hormonal excesses in their bodies. In some Third World countries, children under the age of 10 years who have been exposed to high levels of estrogen have been documented to have developed breasts and even pubic hair. Excessive hormones were found in the milk, eggs, and meat of farm animals raised in those countries.

Recently, the FDA approved the use of radiation in the United States to eliminate *E. coli* and other dangerous bacteria that could be harbored in meat. Radiation can harm the inherent nutrient quality of the meat as well as potentially expose consumers to low levels of radiation. Food poisoning of this nature could pose risks for the young, the elderly, and immunologically suppressed individuals. Better cooking methods would be more appropriate than the mass exposure of the nation's meat supply to radiation.

The purchase of organically grown meat, poultry, eggs, and milk would be a wise decision on the part of the consumer. This will send a message to the mass producers of meat who use antibiotics, hormones and other chemicals in their husbandry methods. Perhaps it may reduce this unhealthy practice. Organic meats, of course, still contain some toxins that are part of the natural setting, but such products are free of antibiotics and hormones, and the chemical pesticides typically found in the grains fed to the animals. The overall quality and taste of the meat is significantly improved when organically grown and processed.

Table 5-1 Meat, Poultry and Exotics

Table 5-1 (a) Low Toxicity—Meat, Poultry and Exotics

Food	Chemical Contaminants	Safest Source	Toxic Source	Toxic Residues
Alligator Meat	Methylmercury	Farm raised	Fresh water	1
Buffalo Meat	Chlordane, DDT, Some Sulfa Antibiotics	Free range	Commercial	6
Chicken	DDT, Dieldrin, Heptachlor, HCB, Penta	Organic	Commercial	42
Duck	Chemical-free	Free range	Commercial	Less than 1
Frog Meat	Chemical-free	Fresh	Commercial	Less than 1
Goose	Chemical-free	Free range	Commercial	Less than 1
Lamb Chops	BHC, DDT, HCB, Octachlor	Organically Raised or Free Range	Commercial	49
Pork Roast	DDT, Penta, HCB	Organic	Commercial	19
Rabbit	Chemical-free	Free range	Commercial	Less than 1
Reptile—Rattlesnake	Chemical-free	Free range	Commercial	Less than 1
Turkey	DDT, Dieldrin, HCB, Penta	Organic	Commercial	9
Turtle Meat	Chemical-free	Farm raised		Less than 1
Venison—Domestic	Chemical-free	Domestic	Imported	Less than 1
Venison—Imported	Radiation	None	Imported	Less than 1

Table 5-1 (b) Intermediate Toxicity—Meat, Poultry and Exotics

Food	Chemical Contaminants	Safest Source	Toxic Source	Toxic Residues
Beef Round Steak	BHC, DDT, HCB, Octachlor	Organic	Commercial	39
Fried Chicken	DDT, Dieldrin, Heptachlor, HCB, Penta, Malathion	Organic	Commercial	44
Ham	HCB, Lindane, Toxifene, diphenyl 2-ethylhexyl phosphate	Organic	Commercial	21
Pork Chops	BHC, DDT, Diazinon, Dieldrin, HCB, Lindane, Sulfamethazine	Organic	Commercial	28

Table 5-1 (c) High Toxicity—Meat, Poultry and Exotics

Food	Chemical Contaminants	Safest Source	Toxic Source	Toxic Residues
Bacon	DDT, Dieldrin, Lindane, Octachlor, Penta, BHC, Heptachlor, HCB, Methoxychlor	None	All	48
Beef Hot Dogs	BHC, DDT, Dieldrin, Heptachlor, HCB, Lindane, Penta, Octachlor	Organic	Commercial	123
Bologna	PCBs, BHC, DDT, Dieldrin, Heptachlor, HCB, Lindane, Octachlor, Penta	None	All	102
Ground Beef	BHC, DDT, Dieldrin, Heptachlor, HCB, Octachlor	Organic	Commercial	82
Liver	HCB, Octachlor, Penta, Dieldrin, Heptachlor, DDT, BHC	Organic	Commercial	49
Pork Sausage	DDT, BHC, Dieldrin, Heptachlor, HCB, Lindane, Octachlor	None	All	71
Roast Beef	BHC, DDT, Dieldrin, Heptachlor, HCB, Octachlor	Organic	Commercial	52
Salami	HCB, Lindane, Octachlor, Heptachlor, BHC, DDT	None	All	98
Top Sirloin Steak	DDT, BHC, Dieldrin, Heptachlor, HCB, Octachlor, Diazinon	Organic	Commercial	49
Veal	HCB, Lindane, Octachlor, PCBs, Toxaphene	Organic	Commercial	47

Dairy Products

Blood Type A and O individuals have sensitivity to dairy products due to a lectin incompatibility. For all types, however, there is potential risk from the high levels of various chemicals and hormones commonly found in dairy. These substances include DDT, dieldrin, heptachlor, HCB, BHC, chlordan, and bovine growth hormone, which are basically passed from the animal into the milk, and of course, then on to our grocery shelves. Many mothers feeding their infants whole milk or evaporated milk instead of human breast milk are doing their tots a serious disservice because of this high level of contamination. I recommend that organically produced milk be used if your blood type allows you to consume dairy products. Cheeses are some of the most toxic foods that are known. The hard cheeses and American cheeses are laced with various chemicals and bacteria.

Table 5-2 Dairy Products

Table 5-2 (a) Low Toxicity—Dairy Foods

Food	Chemical Contaminants	Safest Source	Toxic Source	Toxic Residues
Buttermilk	DDT, Penta	Organic	Commercial	3
Margarine	PCBs, HCBs	None	Domestic	19
Milk (low to nonfat)	DDT, Dieldrin, BHC	Organic	Commercial	19
Yogurt (low to nonfat)	DDT, Penta	Organic	Commercial	6

Table 5-2 (b) Intermediate Toxicity—Dairy Foods

Food	Chemical Contaminants	Safest Source	Toxic Source	Toxic Residues
Ice Milk	BHC, DDT, Dieldrin, HCBs, Heptachlor, Penta	None	Commercial	35
Milk Shakes (commercial)	BHC, DDT, Malathion, Penta	None	Commercial	23
Yogurt with Fruit	DDT, Endosulfan, Vinclozolin	Organic	Commercial	32

Table 5-2 (c) High Toxicity—Dairy Foods

Food	Chemical Contaminants	Safest Source	Toxic Source	Toxic Residues
Butter	BHC, DDT, Heptachlor, HCB, PCBs, Lindane	Organic	Commercial	101
Cheeses (hard)	DDT, Dieldrin, Heptachlor, HCB, Octachlor, Penta	Organic	All Others	100
Cottage Cheese	HCB, Penta, Heptachlor, Dieldrin	Organic	Commercial	49
Eggs	DDT and other various antibiotic residues	Organic	Commercial	Not Available
Ice Cream	DDT, HCB, Heptachlor, Dieldrin	Organic	Commercial	81
Milk (evaporated)	Dieldrin, Heptachlor, HCB, Penta, Malathion	None	Commercial	49
Milk (half and half)	HCB, Octachlor, PCBs, DDT, BHC	Organic	Commercial	66
Milk (whole)	HCB, DDT, BHC, Lindane, Octachlor, Bovine Growth Hormone	Organic	Commercial	29

SEAFOOD

Seafood has rapidly replaced red meat and other meat products as the food of choice over the course of the last 10–20 years because of the concerns about red meat and heart disease. However, many fish contain serious levels of mercury, pesticides and other toxic substances. Agrochemical runoffs have created widespread contamination of rivers, lakes, and other waterways. Toxic elements such as mercury, DDT, PCBs, and dioxins are all found in high levels in certain classes of fish. Differentiating between fish that are safe to eat and the ones that should definitely be avoided is vital if you are concerned about protecting your health.

Seafood in general has many positive attributes. It is high in omega-3 fatty acids, which are vital for improving our cardiovascular system, enhancing our skin and muscle tone, and reducing body fat. It possesses a low amount of Yang energy, and is generally an acceptable food for all blood types, with a few exceptions.

It is especially important to know where the seafood you eat originates. For example, the Great Lakes have had serious troubles with contamination in certain species of fish. Similar hazards have been publicized in relation to fish caught near large cities, such as in Santa Monica Bay or Boston Harbor. Even though these fish may not be listed in the most toxic category, they can still contain high levels of pollutants because of the chemical runoff in coastal waters. The farther offshore the fish are caught, the safer the fish is to eat. Also, fish that are caught off New Zealand, Mexico, and Central and South America all tend to be very safe and clean.

Table 5-3 Seafood

Table 5-3 (a) Low Toxicity—Seafood

Food	Chemical Contaminants	Safest Source	Toxic Source	Toxic Residues
Abalone	Chemical-free	All Sources	None	N/A
Arctic Char	Chemical-free	Canada	Domestic	N/A
Blue Crab	Chemical-free	Puerto Rico	Domestic	N/A
Catfish	Chemical-free	Brazil, Thailand	Midwestern Rivers and Eastern Rivers	N/A
Caviar	Chemical-free	Canada	N/A	N/A
Cod	Chemical-free	New Zealand, Denmark	N/A	N/A
Crab	Chemical-free	N/A	Chesapeake Bay	N/A
Crawfish	Chemical-free	Louisiana	Arkansas	N/A
Dover Sole	Chemical-free	France, Korea, Netherlands	California, Washington	N/A
Flounder	Chemical-free	Netherlands, Mexico, Argentina	N/A	N/A
Grouper	Chemical-free	Argentina, Chile, Mexico	N/A	N/A
Haddock	Chemical-free	United Kingdom, Canada	N/A	N/A
Halibut	Chemical-free	California, Alaska	Los Angeles	N/A
Mahi-Mahi	Mercury Accumulator	Florida, Hawaii	N/A	N/A
Marlin	Mercury Accumulator, otherwise chemical-free	California, Alaska	N/A	N/A
Menpachi	Chemical-free	Hawaii	N/A	N/A
Monkfish	Chemical-free	New Zealand, Thailand	N/A	N/A
Mullet	Chemical-free	Mexico, Thailand	N/A	N/A
Octopus	Chemical-free	Hawaii, California	N/A	N/A
Orange Roughy	Some preservatives which people could be allergic to, otherwise chemical-free	N/A	N/A	N/A
Red Snapper	Chemical-free	N/A	N/A	N/A
Pacific Salmon	Chemical-free	Alaska, California, Oregon	N/A	N/A
Scallops	Chemical-free	N/A	N/A	N/A
Sea Bass	Chemical-free	N/A	N/A	N/A
Sea Urchin	Chemical-free	N/A	N/A	N/A
Shrimp	Chemical-free	N/A	N/A	N/A
New Zealand Mussels	Chemical-free	N/A	N/A	N/A
Sole	Chemical-free	California, Washington	N/A	N/A
Spiny Lobster	Chemical-free	Australia, New Zealand, California	N/A	N/A
Squid	Chemical-free	N/A	N/A	N/A
Tilapia	Chemical-free	California, Puerto Rico	N/A	N/A
Tuna	Basically chemical-free, but is a mercury accumulator	California	N/A	N/A
Wahoo	Chemical-free	Mexico	N/A	N/A
Yellowtail	Chemical-free	Pacific Ocean	N/A	N/A

Table 5-3 (b) Intermediate Toxicity—Seafood

Food	Chemical Contaminants	Safest Source	Toxic Source	Toxic Residues
Angel Shark	DDT, Mercury Accumulator	N/A	N/A	N/A
Barracuda	DDT, PCBs	N/A	Pacific Ocean	N/A
Benito	DDT, PCBs	N/A	California	N/A
Butterfish	BHC, DDT	N/A	Virginia	N/A
Cod	DDT	N/A	California	N/A
Norwegian Salmon	BHC, Lindane, PCBs	N/A	N/A	N/A
Ocean Perch	DDT, PCBs	N/A	California	N/A
Rainbow Trout	DDT, PCBs	N/A	Colorado, Missouri	N/A
Smelt	DDT, PCBs	N/A	Oregon, Canada	N/A
Thresher Shark	DDT, Mercury Accumulator	N/A	Canada	N/A
Trout	BHC, DDT, PCBs	N/A	New Jersey	N/A

Table 5–3 (c) High Toxicity—Seafood

Food	Chemical Contaminants	Safest Source	Toxic Source	Toxic Residues
Black Cod	DDT	N/A	California	N/A
Bluefish	DDT, Chlordan, Monachlor, PCBs	N/A		N/A
Carp	PCBs, BHC, Chlordan	N/A	Arkansas, Michigan, Wisconsin	N/A
Catfish	PCBs, DCPAs, DDT, BHC, Chlordan	N/A	Midwestern and Eastern Rivers, including farm-raised catfish	N/A
Chub	Dieldrin, Dioxin, Endrin, HCB, Heptachlor	N/A	Wisconsin, Michigan, Ohio	N/A
Cod	DDT, PCBs	Imported	Domestic Sources	N/A
Coho Salmon	BHCs, Chlordan, DDT, Dioxin, HCB	N/A		N/A
Croaker	DDT, Dioxin, PCBs	Imported	Domestic Sources	N/A
Eel	BHC, DDT, Dioxin, HCB, Mercury Accumulator	None	New Jersey, New York, Canada, Japan	N/A
Freshwater Bass	PCBs, DDT	N/A	Great Lakes	N/A
Lake Trout	DDT, Chlordan, BHC, PCBs		Great Lakes	N/A
Lobster	Saturated with PCBs	California or Imported	Maine or Massachusetts	N/A
Mackerel	PCBs, BHC, Chlordan, DDT	None	New York	N/A
Northern Pike	Serious Mercury Accumulator	None	Midwestern States	N/A
Sea Herring	DDT, B131 Chlordan, BHC	None	United States	N/A

Shark	Saturated DDT, PCBs, Mercury Accumulator	N/A		N/A
Striped Bass	DDT, BHC, Chlordan, PCBs, Mercury Accumulator	None	Sacramento, San Francisco, Northeastern States	N/A
Sturgeon	BHC, Chlordan, DDT, Dioxin	None	Illinois, Minnesota	N/A
Swordfish	DDT, PCBs, Mercury Accumulator	None	Domestic and Imported	N/A
Wheat Fish	DDT, HCB, Chlordan	None	New York	N/A
Whitefish	Dioxin	None	Pennsylvania, Canada	N/A
Yellow Perch	Dieldrin, Dioxin, Endrin, HCB, Heptachlor	None	Pennsylvania	N/A

Sushi

I enjoy sushi and know many patients and friends who enjoy it as well. However, sushi does contains a number of parasites. There are risks.

The safest bet is to avoid sushi altogether, but this is probably asking too much of sushi aficionados. A good idea is to eat all of the raw ginger that accompanies the sushi. The ginger may kill some of the parasites and bacteria that could be present with your fish. Ginger also helps settle the stomach, and this can be beneficial in case there are any toxins that might irritate the sensitive stomach lining.

How can you tell if you have eaten contaminated sushi? Common reactions include gastrointestinal symptoms that develop the next day or within a week. Symptoms include severe gas, bloating, abdominal cramping, loose stools alternating with constipation, and possibly liver pain. The liver is located in the right upper quadrant of your abdomen. Headaches, fevers, or chills could also occur. I would like to mention that eating ceviche, which is raw fish that has been marinated in lime or lemon juice, can also be a source of parasites. The lime juice does not sufficiently kill parasites that may be present.

Table 5-3 (d) Sushi

Safest Sushi	
Seafood	**Japanese Sushi Term**
Albacore	Maguro
Octopus	Tako
Red Snapper	Tai
Scallops	Hotategai
Sea Urchin	Uni
Shrimp	Ebi
Yellowtail	Hamachi
Sushi to Avoid	
Herring Roe	Kazunoki
Mackerel	Saba
Salmon	Sake

The following Food Toxicity Tables 5-4 through 5-7, Grains, Cereals and Breads; Fruits and Vegetables; Oils; and Condiments are the last of the food groups and provide a thorough listing for each category. For further details on Food Toxicity contact the New Millennium Medicine Institute at (800) 969-9914.

Table 5-4 Grains, Cereals or Breads

Table 5-4 (a) Low Toxicity—Grains, Cereals or Breads

Food	Chemical Contaminants	Safest Source	Toxic Source	Toxic Residues
Corn Bread	DDT, Penta	Organic	None	32
Cornflakes	Malathion, Penta, Diazinon	Organic	None	10
Farina	EDB, Malathion	Organic	None	21
Granola	Chlordane, Heptachlor	Organic	None	27
Grits (Hominy)	Malathion, Tributylphosphate	Organic	None	15
Oatmeal	Tributylphosphate, Diazinon, Malathion	Organic	None	24
Pasta	Malathion, Diazinon, Chlorpyrifos	Organic	None	10
Popcorn	EDB, Penta, Dieldron	Organic	None	12
Rice	Diazinon, Methoxychlor, Penta	Organic	None	18
Rice Krispies, Cereal	Malathion, Tributylphosphate	Organic	None	31
Tortillas	DDT, Diazinon, Malathion	Organic	None	34

Table 5-4 (b) Intermediate Toxicity—Grains, Cereals or Breads

Food	Chemical Contaminants	Safest Source	Toxic Source	Toxic Residues
Rye Bread	BHC, Dicloran, Lindane, Parathion, Penta, Tributylphosphate	Organic	Commercial	49
White Bread	Diazinon, Malathion	Organic	Commercial	44
Whole Grain Muffins	DDT, Malathion, Penta	Organic	Commercial	46
Whole Wheat Bread	Fenitrothion, Malathion, Tributylphosphate	Organic	Commercial	49

Table 5-5 Fruits and Vegetables

Table 5-5 (a) Low Toxicity—Fruits and Vegetables

Food	Chemical Contaminants	Safest Source	Toxic Source	Toxic Residues
Alfalfa Sprouts	Chemical-free	Organic	None	none
Apple Sauce	Carbaryl	Organic	None	13
Asparagus	DDT, Dicloran	Organic	None	minimum
Avocados	Penta	Organic	None	2

Azuki Beans	Chemical-free	Organic	None	none
Bananas	Chemical-free	Organic	None	none
Bean Sprouts	Chemical-free	Organic	None	none
Beets	DDT, Dieldrin	Organic	None	2
Black-eyed Peas	Pentachloroaniline, Parathion, Lindane	Organic	None	18
Brussels Sprouts	Traces of DDT	Organic	None	minimum
Cabbage	Diazinon, Dicloran, Dieldrin	Organic	None	7
Carrots	DDT, Linuron	Organic	None	32
Cauliflower	DDT, Diazinon	Organic	None	3
Chives	Chemical-free	Organic	None	none
Corn	Diazinon	Organic	None	2
Cranberry Juice	Chemical-free	Organic	None	none
Dates	Chemical-free	Organic	None	none
Figs	Malathion	Organic	None	minimum
Grape Juice	Carbaryl, Dimethoate	Organic	None	16
Grapefruit	Ethion, Malathion	Organic	None	16
Guavas	Trace of Dimethoate	Organic	None	minimum
Hazelnuts	Chemical-free	Organic	None	none
Lemons	Chlorpyrifos, Thiabendazole	Organic	None	3
Lentils	Chemical-free	Organic	None	none
Lima Beans	BHC, Penta, Toxaphene	Organic	None	19
Limes	Trace of Ethion	Organic	None	minimum
Mushrooms	BHC, Penta	Organic	None	31
Navy Beans	BHC, Diazinon	Organic	None	2
Onions	Chemical-free	Organic	None	none
Oranges	Carbaryl, Dicofol	Organic	None	23
Papayas	Chemical-free	Organic	None	none
Peaches	Dieldrin, Dimethoate	Organic	None	14
Pears	Methamidophos	Organic	None	1
Peas	Acephate, Diazinon	Organic	None	12
Pecans	Malathion, Diazinon	Organic	None	14
Pineapple Juice	Chemical-free	Organic	None	none
Pineapples	Chemical-free	Organic	Mexico	none
Pinto Beans	BHC, Penta	Organic	None	2
Radishes	DDT, Toxaphene	Organic	None	32
Rapini	Chemical-free	Organic	None	minimum
Red Beans	BHC, Dieldrin	Organic	None	7
Sesame Seeds	Trace of Endosulfan	Organic	None	minimum
Shallots	Chemical-free	Organic	None	none
Snap Green Beans	DDT, Endosulfan	Organic	None	34
Beans	Methamidophos	Organic	None	2
Sunflower Seeds	Chemical-free	Organic	None	none
Tangerines	Ethion, Thiabendazole	Organic	None	minimum
Tomatoes	Carbaryl, Endosulfan	Organic	None	13
Watercress	Chemical-free	Organic	None	none
Watermelon	HCB, Dicloran	Organic	None	10

Table 5-5 (b) Intermediate Toxicity—Fruits and Vegetables

Food	Chemical Contaminants	Safest Source	Toxic Source	Toxic Residues
Apple Juice	Carbaryl, Dimethoate	Organic	Imported	15
Apples	DDT, Dicloran, Dicofol, Phosalane	Organic	Domestic or Imported	80
Apricots	Captan, Carbaryl, Fenthion	Organic	Domestic or Imported	7
Artichokes	Endosulfan	Organic	Domestic or Imported	1
Blackberries	Rovral, Dinclozolin	Organic	Domestic or Imported	4
Blueberries	Captan, DDT, Botran	Organic	Domestic or Imported	4
Cantaloupe	Dicofol, Dimethoate, Toxaphene	Organic	Mexico	58
Celery	DDT, Diazinon, Dicloran	Organic	Domestic or Imported	78
Cherries	2,4-dichloro-6-nitrobenzenamine, Acephate, BHC	Organic	Commercial or Domestic	61
Cherry Tomatoes	Chlorothalonil, Endosulfan	Organic	Domestic	5
Chile Peppers	EBDCs, Parathion	Organic	Commercial	2
Choysum	Malathion	Organic	Commercial	1
Collard Greens	DDT, Dicloran, DCPAs, BHCs	Organic	Commercial	87
Cranberries	Chlorothalonil, Malathion, Parathion	Organic	Commercial	7
Crenshaw	Endosulfan	Organic	Commercial	2
Cucumbers	Dieldrin, Endrin, Heptachlor	Organic	Commercial	67
Eggplant	Dimethoate, Permethrin	Organic	Commercial	4
Escarole	Dimethoate, Permethrin	Organic	Commercial	2
Grapefruit Juice	Chlorobenzilate, Ethion	Organic	Commercial	32
Grapes	Captan, Omethoate, DDT	Organic	Mexico and Chile	63
Green Bell Peppers	Acephate, Chlorpyrifos, Omethoate	Organic	Commercial	83
Honeydew Melon	Dimethoate, Chlorothialonil, Endosulfan, Omethoate	Organic	Commercial	2
Jalapeno Peppers	Acephate, BHC, DDT, Ethion	Organic	Commercial	14
Kale	DCPA, DDT, Permethrin	Organic	Commercial	5
Kiwi	Phosmet, Vinclozolin	Organic	Commercial	3
Leeks	DCPA, Quintozene	Organic	Commercial	2
Lettuce	Acephate, Methamidophos	Organic	Commercial	36
Lima Beans	Dicofol, DDT, DCPA	Organic	Commercial	41
Mung Beans	Lindane, Malathion	Organic	Commercial	5

Nectarines	Diazinon, Dicloran, Phosmet	Organic	Commercial	5
Okra	EBDC, Mevinphos	Organic	Commercial or Mexico	4
Orange Juice	Dicofol, Ethion, DBA	Organic	Commercial	43
Parsley	DCPA, DDT, Disulfotonsulfone	Organic	Commercial	5
Parsnips	Dieldrin, Heptachlor, Tecnazen	Organic	Commercial	5
Peaches	DDT, BHC, Captan, Penta-chloroaniline, Penta	Organic	Commercial	97
Pears	DDT, BHC, Ethion, Dicofol	Organic	Commercial	79
Persimmons	Dicloran	Organic	Commercial	1
Plums	DDT, Dicloran, Endosulfan	Organic	Commercial	68
Poblano Pepper	Acephate, Ethion	Organic	Commercial	6
Pomegranates	Dicloran	Organic	Commercial	1
Potatoes	Chlorpropham, Tetrachloro, Benzene	Organic	Commercial	68
Prunes	DDT, Endosulfan, Malathion, Penta, Phosalone, PCBs	Organic	Commercial	62
Radishes	Chlorpyrifos	Organic	Commercial	1
Raspberries	Captan, Carbaryl	Organic	Commercial	4
Rutabagas	Chlorpyrifos	Organic	Commercial	1
Serrano Chiles	Azinphos-Methyl, Diazinon	Organic	Commercial	6
Spinach	DDT, DCPA, UHC, Permethrin	Organic	Commercial	95
Strawberries	Captan, Carbaryl, DDT, Endosulfan, Methomyl, Mevinphos	Organic	Canada, Mexico, Domestic	86
String Beans	Acephate, Dimethoate, Ethion	Organic	Domestic or Commercial	6
Summer Squash	Dieldrin, Endosulfan, Endrin, Heptachlor	Organic	Commercial	81
Sweet Potatoes	DDT, Dicloran, Dieldrin	Organic	Commercial	43
Swiss Chard	DCPA, Permethrin	Organic	Domestic or Commercial	2
Tomatillos	BHC, DDT, Lindane	Organic	Commercial	5
Tomatoes	BPN, Lindane, Methamidophos, Dicloran	Organic	Commercial	50
Tomato Juice	BHC, Carbaryl, Methamidophos, Dicloran	Organic	Commercial	35
Tomato Sauce	DDT, Endosulfan, DCPA	Organic	Canned or Commercial	36
Turnip Greens	DCPA, EBDC's, Mevinphos	Organic	Commercial	5
Turnips	Chlorpyrifos, DDT, Dieldrin	Organic	Commercial	3
Winter Squash	Chlordane, Monachlor, Endosulfan	Organic	Commercial	48

Table 5-6 Oils

Table 5-6 (a) Low Toxicity—Oils

Food	Chemical Contaminants	Safest Source	Toxic Source	Toxic Residues
Avocado Oil	Chemical-free	Organic if if available	All Others	Less than 1
Olive Oil	PCE, TCE but basically chemical-free	Italian	Domestic or Spanish	Less than 1
Other Organic Oils	Chemical-free	Organic if available	None	Less than 1
Sesame Seed Oil	Chemical-free	All	None	Less than 1

Table 5-6 (b) Intermediate Toxicity—Oils

Food	Chemical Contaminants	Safest Source	Toxic Source	Toxic Residues
Corn Oil	BHC, Diazinon, HCB, Pentachlor, Benzene	Organic if available	Commercial	20

Table 5-6 (c) High Toxicity—Oils

Food	Chemical Contaminants	Safest Source	Toxic Source	Toxic Residues
Cottonseed Oil	DDT, Dieldrin	None	All Others	10
Soybean Oil	BHC, DDT, Heptachlor, PCB's	Organic	Commercial	38

Table 5-7 Condiments

Table 5-7 (a) Least Toxic Condiments

Food	Chemical Contaminants	Safest Source	Toxic Source	Toxic Residues
Honey	BHC, EDB, Penta	Organic	Commercial	8
Mayonnaise	Dieldrin, HCBs, Penta	Vegetarian	Commercial	9
Salt	Aluminum	Sea Salt	Commercial	3
Sugar	Diazinon, Penta	Succanut or Organically Grown Sugar	White Sugar or Commercial	6

Table 5-7 (b) Intermediate Toxicity—Condiments

Food	Chemical Contaminants	Safest Source	Toxic Source	Toxic Residues
Jellies and Jams	Carbaryl, Dimethoate	Organic	Commercial	20
Ketchup	DDT, DCPAs, Dicloran, Penta	Organic	Commercial	38

Table 5-7 (c) Most Toxic Condiments

Food	Chemical Contaminants	Safest Source	Toxic Source	Toxic Residues
Dill Pickles	BHC, Chlordan, DDT, Lindane	Organic	Commercial	65
Peanut Butter	DDT, Heptachlor, Lindane	Organic	Commercial	183

Beverages

Our biggest concern with beverages relates to alcohol. Many alcoholic drinks, including wines and distilled liquors, contain urethane, a highly toxic, cancer-causing compound. The presence of this substance is usually measured in parts per billion, but even such minute amounts can harm the liver. Liquors that contain the highest amounts of urethane are American whiskeys, fruit brandies, port wines, sake, Chinese wines, and various European liquors. Rum, tequila, and vodka are lowest in urethane content. Champagne and various sparkling wines also contain very low levels of urethane. Beer has little or no urethane, or other types of chemicals, industrial pollutants or pesticide residues. So beer is probably one of the best alcoholic beverages to consume.

I recommend that if you decide to drink wine that you make your choices among the organically grown products that are available. Wines contain sulfites, compounds added for preservative purposes. Organic wines do contain naturally occurring sulfites; however, these natural compounds have less harmful effects on the body than do synthetic sulfites.

Coffee drinkers beware. Coffee contains significant amounts of chemical residues. In one study, 35 out of 74 different samples of imported coffee tested positive for pesticide content. In addition, the bleached white paper filters that are typically used in brewing coffee could contain dioxin, a very powerful carcinogen. If you are a regular coffee drinker, my advice is to use the brown unbleached coffee filters or cotton filters. Decaffeinated coffee contains methylene chloride. To avoid chemicals used to decaffeinate coffee, seek products made with so-called water processing methods, such as the Swiss water process. Tea is relatively safe. Organically grown coffee, teas or herbal teas are preferred; in general, they have very few pesticides.

Coke or colas actually contain very few chemical residues. But they are not recommended because of their high sugar content that can cause insulin disturbances.

This concludes our discussion of the hidden toxins in our food supply. Read through the charts carefully to help in your understanding of why certain foods are not good for you. Many foods appear to be safe but are not. Commercial farming techniques as well as widespread pollution in our air and water have significantly affected the way we must begin to look at our food supply. Hopefully, your raised awareness and buying choices will impact the harmful methods of mass food production and chemically based fertilization and insect control that have become the standard in recent times. Hopefully, a return to safer, ecologically sound, organic farming techniques will occur. Not just our health, but the health of future generations, is at stake. ■

The Next Step ...

Chapter 6: Into the New Millennium: Putting the Pieces Together

Part Two

"SET"

How to Use the Program

Stepping into the New Millennium

Putting the Pieces of the Puzzle Together

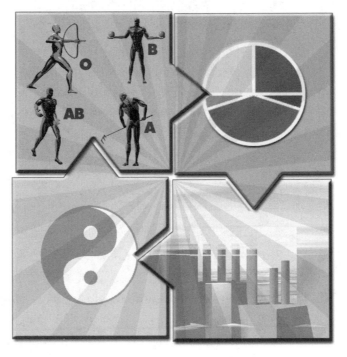

Part One has given you the background information to ready you for the New Millennium Diet. You learned about the components of the program. Here, in Part Two, is the information necessary to put you in the "set" mode, that is, how to use the diet's unique structure in order to make it work most effectively for you.

As we get ready to step forward into the New Millennium Diet, I would first like to quickly review the four basic components of the program which you have read about in the previous chapters. These points must be clearly understood so that you can make maximum use of the program. If you are unclear about anything please refer back to the appropriate chapter.

1. Specific Blood Type (Chapter 2)

The diet utilizes your specific blood type and biological profile to help you make the right lifestyle choices, including food, herbs, supplements, and exercise.

- You need to know *your specific blood type* before you can begin this plan.

- Blood type is critical to understanding how you have evolved, how you have adapted to changing environmental situations, and how food can impact your organs, glands, and cells.

- There are 4 different blood types (antigens) — O, A, B and AB.

- Foods contain special proteins known as lectins that are very similar to the blood type antigens.

- The immune system produces specialized cells known as antibodies which can cause an agglutination reaction against incompatible blood antigens as well as a similar reaction against certain types of foods.

- An understanding of the relationship between food and blood type educates you to which foods are compatible and healing, and which are harmful.

- Understanding how blood type antibodies react to various foods is vital for attaining optimum health and well-being.

2. Macronutrient Balance (Chapter 3)

The diet incorporates the balanced ratio of proteins, carbohydrates and fats according to your specific blood type to achieve optimum health and metabolic efficiency.

- Blood Types *O* and *B* need to follow the macronutrient balance of 30% protein, 40% carbohydrates and 30% fat.

- Blood Types *A* and *AB* need to follow the macronutrient balance of 25% protein, 50% carbohydrates and 25% fat.

- Utilizing the blood type–macronutrient ratio is vital to maintaining your proper hormonal balance. A stable blood sugar level helps to control hunger, allowing you to function on fewer calories.

- Protein should be derived from lean red meats, poultry, seafood, and where appropriate, dairy products.

- Carbohydrate percentages should be derived from low glycemic food sources within the vegetables, grains, beans and fruit groups.

- Fat percentages should be derived from nuts and seeds and unprocessed fats and oils such as olive, hemp seed, linseed and fish oil.

3. Yin and Yang Energy (Chapter 4)

The diet incorporates the Eastern medicine concepts of Yin and Yang to utilize the energy found within food for greater effectiveness in your diet planning.

- We all have natural constitutions that tend towards being either more Yin or Yang.

- Many factors can affect your natural constitution. Foods are a very important factor.

- Most Yin foods tend to be carbohydrate- and fat-based foods.

- Most Yang foods tend to be protein-based foods.

- Foods are rated as having extreme, intermediate or lesser Yin or Yang properties.

- The optimum goal to is eat a balanced diet of Yin and Yang foods.

4. Food Toxicity (Chapter 5)
The New Millennium Diet alerts you to toxicity in foods so that you can select the safest foods to eat.

- The diet has identified many of the hidden toxins in our food and ranked them according to their severity.

- Many foods previously considered as most beneficial, due to a low glycemic index or high blood type compatibility, have been moved to a lesser status in this plan because of their toxic chemical residue content or high glycemic index.

A Quick Preview

Looking ahead now, the following material sets you up to move forward into Chapter 7 and then into Part Three, the "Go" section.

The next chapter, 7, is a simple step-by-step approach to determine the correct amount of proteins, carbohydrates and fats recommended per day and per meal. In Chapter 7, a new unit of measure is introduced called a Portion. Once the amount of necessary Portions per day are determined we can start the program and move into Part Three.

The chapter titles of Part Three are the following:

PART THREE "GO"

PICK YOUR INDIVIDUAL PROGRAM AND START

- **Chapter 8: Blood Type O**
- **Chapter 9: Blood Type A**
- **Chapter 10: Blood Type B**
- **Chapter 11: Blood Type AB**
- **Chapter 12: Special Diet for Candida Sufferers**

The first four chapters of Part Three provide extensive information specific for each blood type. Each of the four blood type chapters consist of a discussion of the personality traits of the specific blood type and its relationship to foods. Food Listings are provided in each of these chapters and when used in conjunction with the Portion calculations determined in Chapter 7, menu planning is simple. Each blood type Food Listing is categorized into four different groups:

1) **Protein Foods**—consisting of meat, poultry, exotics, seafood, and dairy

products.

2) **Carbohydrate Foods**—consisting of beans, legumes, grains, cereals, breads, pasta, flour, vegetables, fruits, and juices.

3) **Fat Foods**—including nuts, seeds, and oils.

4) **Miscellaneous Food**—consisting of beverages, condiments, spices, teas, herbs, and supplements.

Each chapter also contains sample recipes that are compatible for each particular blood type.

The final chapter, 12, is a special chapter for those interested in incorporating the New Millennium Diet into a candida program. A comprehensive amount of information on *Candida albicans* is found in Chapter 12.

Now that we have reviewed the four pieces of our puzzle, chapters 2 through 5, and previewed the remaining chapters 7 through 12, we are ready to proceed. As we begin Chapter 7 we will customize a program that is unique for each participant. You are now ready to create your own program. ■

Chapter 7: The Seven Steps to Individualize Your Diet

Seven Steps to Individualize Your Diet

In this chapter we move to the individual criteria you will need in order to individualize the diet plan. This aspect is somewhat like going into a tailor shop and getting measured. The process facilitates a good fit. This chapter will ensure that you "fit" into the right diet plan and use it with maximum effect. It requires a few simple steps. They are your keys to maintaining healthy eicosanoids levels, hormonal balance, low lectin activity, and Yin-Yang synergy. Once you've covered the steps, you are ready for Part Three — to begin putting the diet plan into action.

Before you begin, you will need to know your blood type. If you don't know already, check with your physician, or you can obtain an inexpensive and easy to use blood type test kit through ProSana. Refer to the information at the end of the book.

To complete the basic calculations in this section, you need a cloth tape measure with which to measure yourself and determine your fat percentage. Also you will want to have access to a bathroom scale, or other weighing device, to monitor your weight. That's all you'll need.

The seven steps we will cover in this chapter are as follows:

Step 1: Determining your daily protein and Portion requirements.

Step 2: Determining your daily carbohydrate requirements.

Step 3: Determining your daily fat requirements.

Step 4: Planning your balanced meals.

Step 5: Determining your Yin and Yang scores.

Step 6: How to go New Millennium grocery shopping.

Step 7: "The Guesstimate method."

The First Step—Determining Your Protein Requirements

Most nutritionists assume that the protein needs of people are similar — that an average man requires 56 grams per day, and an average woman requires approximately 45 grams. However, because of differences in genetics and ancestral diversity, this simple concept has little meaning: 56 grams of protein may be sufficient for a typical sedentary male weighing 153 pounds and who has approximately 23% body fat. But for an active male with less body fat and a higher lean body mass percentage, 56 grams of protein is not nearly enough to prevent protein malnutrition. The same information applies to women who tend to be more active, and larger than average in size.

It is only logical to think that we all have individual needs. We don't wear the same size. We don't take the same strength of a prescription medication. It's the same with food. Every time we eat, the foods we ingest exert certain effects in our body just as medications exert certain effects. Foods influence the way our hormones work during the 4–6 hours after we eat. Determining the proper therapeutic level of a medication is vital for the medication to work. In a similar way achieving therapeutic levels of the important macronutrients on a blood type–specific basis is important for the body to work as it should.

It is not the calories that determine whether or not the ideal therapeutic effect is reached. It is the ratio of macronutrients or Macrobalance™, low-lectin foods, and energetic balancing that create the framework for reaching the effective dietary state.

The type of proteins that can be consumed are dependent on blood type. For example, B blood types cannot use chicken for their protein source, and A blood types do better with vegetable-based proteins than meat-based proteins. After blood type considerations, the amount of protein one needs on a daily basis is dependent upon one's weight, percentage of body fat, and level of physical activity, all of which we will consider now.

Step 1, "Determining Your Protein Requirements," is broken into four parts. They are:

1A—"Calculating Your Body Fat and Lean Muscle Mass";

1B—"Determining Your Physical Activity Level";

1C—"Adding It All Up"; and

1D—"Calculating Your Daily Protein Portions."

Taken step-by-step, determining your protein requirements is a simple process.

The tables required for calculating your body fat and lean muscle mass percentages (Step 1A), as well as your physical activity level (Step 1B), are found in Appendix A for women and Appendix B for men. There you will find detailed instructions, blank worksheets, and sample calculations based on a 130-pound female and a 185-pound male. Refer to the appropriate appendix when you are ready to compute your own specific requirements.

Step 1A — Calculating Your Body Fat and Lean Muscle Mass

The first thing you need to know in order to calculate your daily protein requirements is your body fat and lean muscle mass percentages. We all tend to know our weight but very few of us are familiar with these other vital statistics. These percentages can be determined easily with a tape measure, a pen or pencil, and a bathroom scale. Follow the simple instructions in either appendix A or B, depending on your sex. The body locations for measuring these percentages are different for males and females. You can determine your body percentages at any time without professional assistance. You can monitor decreases in your body percentages on a frequent basis, which will help you to track your progress on the program.

Step 1B — Determining Your Physical Activity Level

Once you have calculated your percentage of body fat and lean muscle mass, the next important measurement is your level of physical activity. The higher the level of physical activity, the higher the amount of muscle tissue that is broken down, and the higher the amount of protein needed for repairing and rebuilding tissue. Remember that proteins make up the bulk of muscle tissue.

Table 7-1 below shows various levels of physical activity as they apply to two blood type groups: O/B and A/AB. Built into the matrix of the table is a *0.1 activity factor* difference between these groups of blood types. You will be using the inherent genetic properties of your blood type to prepare the right dietary plan for you. We know that Type O and B individuals are more carnivorous, that is, they are more meat eaters, whereas Type A and AB individuals are more vegetarians. Therefore, O and B individuals have a somewhat higher protein requirement than A and AB types. The table identifies a range of physical activity factors from sedentary to heavy training. Type O or B individuals leading a sedentary lifestyle need approximately 0.6 grams of protein per pound of lean body mass. Type A or AB individuals need 0.5 grams. If you are involved in intense, heavy workouts, or exercise two times per day, you need twice the amount of protein compared to a sedentary individual. You will need to determine your protein requirement based on your blood type and general level of physical activity.

If you are very overweight, that is, greater than 30% body fat for males and 40% for females, you will need to rank yourself one activity level higher. The reason is this: Even though you may lead a sedentary lifestyle, your body has to work harder and expend more energy to handle the extra weight. This explains why most obese people actually have more lean body mass than thin people. They simply have more body mass, which includes a significant percentage of lean mass or muscle.

Table 7-1 Physical Activity Factors Specific for Blood Type

(Protein Requirements—grams/pound of lean body mass)

Activity Level	O/B Blood Type Factors	A/AB Blood Type Factors
Sedentary	0.6	0.5
Light Activity (Example: Walking)	0.7	0.6
Moderate Activity (30 minutes per day, 3 times per week)	0.8	0.7
Active (1 hour per day, 5 times per week)	0.9	0.8
Very Active (2 hours per day, 5 times per week)	1.0	0.9
Heavy Training (twice-a-day, 5 times per week)	1.1	1.0

Step 1C — Adding It All Up to Figure Your Daily Protein Requirements

Now you will factor together your weight, your lean muscle mass and your activity factor to come up with your daily protein requirement. Remember that this total will apply to you and should be used by no one else.

The best way to help you understand how to make this calculation is to use the standard in the nutritional industry of a male who weighs approximately 153 pounds. Let us assume that this individual has a body fat percent of 23% (this calculation is made in Step 1A), which is considered the average level for an American male. Let us also assume that this male performs very little physical activity and can be put into the sedentary category. Let us also say that our example is an AB blood type. Using these variables, this 153-pound male would have approximately 36 pounds of total fat (153 pounds x 0.23 fat = 36 pounds of fat). Therefore, he would have approximately 118 pounds of lean body mass (153 pounds less 36 pounds of fat = 118 pounds of lean body mass).

Next multiply his lean body mass by 0.5 gram per pound of lean body mass (this is the activity factor for a sedentary individual under the A/AB blood type category). Our calculation now gives us his daily protein requirement of approximately 59 grams of protein (118 pounds x 0.5 gram/pound = 59 grams). This is the number of grams of protein required each day for this 153 lb. male.

Here at a glance is the math involved to get us to the 59 grams of protein:

Weight: 153 pounds

Pounds of Body Fat: 23% (the % of total fat) is multiplied by the total weight: 153 lbs. x 23% = 35 lbs. of total body fat

Total Lean Body Mass/Muscle: Subtract pounds of fat from total weight: 153 lbs. total - 35 lbs. of fat = 118 pounds lean body mass (muscle)

Activity Factor: Blood Type A/AB sedentary lifestyle = .5 gm./lb.

Determine Daily Protein (gms.) Required: Multiply lean body mass (muscle) by the activity factor 0.5 gm./lb.: 118 lbs. lean body mass x .5 gm./lb. = 59 gms. of protein required per day

Grand total: 59 grams daily protein.

Once again, this is the total daily amount of protein (in grams) needed to support a 153 lb., Type AB male, with 23% body fat.

If we had used the activity factor for a sedentary individual under the O/B blood type category the activity factor would be .6. The amount of daily protein required would then be 71 grams (118 pounds x 0.6 gram/pound = 71 grams).

Once you know your individual daily protein requirement, you divide the amount among the meals you eat each day. Using the example of 59 grams over the typical three meals a day, you would eat about 20 grams of protein at each sitting. In the New Millennium diet, however, I recommend spreading your protein over a total of three meals and two snacks per day.

The point to remember is not to consume all of your protein necessarily at one meal because this can overload the body and lead to increased insulin release. Even though protein has more of an effect on glucagon, excess amounts cause increased insulin production, and this will prevent you from achieving balance in the New Millennium Diet.

It is important that the amount of protein be properly balanced. This is going to be based on the ratio of macronutrients for your individual blood type. Usually if you eat too many proteins at one meal, you will not eat enough at other meals. This will lead to higher carbohydrate ratios, imbalances in your glucagon and insulin axis, increased bad eicosanoids levels, and hormonal disarray.

Step 1D — Calculating Your Daily Protein *Portion* Requirements

Now that you understand the importance of spreading your protein over the course of the day, I would like to simplify the task of apportionment of food by introducing you to the **Macrobalance™ Portion Technique.** This concept allows one to think of proteins, carbohydrates, and fats in Portions instead of grams or calories. This approach is a big help in planning your daily and weekly meals. The procedure is simple, and here it is at a glance:

For Blood Types O and B: 7 grams of protein = 1 Portion

For Blood Types A and AB: 5.75 grams of protein = 1 Portion

The conversion from grams to Portions, as you can see, has different values depending on blood type. This difference is another one of the key elements that makes this plan unique from all others.

Now from our earlier example of a 153 lb. male, let's convert the daily protein requirements into the daily protein Portion requirements:

Type A or AB Male

A or AB male 5.75 grams of protein = 1 protein Portion.

We divide 59 grams of daily protein required by 5.75 gms./Portion:

$(59 \div 5.75 = $ approximately 10 Portions)

Type O or B Male

If our example were to use a Type O or B male the Daily Protein Requirement would be 71 grams.

O or B male 7.0 grams of protein = 1 protein Portion.

We divide 71 grams of daily protein required by 7.0 gms./Portion:

$(71 \div 7.0 = $ approximately 10 Portions)

The gram to Portion conversion factors are only needed if you want to use a food not listed in the Food Plan Charts found in Part Three. Otherwise, all foods found in these charts are given in one Portion quantities. This makes meal planning easy.

The next step is to spread the 10 protein Portions over the course of the day. For either of the blood type groups there are 2 options.

Daily Scenario 1:

1st meal containing 2 protein Portions (PP)
2nd and 3rd meals containing 3 protein Portions (PP)
2 snacks with 1 protein Portion (PP) each
Graphically, it looks like this:

Scenario 1

Breakfast	Lunch	Afternoon Snack	Dinner	Late-night Snack
2PP	3PP	1PP	3PP	1PP = 10 protein Portions

Daily Scenario 2:

1st and 3rd meals containing 3 protein Portions (PP)
2nd meal containing 2 protein Portions (PP)
2 snacks with 1 protein Portion (PP)
Graphically, it looks like this:

Scenario 2

Breakfast	Lunch	Afternoon Snack	Dinner	Late-night Snack
3PP	2PP	1PP	3PP	1PP = 10 protein Portions

Try not to go below 2 Portion meals and 1 Portion snack. If your protein Portions at certain meals are higher or lower than the examples shown above, then you would adjust the amount at other meals. Keep in mind, though, that these are intended only as examples of how to apportion approximately 10 protein Portions over the day.

Be flexible. If you only have time for a lesser Portion than what you are supposed to have, you can make up for it at another meal or snack. But try to *maintain the exact number of required proteins on a daily basis* in order to achieve your desired levels.

Meal Spacing

Spreading out your protein Portion requirements throughout the day helps to prevent falls in blood sugar levels and insulin imbalances. The hormonal effects of a meal only last from 4–6 hours. Separating meals and snacks by no more than 4–6 hours will keep you in balance. It is also important to have a snack before you go to bed in order to keep your body in balance while you sleep. Remember, you are only as good hormonally as your last appropriately balanced New Millennium meal. If you eat a meal that is not in Macrobalance™, then you can expect to be in "hormonal disharmony" until you eat your next correctly balanced New Millennium meal.

Refer to Part Three, Food Charts, in your specific blood type chapter for acceptable protein sources as well as the amount per Portion of that specific protein source.

Step 2 — Determining Your Daily Carbohydrate Requirements

Now that you have figured out the number of proteins Portions you need on a daily basis, determining your carbohydrate Portions to balance out the protein is simple. One rule applies:

For all blood types:

Eat 1 Carbohydrate Portion for Each Protein Portion

You don't have to calculate anything. Simply include a carbohydrate Portion at each meal or snack for each protein Portion. If we use 10 protein Portions as the amount of protein that needs to be consumed on a daily basis, then we should have 10 Portions of carbohydrates. While no calculations are required to determine your carbohydrate requirements when using the New Millennium Diet plan and Food Charts in Part Three, you will need to make the following conversion if you use food outside the plan:

For Blood Types O and B: 9 grams of carbohydrates = 1 Portion

For Blood Types A and AB: 11.5 grams of carbohydrates = 1 Portion

Again, these variances have been accounted for in the Portion amount in the specific blood type food charts.

An easy way to look at the relationship between proteins and carbohydrates is that for O and B individuals the correct *ratio* is 7 grams protein to 9 grams of carbohydrates in each meal. This is approximately a 75% relationship, meaning for every gram of protein eaten, Os and Bs should also eat 1 1/2 grams of acceptable carbohydrate.

A and AB individuals should be consuming their correct *ratio* of 5.75 grams of protein to 11.5 grams of carbohydrates. This is approximately a 50% relationship, meaning for every gram of protein eaten, As and Bs should eat 2 grams of acceptable carbohydrate. The "guesstimate" method in Step 7 of this chapter provides a simple manner of approaching these relationships.

Let's now look again at our two meal plan scenarios with carbohydrates added, keeping in mind that the carbohydrate Portions need to be spread throughout the day the same as the protein Portions:

		Scenario 1		
Breakfast	**Lunch**	**Afternoon Snack**	**Dinner**	**Late-night Snack**
2PP	3PP	1PP	3PP	1PP = 10 protein Portions
2CP	3CP	1CP	3CP	1CP = 10 carbohydrate Portions

		Scenario 2		
Breakfast	**Lunch**	**Afternoon Snack**	**Dinner**	**Late-night Snack**
3PP	2PP	1PP	3PP	1PP = 10 protein Portions
3CP	2CP	1CP	3CP	1CP = 10 carbohydrate Portions

Staying in New Millennium balance requires that you try to eat carbohydrates that are of a lower glycemic index. If you aren't clear about the glycemic rating of carbohydrates, refer back to Chapter 3. Carbohydrates with lower ratings enter the bloodstream gradually, preventing a rapid rise in blood sugar levels and a corresponding increase in insulin levels. This maintains a more favorable balance of eicosanoids.

In general, the most favorable carbohydrates are vegetables and most fruits. The most unfavorable carbohydrates include grains, pastas, breads, corn, potatoes, carrots, fruit juices, papayas and bananas. Your specific blood type chapter in Part Three will provide detailed information on acceptable carbohydrates.

Step 3 — Determining Your Daily Fat Requirements

Just as with carbohydrates, the number of fat Portions that you need on a daily basis is the same as the number of protein Portions. The same rule applies:

For all blood types:

For Each Protein Portion Eat One Carbohydrate Portion and

One Fat Portion, a 1:1:1 Ratio

Again, you do not have to calculate anything. A ratio of 1:1:1 is all that is required. Now you can see why using the Macrobalance™ Portion method is so easy. For every protein Portion at a given meal or snack, you will eat a Portion of fat and carbohydrate. If we use 10 protein Portions as the amount of protein that needs to be consumed on a daily basis, then one should have 10 Portions of fats. While no calculations are required to determine your fat requirements when using this diet plan, you will need to make the following conversion if you use food outside the plan.

For Blood Types O and B: 3.0 grams of fat = 1 Portion

For Blood Types A and AB: 2.5 grams of fat = 1 Portion

If you are using the Food Charts in Part Three, these conversions have been used.

The total number of fat Portions for a given day needs to be split evenly across the daily meals, including the snacks. So the number of protein, carbohydrate and fat Portions are always going to be an equal ratio of 1:1:1 for each meal.

There is an exception — if you are a highly trained athlete. In such a case, increase the number of fat Portions to 2 fat Portions for every 1 protein Portions. This would give you a ratio of 1:1:2. The fat should come predominantly from monounsaturated sources. The added fat helps improve the tolerance levels for intense exercise.

There is much discussion regarding saturated fats versus monounsaturated and poly-unsaturated fats. Monounsaturated fats are thought to be the good fats; however, new evidence suggests that saturated fats can also provide some protective capabilities. Balanced fat consumption is the key to good health. Monounsaturates such as olives and olive oil, canola oil, macadamia nuts and avocados must be blood-type accceptable. Most saturated fats are found in animal proteins and whole-fat dairy products. Monounsaturated fats tend to be eicosanoid neutral. They are not converted into any specific good or bad eicosanoid because they have little effect on insulin levels.

Just as there are favorable and unfavorable carbohydrates, there are also good fats and bad fats. Bad fats are those that lead to increased arachidonic acid production in the body, which in turn promotes higher levels of bad eicosanoids. Certain food sources are higher in arachidonic acids than others, including egg yolks, organ meats, and fatty red meat. However, new research indicates that dietary sources of arachidonic acid have little influence on the production of arachidonic acid by the body. Consequently, egg yolks, organ meats and lean red meats are really not unfavorable unless your blood type precludes you from eating these foods.

Fats are a vital aspect in achieving New Millennium balance. You should always include the correct amount of fat at every meal. Fats are the foundation for the production of eicosanoids and certain hormones. In addition, fat is also important in improving the taste of food and causing the release of cholecystokinin from the stomach, which signals the brain that you are full. *Fats do not make you fat; you actually have to eat fat to lose fat, provided they are good fats.* Even though most meats contain fat generally there is not enough to provide the ideal balance of macronutrients required to enter the correct hormonal state.

Step 4 — Planning Your Balanced Meals

Now that you have made all your calculations and know your specific dietary needs, let's move forward and see how easy it is to plan your meals.

The New Millennium Diet calls for eating three meals per day plus two snacks. You should eat every 4 to 6 hours. It is vital that your meals are spread evenly throughout the day in order to maintain proper hormonal levels. Consuming two snacks per day will maximize fat loss efforts. This keeps insulin levels low and prevents the huge swings that occur when the meals are not evenly spaced.

Shown below are the complete scenarios with 10 Portions of proteins, carbohydrates and fats spaced over the course of the day. These equal ratios are designed to help maintain proper hormonal balance by stabilizing insulin and glucagon.

Scenario 1

Breakfast	Lunch	Afternoon Snack	Dinner	Late-night Snack
2PP	3PP	1PP	3PP	1PP = 10 protein Portions
2CP	3CP	1CP	3CP	1CP = 10 carbohydrate Portions
2FP	3FP	1FP	3FP	1FP = 10 fat Portions

Scenario 2

Breakfast	Lunch	Afternoon Snack	Dinner	Late-night Snack
3PP	2PP	1PP	3PP	1PP = 10 protein Portions
3CP	2CP	1CP	3CP	1CP = 10 carbohydrate Portions
3FP	2FP	1FP	3FP	1FP = 10 fat Portions

The concept is to eat equivalent numbers of protein, fat and carbohydrate Portions at every meal based on your individually calculated requirements. This will put you into balance. If you increase your level of activity you will have to consume more protein. Simply recalculate your protein Portions based on your new activity level and balance it out with an equal amount of carbohydrate and fat Portions. Also, recalculate your lean muscle mass every three months as you become more fit. More than likely, you will require additional protein to sustain your weight loss.

It is very important not to eat excessive amounts of protein, since this will stimulate your insulin levels and cause excess protein to be turned into fat. Excess protein will increase the amount of calories that you consume. More calories will increase the amount of insulin that is secreted to deal with the extra calories. It is a good idea not to consume more than six protein Portions per meal and to keep the number of calories to 600 or less per meal. Snacks shouldn't exceed 200 calories.

If you eat a five-Portion meal with balanced proteins, carbohydrates and fats, you would consume less than 500 total calories. This will keep you in a Macrobalanced™ state for the next four to six hours. By referring to the recipes in your blood type chapter, you will see how easy it is.

So in order to determine the actual amount of food required to eat, multiply the number of portions required for proteins, carbohydrates and fats against the one portion amounts listed under the raw or cooked section of your blood type specific food chart. In other words, pick the food you want and listed horizontally across from it is the quantity of food that equals one portion. Then multiply that quantity which is usually listed in ounces, cups, teaspoons, etc. by the total number of portions required to meet your individual protein, carbohydrate or fat portion requirements. So, as an example, if you were Type O, one portion of red meat equals 1 oz of red meat. If as in scenario 2 above, 3 protein portions are required for breakfast, then 3pp x 1 oz means that 3 oz of red meat will satisfy your protein requirements for that meal. Looking at the carbohydrate and fat portion requirements for that same meal requires a similar calculation, except the portion amounts will be different depending on the type of carbohydrate or fat you choose.

If you chose grapes for your carbs and sunflower seeds for your fat, then 3 cp x 1/2 cup of grapes and 3 fp x 3/4 tsp of sunflower seed per portion equals 1-1/2 cups of grapes and 2-1/4 tsp of sunflower seeds. This would have to be eaten with the 3 oz of red meat to correctly complete this New Millennium meal. Once you have taken the time to familiarize yourself with the most frequently eaten foods and their 1 portion quantities, these calculations become routine which improves the ease of use of this program.

Step 5 — Determining Your Yin and Yang Scores

The next step into the New Millennium is Yin/Yang balance and the energetics of food. It is an easy step to incorporate Yin/Yang balance into your program. However, it is important that you do so *only after you are quite comfortable with the previous steps.*

When you consider these energy concepts it will refine your food choices even further. In Chapter 4, Graph 4-1, I scored food according to its Yin/Yang properties. You will recall that the ultimate goal of the Yin and Yang concept is to balance out the amount of Yin food and Yang food eaten at each meal.

In Part Three of the book, the specific blood type food charts provide the Yin/Yang scores for each food listed. To calculate the total amount of Yin or Yang at a meal multiply the number of Portions of proteins, carbohydrates and fats eaten by the Yin Yang score assigned to the listed food. The best way to explain this calculation is again through an example. So, let's say you have a simple 4-Portion meal which consists of the following:

- 4 Portions of lamb (protein)

- 4 Portions of Sauerkraut (carbohydrate)

- 4 Portions of olive oil (fat)

This meal is balanced according to the Macrobalance™ Portion technique, *but* is it balanced according to the Yin and Yang nature of food? Well, let's find out! Go to the food charts in your specific blood type chapter.

- Under PROTEINS, subgroup Meats • Poultry • Exotics and in the ***Most Beneficial*** category you will find ***Lamb*** with a Yang score of +2.

- Under CARBOHYDRATES, subgroup Vegetables and in the ***Neutral*** category you will find ***Sauerkraut*** with a Yin score of -2.

- Under FATS, subgroup Oils and Other Fats and in the ***Most Beneficial*** category you will find ***Olive Oil*** with a Yin score of -2.

As shown in Table 7-3, you now multiple the number of Portions of each food by its Yin or Yang score to get the total score for that specific food. These scores are then added up to determine the final Yin or Yang excess for the meal. This excess rating tells you whether you have eaten too much Yin or Yang foods at a given meal.

Table 7-2 Yin/Yang Rating System

- Excellent: 0 to 3 (positive or negative)
- Good: 4 to 6 (positive or negative)
- Poor: 7 or over (positive or negative)

Table 7-3 Calculating Yin and Yang Score For Meals

	Number of Portions	Yin/Yang Score	Total Yin/Yang Score
Proteins			
Lamb	4 x	+2	= +8
Carbohydrates			
Sauerkraut	4 x	-2	= -8
Fats			
Olive Oil	4 x	-2	= -8
Total Yin/Yang Excess			**-8**

In our example, we have an excess Yin of -8. This is a poorly balanced meal according to our excess Yin/Yang rating system shown above in Table 7-2. The use of chicken instead of lamb would have given us an excess Yin score of - 4, a much better level. Of course, you could only eat chicken if it is acceptable for your blood type.

	Number Portions	Yin/Yang Score	Total Yin/Yang Score
Proteins			
Chicken	4 x	+3	= +12
Carbohydrates			
Sauerkraut	4 x	-2	= -8
Fats			
Olive Oil	4 x	-2	= -8
Total Yin/Yang Excess			**-4**

If you carefully plan your meals, you may be able to completely balance Yin and Yang. Your goal is zero for every meal and snack. This may be a difficult target to achieve, but try to stay below 6 (positive or negative). Whether your overall diet should be more Yin (negative) or Yang (positive) depends on your *constitution* which you determined in Chapter 4.

Once again, I recommend that you incorporate the Yin and Yang scoring into your meal planning after you are comfortable with following your blood type–specific food list. It is essential that you first learn to correctly balance out the proteins, carbohydrates and fats at every meal and snack before progressing to Yin/Yang balance. If you are trying to achieve a faster fat loss or to heal a sickness or disease, then, incorporate this concept into your meals as soon as possible.

Let me add a few tips to make this concept easier to use. Fats are easier to control from a Yin-Yang standpoint than the types of proteins and carbohydrates available at each meal, especially in restaurants. Therefore, use nuts (score -2) if you need more Yin or use seeds (score -1) if you need less Yin to balance your meal. Also, try not to eat many grain type foods with chicken or other poultry because they tend to be neutral and not counterbalancing. Also, avoid eating fruit with fish for the same reason.

Once you get familiar with this part of the diet, you will find yourself easily balancing your foods energetically while maintaining Macrobalance™. Give yourself some time and be patient. As with most things in life, a little work can go a long way and is definitely worth the effort.

Step 6 — New Millennium Grocery Shopping

Be a smart shopper. Look for blood type–compatible foods. It is particularly important now to be alert to the content of canned or packaged items on the grocery shelves. They are usually very high in carbohydrate. Be sure to read the nutritional information on the labels to help you calculate the amount of protein Portions, carbohydrate Portions and fat Portions in a single serving. Remember the following conversion factors mentioned earlier:

For Blood Type O and B

- **One Protein Portion = 7 grams**

- **One Carbohydrate Portion = 9 grams**

- **One Fat Portion = 3.0 grams**

For Blood Type A and AB

- **One Protein Portion = 5.75 grams**

- **One Carbohydrate Portion = 11.5 grams**

- **One Fat Portion = 2.5 grams**

Always eat an equal number of Portions of proteins, carbohydrates and fats at each meal. What is different is the amount, usually ounces, teaspoons cups, etc., of the particular macronutrient in a Portion. When you are shopping, and a particular food does not contain a ratio of macronutrients that fits into the Portion size, you can make corrections at home when you are preparing meals by either adding more protein, carbohydrates or fat. Have fun, be creative.

Keep in mind that one protein Portion, 7 grams, will vary in quantity depending upon the food. For example, 7 grams of beef is one ounce, 7 grams of fish is about one and one-half ounces. I have provided some quick shopping guides to help simplify the quantity of food to buy.

- Four ounces of meat usually contain approximately four Portions of protein for an O and B, and five Portions for an A and AB.

- Six ounces of fish contain approximately four Portions of protein for an O and B, and approximately five Portions of protein for an A and AB.

- Two cups of raw vegetables contain approximately one Portion of carbohydrates for an O and B. Two and a half cups of raw vegetables contain approximately one Portion of carbohydrates for an A or AB.

- One piece of fruit provides approximately two Portions of carbohydrates for O or B. One and a half pieces is approximately two Portions of carbohydrates for an A or AB.

- One cup of cooked beans, pasta or rice contains approximately four Portions of carbohydrates for an O or B, and it contains approximately three Portions of carbohydrates for an A or AB.

Step 7 — "The Guesstimate Method"

The practice of reading labels and attempting to calculate the amount of food needed to buy for the New Millennium diet may be difficult for some people to follow. However, you can still adhere to the blood type–based diet lists and make a close estimate of the amount of foods that you are consuming. The cupped palm of the hand is a good measure to use for calculating the amount of food one should eat. The palm holds about four Portions of protein for an O or B and five Portions of protein for an A or AB. This is equivalent to about 4 ounces of meat, chicken or turkey.

If you are eating favorable low-glycemic carbohydrates, there should be about two times as much carbohydrates as there is protein on your plate for O and B individuals, and about three times as much carbohydrates compared to protein for the A and AB folks. If you are eating a low-fat protein source, you definitely need to add some additional fat to your meal. You can do that with a good oil in your salad or maybe a few macadamia nuts. Approximately one macadamia nut is equivalent to one fat Portion. For example, if you are consuming four protein Portions, you need to have four additional macadamia nuts added to your meal.

I usually carry a bag of macadamia nuts and a bag of sunflower seeds when I eat out. I can use these nuts and seeds to adjust my Yin/Yang requirements. If I need a lot more Yin I eat the macadamia nuts because they have a -2 Yin score. If I only need a small amount of Yin to balance out my meal then I use the sunflower seeds which have a -1 Yin score.

While eating out at restaurants, use the same approach in terms of "guesstimating" the amount of proteins, carbohydrates and fats that you need to consume. If you can see that there is more food on your plate than you need, only eat the correct amount. Do not overeat just because the food is on your plate. Take the food home for another meal. *It is always better to undereat than overeat.*

A special note on wine or beer. They are concentrated carbohydrate drinks. If you drink alcohol with your meal, reduce the amount of carbohydrates you eat, or choose more protein and fat in order to keep in balance.

If you plan on having dessert, make sure the dessert fits into your appropriate blood type chart. For example, O individuals do poorly with dairy and wheat. Therefore, a dessert made from either soy or rice would be more beneficial. Wheat is a highly allergenic food for blood Type O. Type B and A individuals have some compatibility with wheat. If you eat in fast-food restaurants, try to avoid the muffins or the rolls as they tend to be highly glycemic foods. Muffins and rolls may cause disturbances not only in your hormonal balance, but also in the amount of lectins that are circulating in the blood.

Illustration 7.1

The relative distribution of protein to carbohydrates for each blood type using a typical plate of food.

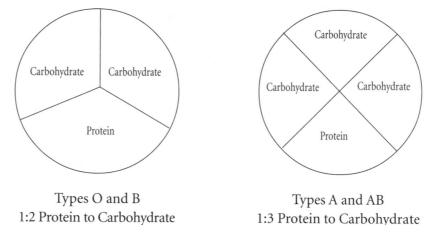

Types O and B
1:2 Protein to Carbohydrate

Types A and AB
1:3 Protein to Carbohydrate

Ten Key Points to the New Millennium Diet

As with any new program, there are always certain guidelines that need to be emphasized. Here is a list of them that will serve you well as you step forward now into the New Millennium Diet.

1. **Try to Incorporate All Systems of the Diet.** As stated earlier, the Macrobalance™, blood type compatibility and the Yin/Yang concept are three different systems, each of which can be manipulated to some degree in the overall diet. Ideally, I like patients to adhere to all three of them at the same time for maximum re-

sults. If you are unable to incorporate all three systems at one time, then apply the blood type–specific system and the Macrobalance™ concept first. Postpone the Yin and Yang concept if you find the going too complicated. You may find that one particular system works better for you than the others. You may also find that initially, while you are learning these systems, that when one system has been mastered, you to will find it easier to understand the next system. You can build upon the foundation of knowledge that you are creating by understanding these three different systems separately and then working them as a team. **Take it slow. Do it in your own good time.**

2. **1:1:1 Ratio**. Be sure to eat the proper 1:1:1 ratio of protein Portions, carbohydrate Portions and fat Portions for your specific blood type. If it is not possible to get it as exact as I am recommending, then either a slightly higher or lower amount of protein or carbohydrates will still be sufficient as long as you are able to maintain a high level of blood type compatibility and Yin/Yang balance.

3. **This Is Not a Low-Calorie Program.** If you go below 1,000 calories a day, you should do it under the guidance of your physician. Good carbohydrate foods usually occupy a large amount of space on the plate because of their fiber (bulk) content. Consequently, you may find it difficult to eat all the food that is on your plate because of the change in serving Portions relative to your old diet. Please attempt to eat all of the carbohydrates because they provide important fiber, the roughage that promotes healthy elimination and which also helps to stabilize blood sugar levels. Moreover, fiber helps to reduce the possibility of developing the so-called "leaky gut syndrome," where damage to the intestinal lining allows allergenic food substance to easily enter the bloodstream and cause problems.

4. **Try to Eat 100% Blood Type–Compatible Foods.** In any case, do not eat less than 70% of your diet that is specifically blood type–beneficial or neutral to you.

5. **Stay in Dietary Balance.** Be diligent about the times of the day that you eat in order to maintain proper hormonal balance.

6. **Never Skip a Meal.** This is particularly important in the morning. Breakfast means you are breaking a fast. Be sure you eat within one hour of waking. Don't miss your snacks, either.

7. **Drink Enough Liquids.** That means at least eight 8-ounce glasses of water a day. I recommend purified water in order to reduce the amount of toxins entering the body. If you are O, do not drink coffee because it is not compatible with your blood type. Try a herbal coffee substitute instead. However, if you are B, A or AB, one cup of coffee a day is acceptable and it helps to promote improved digestion and hormonal balance.

8. **Eat Extra Fat If You Crave Sweets or Find That You're Losing Too Much Weight.** If you find yourself having sweet cravings while on the New Millennium Diet, eat an additional fat Portion for every protein Portion. If, for instance, you are

eating one protein and one carbohydrate Portion, then add a second fat Portion. This helps to reduce the rate at which sugar is released into the blood and helps to cause secretion of cholecystokinin, the hormone that reduces appetite and craving. If you still experience cravings on the New Millennium Diet, assess the last meal you ate in regard to proper Macrobalance™ and blood type compatibility. Failing to meet these two criteria can lead to sugar cravings. If cravings persist and your macronutrient balance and blood compatibility criteria are OK, then you need to turn your attention to the Yin and Yang principles. If you are consuming too many Yang foods, then the body in its wisdom tries to tell you to eat more Yin foods. The foods with the most Yin properties are sugars. That's why you are having those dreaded sweet cravings. The message is to be more conscientious about balancing Yin and Yang at every meal. If you are losing weight or want to gain weight on the diet, add a second or third fat portion to every protein and carbohydrate portion consumed.

9. **Avoid Simple Sugars Which Are Highly Glycemic.** This includes not just refined sugar (sucrose), but foods such as white rice and white flour products (bagels, cookies, cakes, etc.). Such foods are high in Yin qualities and can throw your body out of Yin and Yang balance.

10. **Exercise Regularly.** Refer to your blood type exercise routine in Part Three for the type of exercise and frequency that you should follow.

The New Millennium Diet may appear somewhat complicated when you first get into it. Go slow. Don't be discouraged. As you pick up steam you'll start feeling the benefits. Soon you will become a pro at balancing your diet, just like many of my patients.

You will make mistakes while you are learning. It's OK. Don't worry. Just stick with it. This program brings into play well-documented dietary systems along with principles that have been followed for thousands of years. The combination has a huge potential for lifting you to optimum health and keeping you there, preventing the onslaught of degenerative diseases ravishing our modern industrialized societies.

If you fall out of the Macrobalanced™ state, remember that you are only one meal away from reentering it again. You simply need to become more accurate in the next meal. That will put your body and hormones back into the correct physiologically balanced state.

You now have the structure, the basics and the guidelines for entering and following the New Millennium Diet. This is a diet for life, not a fad diet. It is based on both ancient and modern wisdom, and should provide you with a lifetime of health and well-being. Select your specific blood type chapter in Part Three. It is packed with the compatible Food Charts, meal recipes and guidelines that *will* transform you. ■

Let's Take Our Individual Program and Move to the "GO" Section

Part Three

"**GO**"

Pick Your Individual Program and Start

Chapter 8

Blood Type O: The Hunter

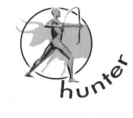

Health and Dietary Characteristics

- 30% Protein
  40% Carbohydrate
  30% Fat
- Strong Digestive Tract
- Overreactive Immune System
- Poor Dietary and Environmental Adaptation
- Requires Intense Physical Exertion for True Health

Personality Characteristics

- Strong Survival Instincts
- Strong Leadership Qualities
- Self-Confident
- Good Business Managers

BLOOD TYPE O—CHARACTERISTICS

PERSONALITY CHARACTERISTICS

Blood Type O is the most common blood type, making up 45% of the world population. Type O individuals display self-confidence and strength. They have strong survival instincts, making them very competitive in life, especially in the business arena. The instinctual drive to survive and persevere in prehistorically harsh environments allows the O type to overcome most obstacles. Type O is best suited for leadership or managerial positions.

PHYSIOLOGY AND DIETARY CHARACTERISTICS

Type Os require a higher protein, meat-based dietary plan for optimum efficiency. In the Stone Age, when primitive man had to hunt and kill for food, most calories came from animal protein. Only a small quantity of carbohydrates were mixed with protein.

Humans of that day were lean and fit with a very low fat percentage. Intense physical exertion, climbing, lifting and running, all contributed to their physical fitness. Consequently, daily physical exertion is necessary for Type O's optimum fat metabolism and health.

Chemical additives were, of course, nonexistent during that time period. There were no steroids, hormones, pesticides, fertilizers, or antibiotics in food. Today, however, millions of tons a year of chemicals end up in our food and water. This makes it impossible to truly follow our nature-based diets of old. Organic foods, when available, offer the closest resemblance to the foods our ancestors ate.

Weight Management and Lectins

Type O individuals can enhance their fat loss efforts by reducing the consumption of breads, legumes, beans, grains, and dairy products. Wheat and gluten, one of many lectins found in wheat, are major offenders. These lectins can have a tremendous inhibiting factor on blood Type O metabolic function. Lectins in wheat bind to the internal digestive organs and reduce the body's ability to digest and assimilate food. In the United States today, grains are the foundation of the recommended food pyramid. If you are Type O, these recommendations may seriously disturb your organs and digestion.

Lentils, kidney beans, and a number of other beans and legumes contain lectins that can inhibit proper muscle functioning. These lectins lead to alkalinity in the muscle tissue, which makes the muscles function inefficiently. The muscles of Type O individuals function better in a slightly acidic state.

Weight Management and Thyroid Function

Blood Type Os also have sluggish thyroid function because of their improper assimilation of iodine, which is a mineral. Reduced thyroid hormone production leads to hypothyroidism. What's confusing about hypothyroidism is that many times just utilizing the standard thyroid function studies available through your doctor's office or laboratory (which include thyroid-stimulating hormone, T_4, free T_3, and T_3 index) sometimes is not an accurate enough method to determine whether or not you have low thyroid gland function.

As an example, in one study 100 women were given thyroid function tests. This group of women had been reporting symptoms that could be associated with low thyroid function, such as fatigue, hair loss, constipation, chilliness, depression, infertility, dry skin and weight gain. Ninety-five of the women had normal thyroid tests indicating that they had no problem with their thyroid. The physicians conducting the study went ahead and placed these patients on thyroid medication regardless of the test results. All of the women who tested normal reported significant improvements in their symptoms after starting the thyroid medications.

This led the researchers to the conclusion that thyroid tests alone may not be a sufficient enough indicator for determining low thyroid function. I believe the normal range for TSH levels should be lowered. In my clinic, if patients have a TSH higher than 3.5, there is a possibility that they may be running into subclinical hypothyroidism. Type Os have the most problems with low thyroid function compared to all the other blood types. Any physician reading this book should be aware of this weakness in their Type O patient population.

Foods Encouraging Fat Gain:

Gluten, wheat, corn, navy beans, kidney beans, lentils, cabbage, brussels sprouts, cauliflower, and mustard greens.

Foods Encouraging Fat Loss:

Kelp, seafood, iodized salt, red meat, kale, spinach, and broccoli.

Exercise

Blood Type O individuals need intense physical exertion to stay healthy and fit. Their ancestral instincts for running, jumping, and pursuing prey dictates an ongoing need for intense physical activity. Their hormones and enzymes, their emotional and mental stability, all depend on movement and exertion.

Type O bodies usually are more muscular and heartier than many of the other blood types. As a result, they are more suited for intense activities. Aerobics, swimming, jogging, weight training, cycling, calisthenics, and dancing are examples of activities providing Type O individuals with the kind of exercise stimuli they need.

In order to increase fat loss and muscle mass production, more physical intensity is required of this blood type. However, it is not advisable to go above the target heart rate range. The target heart rate is the level of heart beats per minute needed to maintain an ideal aerobic exercise level, usually 70–80% of the maximum heart rate. Maximum heart rate is determined by subtracting your age from 220 and then taking 75% of that number.

The Type O person should exercise a minimum of 30–60 minutes, 3–4 times a week for proper balance of mind, body, and spirit. If you're just starting out on an exercise program, begin slowly and build up gradually. My recommendation to many of my Type O patients is to start with something simple, such as walking for 10–20 minutes a day. Slowly and comfortably, extend the activity so that eventually you are striding out briskly for up to an hour a day.

The same slow start approach applies to weight lifting. Start with a light set of 10 or 15 repetitions, targeting each body part or muscle group. Build up to 2–3 sets per body part once you have developed sufficient strength, balance, and flexibility. Weight lifting is a good exercise because it emphasizes weight-bearing movements, which place stress on the bone. This stress induces the development of greater bone density and a reduction in osteoporosis.

Hatha yoga, in a heated room, is also an excellent health building system that can be performed after weight lifting or aerobic activity. The heated room, up to 105° F, helps to open the sweat glands, warm the muscles, ligaments, tendons and organs, facilitating detoxification and flexibility. Hatha yoga is acceptable for all blood types including Type O.

DIETARY SPECIFICS

PROTEIN

MEATS AND POULTRY

The New Millennium blood Type O diet emphasizes high-quality beef, lamb, turkey, chicken, and acceptable fish. If it puts no strain on your budget, try to eat organic. Meat can be consumed as frequently as desired as long as it is balanced according to the correct macronutrient percentages.

Poultry is one of the most Yang foods. Red meats and other types of game have fewer Yang qualities. It is easier to balance the Yang of red meat than it is the highly Yang qualities of poultry. Red meat balances well with foods such as fruits, vegetables, and nuts.

The carbohydrates in fruits and vegetables and the fat in nuts and seeds is balanced by protein in the 30:40:30 plan both macronutriently and energetically (to a limited degree). However, excess amounts of Yang, such as eating high levels of poultry, can disrupt the energetic systems of the body.

Type O individuals have more stomach acid than any of the other blood types because of their genetic meat-eating heritage. Meat is a difficult food to break down and digest, but the Type O digestive tract is geared to handle meat protein. However, Type O individuals have a much higher incidence of gastritis, peptic ulcers, and other digestive disturbances because of the increased stomach acid production. This is why it's so important to understand and follow these concepts. Eating according to your body's genetic makeup minimizes your risk of disease.

The Type O of African descent should avoid fattier meats, such as chicken and lamb, and emphasize instead red meats and game. Such an individual's ancestors ate predominantly wild game and birds, which possessed much less fat than the commercially raised meat of today.

PROTEIN

DAIRY

Avoid most dairy products. Blood Type O people do not handle dairy well. Limit your intake to small amounts consumed on an infrequent basis. The lactose and lectins found in these products are not digestible. When eaten too frequently, dairy and eggs cause increased fat deposition and organ dysfunction.

O negative blood types can tolerate more dairy in their diet. The lack of the Rh factor allows O negatives some leeway in the use of these products in their diets. Most yogurts are considered to be a neutral food for O negative blood types. O positives, however, still must avoid all cow yogurts and most dairy foods; however, goat yogurt is acceptable.

Type O individuals of African descent should completely avoid dairy. They are lactose intolerant. Such foods were not typically available in Africa until much later in recorded history.

Dairy frequently triggers digestive disturbances because lactose, which is a milk sugar, is not properly broken down by the body. Among the disturbances is something known in the holistic medical field as intestinal permeability or "leaky gut syndrome." This is a condition in which small holes are created in the mucous lining of the intestines. The lining can be broken down further from excessive lectins in foods, which actually attack and damage this protective coating of the gut. When this develops, large molecules of undigested food particles, proteins, carbohydrates, lectins, or other types of antigens pass through into the bloodstream, where they can cause severe allergic reactions. This scenario helps explain why many people develop food allergies by eating the wrong foods.

Repairing this damage is imperative if you want to completely regain health and gain maximum benefit from the New Millennium dietary system. To facilitate the repair process, I recommend L-glutamine, an amino acid supplement, along with a type of sugar known as fructo-oligosaccharide. This sugar is not assimilated by the body, so you do not have to worry about hormonal swings. Known as FOS for short, the sugar provides a source of nourishment for the good bacteria in the gut, such as acidophilus and bifidus bacteria, which perform important functions for the body. When taken as supplements, FOS and L-glutamine can significantly enhance the normal bacteria in the gut, which helps to heal damaged intestinal tissue and symptoms of the "leaky gut syndrome." If you suffer with food allergies or other types of immune system dysfunction, such as psoriasis, candida, and chronic fatigue syndrome, you probably have a "leaky gut" component to your problem.

Dairy is a major source of calcium in the diet. When you reduce your intake of dairy products, it is important to replace the lost calcium. I recommend a supplement called microcrystalline hydroxyapatite, a highly bio-available form of calcium. Calcium and magnesium work together in the body to make and maintain strong bones. For that reason, I like to combine calcium with magnesium glycinate, the most bio-available form of that important mineral. I suggest calcium and magnesium in a 2:1 ratio. In other words, if you take 1,000 milligrams of calcium daily, be sure to take 500 milligrams of magnesium. Take these supplements at bedtime for best results. At night there are lower circulating levels of magnesium and calcium in the bloodstream. Supplementing at night prevents the body from pulling the calcium from the bones in an attempt to compensate for the lower than normal calcium levels in the blood. If adequate amounts are taken at night, then the body has no need to pull minerals from the bones. Also, there are many calcium–enriched soy and rice milks available in the marketplace today if you prefer not to take supplements.

A second benefit to taking these supplements prior to bedtime: they relax the muscles, calm the nerves, and help you fall asleep. It's vital that calcium be taken by both men and women.

PROTEIN

SEAFOOD

Most fish is excellent for blood Type O. Seafood is a highly concentrated source of protein, especially for those of European and Asian descent because of the coastal habitation of their ancient ancestors.

Seafood in particular contains a high level of omega-3 essential fatty acids, vital for good eicosanoid production. These fatty acids contain linoleic acid, one of the main building blocks of eicosanoids. Linoleic acid is converted by the body to gamma linoleic acid (GLA), the most metabolically active form of the essential fatty acid. GLA is not found in food; however, mother's milk does contain high concentrations of GLA. GLA has been linked to increased intelligence in babies who are breast fed. Such babies are also healthier and tend to be leaner than babies fed infant formulas that typically contain high amounts of processed carbohydrates and lower amounts of GLA. Breast-fed infants also have higher muscle mass and lower fat percents.

The body cannot make fatty acids, and this is why we have to obtain them from food. GLA is the activated essential fatty acid that is required for proper body function and optimum metabolism. Having high amounts of GLA promotes fat loss. Seafood, especially cold water fish such as mackerel and cod, is an excellent source of fatty acids which are necessary to make GLA.

It is known that blood Type O individuals have thinner blood than the other blood types. Consequently, fish oils should be used according to the dosages recommended on the label; otherwise, unwanted blood thinning could occur. Eating a great deal of fish will not cause excessive blood thinning. Fish oil-induced blood thinning could only occur by consuming an excessive amount of concentrated fish oil which is usually sold in capsule form.

GLAs and the essential fatty acids found in fish can help improve conditions such as irritable bowel syndrome, Crohn's disease and diverticulitis. Certain seafoods also contain large amounts of iodine, a mineral necessary for proper thyroid function.

When seafood becomes a regular part of the diet, try not to eat excessively Yin foods. You can eat fish with rice and other types of grains that are acceptable for O blood types, but you must be careful about consuming too many Yin foods, such as sugar products or fruits along with fish. Fruits and sugars will throw you energetically right out of your Macrobalanced™ state if eaten with fish.

CARBOHYDRATES

BEANS AND LEGUMES

The Type O person doesn't do well with beans and legumes because they have high levels of lectins, which can inhibit proper intestinal tract function. The lectins can target thyroid, adrenal, and other glandular tissue causing a slowdown in your metabolism. Type O negatives can tolerate green and red lentils, which for them are considered a neutral food group.

CARBOHYDRATES

BREADS

Wheat breads should be avoided. Not only are they high-glycemic foods, which disrupt the insulin-glucagon balance within your bloodstream, but they also contain high levels of lectins. If you are going to eat bread, it should be either Ezekiel or Essene bread, which are sprouted wheat and seed breads that contain very few lectins or glutens. These particular products are widely available in health food stores, and even in some supermarkets.

Candida patients need to eat yeast-free and wheat-free breads until their condition is cleared up. It's vital that these breads be appropriately balanced on a Yin-Yang basis as well as on a protein, carbohydrate, and fat basis in order to minimize blood sugar swings and to prevent the overgrowth of yeast. Spelt and rice breads are acceptable.

CARBOHYDRATES

FRUITS

Many fruits thought of as a healthy part of the American diet may not be so healthy when considered in light of the blood type diet. Fruits such as oranges, strawberries, tangerines, and certain melons are not tolerated well by Type O individuals. Oranges, tangerines, and strawberries are much higher in acid and can exacerbate the acid balance, leading to ulcers and other types of inflammatory conditions. Grapefruit is acceptable because it is converted into a more alkaline state in the body. Plums, prunes, and figs are much better because of their high alkaline content which helps to balance out the high acidic content in most blood Type O digestive systems. Avoid blackberries as they have a very powerful lectin that disturbs the intestinal tract.

Fruit is a highly Yin food. The larger the fruit, or if the fruit comes from a tree as opposed to a bush or a plant, the more Yin qualities it possesses. Remember that Yin and Yang are relative terms. Tropical fruits are more Yang than fruits that come from more temperate or colder climates. This does not mean that tropical fruits are a Yang food. It simply means that the fruit is not as Yin as a fruit that comes from a colder climate.

You will notice that fruits such as bananas, dates, figs, mangoes, papaya, and prunes have an asterisk next to them in the food listings. This is to indicate that they are high glycemic index foods. They have been placed on the neutral food list because they have certain beneficial characteristics that outweigh their glycemic ratings. However, if you have diabetes or are still finding it difficult to lose fat, then these fruits should be eaten only in moderation. It's always important when consuming these beneficial fruits to balance them out in the 30:40:30 approach in order to minimize their conversion into sugar.

Type O negatives can tolerate honeydew, cantaloupe, and strawberries.

CARBOHYDRATES

GRAINS AND CEREALS

Most of the commercially available cereals spell trouble for blood Type O. Avoid all forms of wheat and corn because they lead to excess fat storage due to lectin incompatibilities. The grains that are acceptable include amaranth, kamut, and spelt. These cereals can now be found in many supermarkets, whereas up until a couple of years ago they had to be searched for in the aisles of health food stores. Blood Type O negatives tolerate oat bran, which for them is considered to be a neutral food group.

CARBOHYDRATES

JUICES

Juices are usually highly glycemic and are rapidly converted into sugar. Even if you do balance them with proteins and fats, they rapidly move through the digestive tract and enter the bloodstream. If you are attempting to reduce your level of body fat, I recommend that juices be limited.

CARBOHYDRATES

VEGETABLES

Not all vegetables are created equal. Many vegetables, because of their lectin content or other active compounds, can interfere with the proper functioning of blood Type O systems. Avoid cabbage, brussels sprouts, cauliflower, and mustard greens. They can all disrupt the utilization of iodine. Vegetables from the nightshade family, which include eggplants and potatoes, contain levels of lectins that can harm the intestinal lining.

I do not recommend mushrooms, either domestic or imported. They contain molds that will trigger reactions in the immune system and cause food allergies and fatigue. Corn and potatoes should be limited. They are high in lectins and high on the glycemic scale.

Tomatoes are tolerated even though they belong to the nightshade family and contain lectins known as panhemoglutinins, which usually agglutinate all blood types. Blood Type O individuals have the ability to neutralize these substances readily without any type of ill effect on the system.

Vegetables tend to be a Yin-based food. Leafy, round vegetables are more Yin than the root vegetables.

CARBOHYDRATES

PASTAS AND FLOURS

Most pastas contain wheat, specifically semolina, which has a large amount of gluten and lectins. In addition, pastas are very high-glycemic foods, which can disrupt hormonal balance, leading to increased fat deposition. Try to choose pastas made from Jerusalem artichoke, rice, spelt, kamut, or other types of nonwheat grains. Type O negatives can include oat flour as a neutral food group.

OILS AND OTHER FATS

OILS

Oils and fats have a very profound effect on blood Type O. Monounsaturated oils, such as olive, flaxseed, and fish oils, have a protective effect on the lining of the arteries and the heart. They help to reduce inflammation in the intestinal tract and are important for healthy cell membranes. However, when excessive amounts of the least beneficial oils are consumed, they will be incorporated into the membranes themselves and disrupt the cell's ability to repel damaging free radicals, which are molecules that lead to aging and disease.

The omega-3 and omega-6 essential fatty acids, which include EPA, GLA, and DHA, are vital for optimum health for blood Type O individuals. Type O negatives can utilize safflower oil as a neutral oil. However, blood Type O positives must still avoid it. The oil content of food increases its Yin state. The more oil in a food, the more it has Yin qualities.

Certain saturated fats may not be as harmful as once thought. Many societies living in tropical regions of the world have traditionally consumed large amounts of coconut and palm oils but have little if any heart disease. This goes against the traditional view that saturated fats are bad fats. Just to be on the safe side try to use monounsaturated and polyunsaturated fats such as olive, flax seed, and canola oils.

FATS

NUTS AND SEEDS

Nuts and seeds are important foods in the 30:40:30 dietary plan. You want to especially use those nuts or seeds that contain high amounts of the mono and polyunsaturated fats when balancing out the protein and carbohydrates in the diet. I recommend macadamia nuts because one large macadamia is equivalent to approximately one portion of fat. Nuts are given a -2 Yin score, while seeds are given a -1 Yin score. Use seeds if you only have a small amount of Yang to balance and use nuts if you have larger amounts of Yang to balance.

MISCELLANEOUS

BEVERAGES

The excess acid in Type O digestive tracts can be slightly neutralized with club soda or seltzer water. Don't drink them at meal time because you need to maintain a higher level of acid for proper digestion. Cokes and coffee are not recommended. Cokes and other soda pop contain too much refined sugar, which upsets the body's hormonal balance. The caffeine in coffee interferes with adrenal gland function by overstimulating these glands to produce adrenaline, causing the fight or flight response. Moreover, coffee is also very acidic. This can promote acid indigestion because Type O individuals already have a high acid level. Black teas have the same type of effect as coffee on the digestive tract, and should be avoided.

A new product available called "Acid Tamer" can be added to decaffeinated coffee and orange juice, or to any acid drink. The product neutralizes the acid and allows Type O individuals to indulge in decaf now and then.

If you are a heavy coffee drinker, eliminating the habit can be difficult. You may suffer withdrawal reactions such as headaches, irritability, and flulike symptoms. A good homeopathic remedy that can quickly remedy the symptoms is nux vomica at the 30 C potency. Take two or three pellets, 2–3 times a day for the first two or three days after stopping coffee. It is like a "miracle cure." I also recommend taking some activated charcoal, usually 2–4 capsules three times per day. These remedies also apply to withdrawal from caffeine found in soda pop or other caffeinated products.

Distilled liquors contain urethanes and alcohol, substances that are toxic to the liver. Beer and wine are acceptable in limited amounts. These beverages are highly glycemic, so be sure to account for them when you are balancing your macronutrients.

MISCELLANEOUS

CONDIMENTS

Most condiments are not well tolerated by Type O people. They contain certain ingredients and spices that are often incompatible. If you use condiments in your meal preparation, try to use the health food store varieties which utilize natural ingredients free of artificial and processed compounds. For example, if you like mayonnaise, obtain the nondairy vegan mayonnaise. Remember that Type O folks do not do well with dairy. The same standard works well for jams and mustards. Buy organic, if you can.

MISCELLANEOUS

SPICES

Important spices for the Type O include curry, cayenne pepper, ginger, turmeric, and deglycyrrhizinated licorice, all of which have powerful protective and healing effects for their digestive tract lining. Avoid products with corn syrup for two reasons: their lectin content and high glycemic rating. As do most sugars, they have a very negative effect on the immune and glandular systems, including the adrenal and thyroid glands. O negatives can consume small amounts of white vinegar, vanilla, and nutmeg. O positives, of course, still need to avoid them if possible.

MISCELLANEOUS

TEAS AND HERBS

Many of the beneficial teas improve immune and digestive function. They help normalize the immune system as opposed to stimulating it. They also help repair damage to the mucosal membranes of the intestine. Especially good for this are parsley, rosehips, and deglycyrrhizinated licorice, also known as DGL. You can make DGL into a tea by taking 4–6 tablets and boiling them in water. The tablets break down into a nice tea that can be very effective in helping to heal stomach ulcers, indigestion, esophagitis, and reflux. DGL is a highly effective herb and can be used as a replacement for common antacids that are taken by people to lower their stomach acid.

Antacids increase the probability of bacteria, fungi, and parasites surviving the typically fiery road through the stomach to the intestines. Their survival means a greater chance to proliferate, causing more serious problems. We evolved with a high level of stomach acid to deal with the numerous organisms that accompanied food. Suppression of this initial defense mechanism can lead to problems, including opening the door to a particular strain of bacteria known as *H. pylori*, which has been associated with stomach ulcers, inflammatory conditions, and the development of stomach cancer. Many resistant strains of bacteria, fungi, and parasites are now present in our world, so keeping your body's defense mechanisms as finely tuned as possible is becoming a matter of life or death.

It's critical that we all maintain high immune system function, and any type of natural protective barriers we possess, that are specific to our blood type, need to be supported and not suppressed. That's why DGL is so important as a replacement for antacids and other types of stomach acid–suppressing drugs.

Herbs such as aloe vera, burdock, cornsilk, alfalfa, echinacea, and yellow dock can be too stimulating to the immune system. The key to using any herb is balance. Echinacea, for instance, may cause hyperstimulation of the immune system. Most people think of it, along with goldenseal, as the herb of choice at the first sign of a cold or flu. However, blood Type O individuals need to use it cautiously. Other natural substances, such as colloidal silver, olive leaf extract, and homeopathic remedies, are just as a effective, if not more so, than echinacea.

Kelp, the well-known health boosting seaweed, is considered one of the most powerful herbs for Type O because it contains many vital minerals, especially iodine, a key nutrient for good thyroid gland function. Another important seaweed, one you probably haven't heard of, is bladderwrack. It also contains iodine and enhances thyroid function, which in turn promotes fat loss and improves metabolic function. Bladderwrack is known also for its beneficial effect on the digestive tract. It contains fucose, a sugar that exerts a protective influence on the stomach lining. The sugar binds to receptors within the digestive tract helping to heal the tissue and repair "leaky gut syndrome." It helps prevent bacteria, parasites, and other harmful organisms from attaching to the wall of the stomach or the intestinal tract. Fucose works in a similar protective way in the lining of the bladder. It actually attaches to the same receptors that the bacteria attach to in the bladder lining, preventing the binding of the bacteria.

Colloidal silver is known for its reliability in killing over 650 different viral, parasitic, fungal, and bacterial organisms. I have used it for years for all types of infections. Olive leaf extract also has a powerful anti-infective property and can be used in place of stimulating herbs to heal infections.

MISCELLANEOUS

SUPPLEMENTS

Multivitamins

Supplements are a mainstay of modern-day life because of the reduction in the amount of minerals and vitamins found in our foods. Even if you are eating blood type specific foods that are organically grown, a significant amount of nutrient loss occurs because of the distance and time that it takes for food to be transported from the farm to your household.

I have designed a multivitamin that is blood type specific. All of the nutrients have been appropriately adjusted to meet specific blood type needs. Type O people require large amounts of B vitamins in order to meet their high metabolic requirements. In addition, B vitamins are important for proper brain and nerve function. They also help reduce the amount of age-related wear and tear on the body's cells.

Vitamin C

Vitamin C is an important free radical scavenger. It tends to be utilized rapidly by the body, so ample amounts of this water-soluble vitamin are needed for replacement purposes. Vitamin C also helps to repair connective tissues, such as the gums and mucosal membranes in the gut. It is very effective at stabilizing and regulating immune system problems commonly found in Type O individuals.

Vitamin D

New research on vitamin D indicates that this vitamin is much more widely deficient in the American diet than previously recognized. A daily dosage of around 600 International units (IU) is recommended.

Vitamin E

I recommend the tocotrienol version of vitamin E over the tocopherol variety. The daily dosage should be 400 IU to 800 IU.

Calcium

Refer to the dairy section earlier in this chapter where I discussed the issue of calcium in relation to the blood Type O individual. Avoiding dairy, as we have seen, requires finding an alternative source of calcium, which is a critical mineral for the health of bones, teeth, and nerves.

Iodine

Iodine is important for proper thyroid gland function as it is involved in the production of thyroid hormones. Some of the symptoms associated with low thyroid function (hypothyroidism) include fatigue, weight gain, bloating, hair loss, dry skin, cold hands and feet, and a lowered body temperature. The blood type–based vitamins I have developed contain small amounts of kelp to help prevent deficiency. I do not recommend that you take iodine supplements unless under the advice of a physician.

Standard thyroid function tests do not accurately determine whether or not you have hypothyroidism. For this reason I recommend an alternative method that has been proven over decades and which involves simply checking your body temperature daily under the arm before arising from bed. This is done for several days. Generally, if your armpit temperature is less than 97.2 degrees Fahrenheit, there's a strong possibility that you have subclinical hypothyroidism. When you take your temperature in this manner, be sure to do so before any activity. Shake down your thermometer the night before and place it on a nightstand beside your bed.

Manganese

Manganese is a mineral nutrient that is deficient in Type O individuals. It is commonly found in whole grains and legumes, but because these foods are not recommended, additional manganese should be included in any multivitamin/mineral formula used by blood Type O individuals.

MSM

I recommend MSM (methylsulfonylmethane), a source of dietary sulfur, for all blood types. It provides relief for many pain and allergic conditions. I recommend starting with 2 grams a day and slowly adding more as needed. It is best taken with meals. Sulfur is known as nature's fountain of youth mineral. MSM has a profound effect on strengthening hair, skin, and nails.

Fish Oils

Fish oils and other types of essential fatty acids are recommended for blood Type O individuals. Omega-3 and omega-6 essential fatty acids are vital for the production of good eicosanoids, which are the key to reaching a New Millennium state of health. Vitamin A derived from fish oils is recommended over the synthetically derived versions.

Enzymes

Pancreatic enzymes aid in proper digestion. If you are a vegan who is an O blood type, and you want to begin incorporating meat back into your diet, it is a good idea to take digestive enzyme supplements with meat meals. Do this until the body adjusts and can handle the meat on its own. The enzymes help promote the breakdown of proteins, carbohydrates, sugars, and fats. Taking 2-3 capsules 10 minutes before a meal usually is sufficient to achieve the desired effect. I recommend using an aspergillus-based digestive enzyme.

As with any supplement or medication, if you take too many digestive enzymes, you could potentially suppress your body's own pancreatic enzyme production. However, the aspergillus-derived enzymes have a less suppressive effect on pancreas enzyme production. This is why I use them over animal-derived pancreatic enzymes. Especially avoid pancreatic enzymes that are derived from pork.

Blood Type O Food Chart

30% Protein—40% Carbohydrate—30% Fat

Proper Food Ratio

The proper macronutrient ratio for blood Type O is 30% protein, 40% carbohydrate and 30% fat. One Portion of protein equals 7 grams, one Portion of carbohydrates equals 9 grams and one Portion of fat equals 3.0 grams. You will only use this information if you want to use a food not listed in the food groups. Otherwise, all food listings are designated in their appropriate Portion requirements.

Classification of Foods

Three (3) food classifications are used in the New Millennium Diet Plan. They are most beneficial, neutral and least beneficial foods. These classifications are based on blood type compatibility, glycemic index, toxicity levels and other food characteristics.

These factors have been carefully analyzed and weighed against each other to determine their appropriate designation within the food classifications. For example, swordfish has been considered as a *favorable food* by other diet plans. In this diet plan, it has been rated as *least beneficial*, due to the fact that it contains numerous chemical residues. Similar reclassifications of foods have been made on this basis.

It is important that you realize this distinction in your meal planning to achieve maximum results.

Most Beneficial Foods

These foods demonstrate optimum blood type compatibility and contain the lowest level of toxic chemical residues. They should be selected as your first choice in diet planning.

Neutral Foods

These foods are neutral in their blood type compatibility, but may contain slightly higher levels of toxic chemical residues. They should be selected as your second choice in diet planning.

Least Beneficial Foods

These foods demonstrate the least blood type compatibility and may contain the highest levels of toxic chemical residues. They should be considered as the last choice in diet planning and be consumed only on a very limited basis, if at all.

Rh Factor—Type O Positive and Type O Negative

The Type O positive and Type O negative diets are very similar except for certain foods that are in **bold type** in the Least Beneficial section of the different food classifications. Type O negatives can consider the **bold type** foods as neutral foods unless you have a known allergic reaction to the food. However, Type O positives must look at those bold types in the chart as a Least Beneficial food. This system applies to all blood types. This is the only pertinent difference between Type O negatives and Type O positives.

FOOD GROUPS USED IN THE CHART

PROTEINS
- MEAT • POULTRY • EXOTICS
- SEAFOOD
- DAIRY PRODUCTS

CARBOHYDRATES
- BEANS and LEGUMES
- GRAINS and CEREALS
- BREADS
- PASTAS and FLOURS
- VEGETABLES
- FRUITS
- JUICES

FATS
- NUTS and SEEDS
- OILS and other Fats

MISCELLANEOUS
- BEVERAGES
- CONDIMENTS
- SPICES • TEAS • HERBS

FOOD CHART LEGEND

+ Organic Is Preferable

* Highly Glycemic

⊕ Acid Neutralized

■ Acceptable Fruits & Vegetables Only

< This food possibly has a Yin or Yang energy, but for our diet planning is considered negligible

1P 1 Protein Portion

1C 1 Carbohydrate Portion

1F 1 Fat Portion

*1P/1C/1F This food contains 1 Portion of protein, 1 Portion of carbohydrate and 1 Portion of Fat in the serving size listed

* Note: The number before the letter will always signify the amount of Protein-Carbohydrates-Fat Portions in the serving size listed

PROTEINS

MEAT • POULTRY • EXOTICS

Most Beneficial:	1 Portion =		Yin	Neutral	Yang	Yin/Yang Score
	Raw	Cooked				
Beef (Lean cuts) +		1 oz.			X	+2
Beef Ground (10–15 % fat) +		1 1/2 oz.			X	+2
Buffalo		1 oz.			X	+2
Heart (Beef) +		1 oz.			X	+2
Lamb		1 oz.			X	+2
Mutton		1 oz.			X	+2
Ostrich		1 1/2 oz.			X	+2
Tripe		1 1/2 oz.			X	+2
Veal +		1 oz.			X	+2
Venison (Domestic)		1 oz.			X	+2

Neutral:	1 Portion =		Yin	Neutral	Yang	Yin/Yang Score
	Raw	Cooked				
Chicken (Breast, skinless) +		1 oz.			X	+3
Chicken (Breast, deli, ground) +		1 1/2 oz.			X	+3
Chicken (Dark, skinless) +		1 oz.			X	+3
Chicken (hot dogs)		1 link			X	+3
Cornish Hens		1 oz.			X	+3
Duck		1 1/2 oz.			X	+3
Partridge		1 1/2 oz.			X	+3
Pheasant		1 1/2 oz.			X	+3
Rabbit		1 oz.			X	+2
Rattlesnake		1 1/2 oz.			X	+2
Soy Burger		1/2 patty			X	+1
Soy (hot dog)		1 link			X	+1
Soy Sausage		2 links			X	+1

+ Organic Is Preferable   * Highly Glycemic   ⊕ Acid Neutralized   ■ Acceptable Fruits & Vegetables Only

Neutral: (continued)	1 Portion =		Yin	Neutral	Yang	Yin/Yang Score
	Raw	Cooked				
Soy sausage patty		1 patty			X	+1
Tempeh		1 1/2 oz.	X		X	+1/-1
Tofu (soft or regular)		3 oz.	X		X	+1/-1
Tofu (firm or extra firm)		3 oz.			X	+2
Turkey		1 oz.			X	+3
Turkey Breast (skinless)		1 oz.			X	+3
Turkey Breast (deli, ground)		1 1/2 oz.			X	+3
Turkey (hot dog)		1 link			X	+3
Turkey (bacon)		3 strips			X	+3
Quail		1 1/2 oz.			X	+3

Least Beneficial:	1 Portion =		Yin	Neutral	Yang	Yin/Yang Score
	Raw	Cooked				
Alligator		1 1/2 oz.			X	+2
Bacon		3 strips			X	+1
Bacon (Canadian)		1 oz.			X	+1
Beef (hot dog)		1 link			X	+2
Goose		1 1/2 oz.			X	+3
Ham (Deli)		1 1/2 oz.			X	+1
Ham (Lean)		1 oz.			X	+1
Kielbasa		2 oz.			X	+2
Kidney (Beef)		1 oz.			X	+2
Liver (Beef)		1 oz.			X	+2
Pepperoni		1 oz.			X	+2
Pork		1 oz.			X	+1
Pork (Chop)		1 oz.			X	+1
Pork (Hot dog)		1 link			X	+1
Pork (Sausage)		2 links			X	+1
Salami		1 oz.			X	+2
Venison (imported)		1 1/2 oz.			X	+2

+ Organic Is Preferable   * Highly Glycemic   ⊕ Acid Neutralized   ■ Acceptable Fruits & Vegetables Only

PROTEIN

DAIRY PRODUCTS

(Protein-rich dairy sources unless otherwise noted)

Most Beneficial:	1 Portion =		Yin	Neutral	Yang	Yin/Yang Score
None						

Neutral:	1 Portion =		Yin	Neutral	Yang	Yin/Yang Score
	Raw	Cooked				
Cheese (Almond)	1 oz.				X	+2
Cheese (Goat)	1 oz.				X	+2
Cheese (Soy)	1 oz.				X	+2
Eggs, White	2 (large)				X	+3
Eggs	1 (large)				X	+3
Farmer	1 oz.				X	+2
Feta	1 oz.				X	+2
Ice Cream, Soy (1C)	1 cup		X			-3
Ice Cream, Rice (1C)	1 cup		X			-3
Milk, Almond (1C)	3/4 cup		X			-2
Milk, Rice (1C)	3/4 cup		X			-2
Milk, Soy (1C)	3/4 cup		X			-1
Mozzarella	1 oz.				X	+2
Yogurt, Goat (plain) (1P/1C/2F)	1/2 cup		X		X	+1/-1/-1
Yogurt, Soy (plain) 1P/1C	1/2 cup		X		X	+1/-1

Least Beneficial:	1 Portion =		Yin	Neutral	Yang	Yin/Yang Score
	Raw	Cooked				
American Cheese	1 oz.				X	+2
Blue Cheese	1 oz.				X	+2
Brie	1 oz.				X	+2
Buttermilk (1P/1C/2F)	1 cup		X		X	+1/-1/-1
Camembert	1 oz.				X	+2
Casein	1 oz.				X	+2
Cheddar	1 oz.				X	+2
Colby	1 oz.				X	+2
Cottage Cheese	2 oz.				X	+2
Edam	1 oz.				X	+2
Egg (Substitute)	1/4 cup				X	+2
Emmenthal	1 oz.				X	+2
Gouda	1 oz.				X	+2
Gruyere	1 oz.				X	+2
Ice Cream (1C)	1/4 cup		X			-3
Ice Milk (1C) *	1/4 cup		X			-3
Jarlsberg	1 oz.				X	+2

+ Organic Is Preferable   * Highly Glycemic   ⊕ Acid Neutralized   ■ Acceptable Fruits & Vegetables Only

Least Beneficial: (cont.)	1 Portion =		Yin	Neutral	Yang	Yin/Yang Score
	Raw	Cooked				
Kefir (1P/1C)	1 cup		X		X	+1/-1
Milk (Evaporated)	1/4 cup				X	-1
Milk (Goat) (1P/1C/2F)	1 cup		X		X	+1/-1/-1
Milk (Lowfat) (1P/1C)	1 cup		X		X	+1/-1/
Milk (Whole) (1P/1C/2F)	1 cup		X		X	+1/-1/-1
Milk, Oat (1C)	3/4 cup		X			-2
Milk shake (1C) *	1/4 cup		X			-3
Monterey Jack	1 oz.				X	+2
Muenster	1 oz.				X	+2
Parmesan	1 oz.				X	+2
Provolone	1 oz.				X	+2
Neufchatel	1 oz.				X	+2
Ricotta	2 1/2 oz.				X	+2
Sherbet	1/4 cup		X			-3
Skim Milk (1P/1C)	1 cup		X		X	+1/-1
String Cheese	1 oz.				X	+2
Swiss	1 oz.				X	+2
Whey	1/3 oz.				X	+2
Yogurt, Frozen (1C)	1/3 cup		X			-3
Yogurt, Plain (lowfat) (1P/1C)	1/2 cup		X		X	+1/-1
Yogurt with fruit (1C) * ■	1/4 cup		X			-3

PROTEINS

SEAFOOD

Most Beneficial:	1 Portion =		Yin	Neutral	Yang	Yin/Yang Score
	Raw	Cooked				
Butterfish (Imported)		1 1/2 oz.			X	+1
Bonito		1 1/2 oz.			X	+1
Cod (Imported)		1 1/2 oz.			X	+1
Hake		1 1/2 oz.			X	+1
Halibut		1 1/2 oz			X	+1
Mullett (Domestic)		1 1/2 oz.			X	+1
Mullet (Imported)		1 1/2 oz.			X	+1
Pollock		1 1/2 oz.			X	+1
Salmon (Pacific)		1 1/2 oz.			X	+1
Sardine		1 oz.			X	+1
Shad		1 1/2 oz.			X	+1
Snapper		1 1/2 oz.			X	+1
Snapper (Red)		1 1/2 oz.			X	+1
Sole		1 1/2 oz.			X	+1
Tilefish		1 1/2 oz.			X	+1
Trout (Imported)		1 oz.			X	+1
Tuna (Canned)		1 oz.			X	+1
Tuna (Steak)		1 oz.			X	+1
White Perch		1 1/2 oz.			X	+1
Yellowtail Tuna		1 1/2 oz.			X	+1

Neutral:	1 Portion =		Yin	Neutral	Yang	Yin/Yang Score
	Raw	Cooked				
Abalone		1 1/2 oz.			X	+1
Albacore (Tuna)		1 oz.			X	+1
Anchovies		1 oz.			X	+1
Angle shark		1 1/2 oz.			X	+1
Arctic char		1 1/2 oz.			X	+1
Belt fish		1 1/2 oz.			X	+1
Beluga		1 1/2 oz.			X	+1
Bluegill Bass		1 oz.			X	+1
Bream		1 1/2 oz.			X	+1
Clam		1 1/2 oz.			X	+1
Crab		1 1/2 oz.			X	+1
Crayfish		1 oz.			X	+1
Flounder		1 1/2 oz.			X	+1
Frog		1 1/2 oz.			X	+1
Gray sole		1 1/2 oz.			X	+1
Grouper		1 1/2 oz.			X	+1
Haddock		1 1/2 oz.			X	+1
Lobster (Spiny)		1 oz.			X	+1
Mackerel		1 1/2 oz.			X	+1
Mahi Mahi		1 1/2 oz.			X	+1
Marlin		1 1/2 oz.			X	+1
Menpachi		1 1/2 oz.			X	+1
Monkfish		1 1/2 oz.			X	+1
Mud fish		1 1/2 oz.			X	+1
Mussels		1 1/2 oz.			X	+1
Ocean Perch		1 1/2 oz.			X	+1
Oysters		1 1/2 oz.			X	+1
Palani		1 1/2 oz.			X	+1
Pickerel		1 1/2 oz.			X	+1
Porgy		1 1/2 oz.			X	+1
Ribbonfish		1 1/2 oz.			X	+1
Sailfish		1 1/2 oz.			X	+1
Scallop		1 1/2 oz.			X	+1
Sea Bass (Imported)		1 oz.			X	+1
Sea Urchin		1 oz.			X	+1
Shrimp		1 1/2 oz.			X	+1
Silver Perch		1 1/2 oz.			X	+1
Smelt		1 1/2 oz.			X	+1
Snail		1 1/2 oz.			X	+1
Squid (calamari)		2 1/2 oz.			X	+1
Talapia		1 1/2 oz.			X	+1

+ Organic Is Preferable   * Highly Glycemic   ⊕ Acid Neutralized   ■ Acceptable Fruits & Vegetables Only

Neutral: (continued)	1 Portion =		Yin	Neutral	Yang	Yin/Yang Score
	Raw	Cooked				
Thresher Shark		1 1/2 oz.			X	+1
Trout, sea		1 oz.			X	+1
Turtle		1 1/2 oz.			X	+1
Wahoo		1 1/2 oz.			X	+1
Whitefish		1 1/2 oz.			X	+1
Whiting		1 1/2 oz.			X	+1

Least Beneficial:	1 Portion =		Yin	Neutral	Yang	Yin/Yang Score
	Raw	Cooked				
Barracuda		1 1/2 oz.			X	+1
Black Cod		1 oz.			X	+1
Bluefish		1 1/2 oz.			X	+1
Buffalo fish		1 1/2 oz.			X	+1
Carp		1 1/2 oz.			X	+1
Catfish		1 1/2 oz.			X	+1
Caviar	1 1/2 oz.				X	+1
Cod (Domestic)		1 1/2 oz.			X	+1
Coho Salmon (Great Lks.)		1 1/2 oz.			X	+1
Conch		1 1/2 oz.			X	+1
Croaker		1 1/2 oz.			X	+1
Eel		1 1/2 oz.			X	+1
Herring		1 1/2 oz.			X	+1
Herring (Pickled)		1 1/2 oz.			X	+1
Lobster		1 oz.			X	+1
Lox (smoked salmon)		1 1/2 oz.			X	+1
Milkfish		1 1/2 oz.			X	+1
Octopus		1 1/2 oz.			X	+1
Orange Roughy		1 1/2 oz.			X	+1
Pike		1 1/2 oz.			X	+1
Sand dabs		1 1/2 oz.			X	+1
Sea Bass (domestic)		1 oz			X	+1
Sea Herring		1oz.			X	+1
Shark		1 1/2 oz.			X	+1
Sheephead		1 1/2 oz.			X	+1
Spot Fish		1 1/2 oz.			X	+1
Striped Bass		1 oz.			X	+1
Sturgeon		1 1/2 oz.			X	+1
Swordfish		1 1/2 oz.			X	+1
Tarpon		1 1/2 oz.			X	+1
Trout, Rainbow (domestic)		1 oz.			X	+1
Walleye		1 1/2 oz.			X	+1
Weakfish		1 1/2 oz.			X	+1
White Bass		1 oz.			X	+1
Yellow Perch		1 1/2 oz.			X	+1

+ Organic Is Preferable   * Highly Glycemic   ⊕ Acid Neutralized   ■ Acceptable Fruits & Vegetables Only

CARBOHYDRATES

BEANS AND LEGUMES

Most Beneficial:	1 Portion =		Yin	Neutral	Yang	Yin/Yang Score
	Raw	Cooked				
Aduke Beans		1/6 cup	X			-1
Adzuki Beans		1/6 cup	X			-1
Black-eyed Peas		1/3 cup	X			-1
Pea, Pods		1/3 cup	X			-1

Neutral:	1 Portion =		Yin	Neutral	Yang	Yin/Yang Score
	Raw	Cooked				
Bean Sprouts	10 cups		X			-1
Black Beans		1/3 cup	X			-1
Broad Beans		1/2 cup	X			-1
Cannellini Beans		1/3 cup	X			-1
Fava Beans		1/3 cup	X			-1
Garbanzo Beans		1/4 cup	X			-1
Green Beans		1 cup	X			-1
Green Peas		1/3 cup	X			-1
Jicama Beans		1/2 cup	X			-1
Lima Beans *		1/4 cup	X			-1
Northern Beans		1/3 cup	X			-1
Pinto Beans +		1/3 cup	X			-1
Snow Peas		1/3 cup	X			-1
Red Beans		1/3 cup	X			-1
Red Soy beans		1/3 cup	X			-1
Snap Beans		1/3 cup	X			-1
String Beans		1 cup	X			-1
White Beans		1/3 cup	X			-1

Least Beneficial:	1 Portion =		Yin	Neutral	Yang	Yin/Yang Score
	Raw	Cooked				
Copper Beans		1/3 cup	X			-1
Kidney Beans		1/3 cup	X			-1
Mung Beans		1/3 cup	X			-1
Navy Beans		1/4 cup	X			-1
Refried Beans		1/4 cup	X			-1
Tamarind Beans		1/3 cup	X			-1
Domestic Lentils	1/3 cup	1/4 cup	X			-1
Green Lentils	1/3 cup	1/4 cup	X			-1
Red Lentils	1/3 cup	1/4 cup	X			-1

+ Organic Is Preferable   * Highly Glycemic   ⊕ Acid Neutralized   ■ Acceptable Fruits & Vegetables Only

CARBOHYDRATES

BREADS

Most Beneficial:	1 Portion =		Yin	Neutral	Yang	Yin/Yang Score
None						

Neutral:	1 Portion =		Yin	Neutral	Yang	Yin/Yang Score
	Raw	Cooked				
Brown Rice Bread		1/2 slice		X		0
Brown Rice Cakes		1 cake		X		0
Fin Crisp		2 pieces		X		0
Essene Bread		2 oz.		X		0
Ezekiel Bread		3/4 slice		X		0
Gluten-Free Bread		1/2 slice		X		0
Ideal Flat Bread		2 pieces		X		0
Kamut		1 slice		X		0
Millet Bread		1/2 slice		X		0
Rye Bread (100%)		3/4 slice		X		0
Soya Flour Bread		1 slice		X		0
Spelt Bread		1/2 slice		X		0
Wasa Bread		1 slice		X		0

Least Beneficial:	1 Portion =		Yin	Neutral	Yang	Yin/Yang Score
	Raw	Cooked				
Bagels, Wheat		1/4 bagel		X		0
Bread Sticks (hard)		1 stick		X		0
Bread Sticks (soft)		1/2 stick		X		0
Cake		1/2 slice	X			-2
Corn Muffins		1/4 muffin		X		0
Doughnut		1/3	X			-2
Durum Wheat		1/2 slice		X		0
Graham Crackers		1 1/3 cracker	X			-2
High Protein Bread		1/2 slice		X		0
English Muffins		1/4 muffin		X		0
Matzo Wheat		1/3 board		X		0
Melba Toast		1/2 slice		X		0
Multi-Grain Bread		1/2 slice		X		0
Oat Bran Muffins		1/3 muffin		X		0
Pancakes, Wheat (4")		1/2		X		0
Pita Bread (Pocket)		1/4 pocket		X		0
Pumpernickel		2/3 slice		X		0
Rice Crackers		6 crackers		X		0
Rye Crisp		3 pieces		X		0
Rice Cake, white		1 cake		X		0
Saltine Crackers		3 crackers		X		0
Sprouted Wheat Bread		1/2 slice		X		0
Waffle, Wheat		1/2		X		0
Wheat Bran Muffins		1/4 muffin		X		0
Whole Wheat Bread		1/2 slice		X		0
Vita, Rye		3 pieces		X		0

CARBOHYDRATES

FRUITS

Most Beneficial:	1 Portion =		Yin	Neutral	Yang	Yin/Yang Score
	Raw	Cooked				
Cactus	1/3 cup		X			-3
Figs, Fresh *	1 piece		X			-3
Plums, Dark +	1		X			-3
Plums, Green +	1		X			-3
Plums, Red +	1		X			-3
Pineapple	1/2 cup		X			-3

Neutral:	1 Portion =		Yin	Neutral	Yang	Yin/Yang Score
	Raw	Cooked				
Apples +	1/2		X			-3
Apricots +	3		X			-3
Bananas *	1/3		X			-3
Blueberries +	1/2 cup		X			-3
Boysenberries	1/2 cup		X			-3
Cherries +	8		X			-3
Cranberries +	3/4 cup		X			-3
Currants, Black	3/4 cup		X			-3
Currants, Red	3/4 cup		X			-3
Currants, White	3/4 cup		X			-3
Dates +	2		X			-3
Elderberries	1/2 cup		X			-3
Feiojas (Medium) +	2		X			-3
Figs, Dried *	1 piece		X			-3
Gooseberries	1 cup		X			-3
Grapefruit	1/2		X			-3
Grapes, Black +	1/2 cup		X			-3
Grapes, Concord +	1/2 cup		X			-3
Grapes, Green +	1/2 cup		X			-3
Grapes, Red +	1/2 cup		X			-3
Guava	1/2 cup		X			-3
Kiwi	1		X			-3
Kumquat	3		X			-3
Lemons	1		X			-3
Limes	1		X			-3
Loganberries	3/4 cup		X			-3
Mangoes *	1/3 cup		X			-3
Melons, Canang	2/3 cup		X			-3
Melons, Casaba +	2/3 cup		X			-3

+ Organic Is Preferable   * Highly Glycemic   ⊕ Acid Neutralized   ■ Acceptable Fruits & Vegetables Only

Neutral: (continued)	1 Portion =		Yin	Neutral	Yang	Yin/Yang Score
	Raw	Cooked				
Melons, Crenshaw +	2/3 cup		X			-3
Melons, Christmas	2/3 cup		X			-3
Melons, Musk	2/3 cup		X			-3
Melons, Spanish	2/3 cup		X			-3
Watermelons	3/4 cup		X			-3
Nectarines (Medium)+	1/2		X			-3
Papaya *	3/4 cup		X			-3
Peaches (Medium) +	1		X			-3
Peaches (Canned) +	1/2 cup		X			-3
Pears (Medium) +	1/2		X			-3
Pears (Canned) +	1/2 cup		X			-3
Persimmons (Medium)+	1		X			-3
Prunes *	2		X			-3
Pomegranates (Medium)+	1/3		X			-3
Prickly Pears	3/4		X			-3
Raisins (Organic only)	1 tbsp.		X			-3
Raspberries	1 cup		X			-3
Star Fruit (Medium)	1 1/3		X			-3

Least Beneficial:	1 Portion =		Yin	Neutral	Yang	Yin/Yang Score
	Raw	Cooked				
Blackberries +	3/4 cup		X			-3
Coconut	5 1/3 oz.		X			-3
Melon, Bitter	1/4		X			-3
Melon, Cantaloupe +	1/4		X			-3
Melon, Honeydew +	1/4		X			-3
Oranges	1/2		X			-3
Plantains	1 oz.		X			-3
Raisins (commercial)	1 tbsp.		X			-3
Rhubarb	2 1/2 cups		X			-3
Strawberries +	1 cup		X			-3
Tangerines	1		X			-3

+ Organic Is Preferable   * Highly Glycemic   ⊕ Acid Neutralized   ■ Acceptable Fruits & Vegetables Only

CARBOHYDRATES

GRAINS & CEREALS

Most Beneficial:	1 Portion =		Yin	Neutral	Yang	Yin/Yang Score
None	N/A				N/A	

Neutral:	1 Portion =		Yin	Neutral	Yang	Yln/Yang Score
	Raw	Cooked				
Amaranth (Flakes)	1/2 oz.			X		0
Barley (Dry)	1/2 tbsp.			X		0
Buckwheat (Dry)	1/2 oz.			X		0
Cream of Brown Rice *		1/3 cup		X		0
Kamut (Flakes)	1/2 oz.			X		0
Kasha	1/2 oz.			X		0
Millet *	1/2 oz.			X		0
Rice Bran	1/3 cup			X		0
Rice, Brown (Puffed) *	1/3 oz.			X		0
Spelt (Flakes)	1/2 oz.			X		0

Least Beneficial:	1 Portion =		Yin	Neutral	Yang	Yin/Yang Score
	Raw	Cooked				
Cornflakes *	1/3 oz.			X		0
Cornmeal *	1/2 oz.			X		0
Cream of Wheat *	1/2 oz.	1/3 cup		X		0
Cream of White Rice *	1/2 oz.	1/3 cup		X		0
Familia	1/2 oz.	1/3 cup		X		0
Farina	1/2 oz.	1/3 cup		X		0
Grapenuts	1/2 oz.			X		0
Granola	1/2 oz.			X		0
Grits	1/2 oz.	1/3 cup		X		0
Oat Bran	1/3 oz.			X		0
Oatmeal	1/2 oz.	1/3 cup		X		0
Rice, White (Puffed)	1/5 cup			X		0
Seven Grain *	2/3 cup			X		0
Shredded Wheat *	1/2 oz.			X		0
Wheat Bran	1/2 oz.			X		0
Wheat Germ	1 oz.			X		0

+ Organic Is Preferable   * Highly Glycemic   ⊕ Acid Neutralized   ■ Acceptable Fruits & Vegetables Only

CARBOHYDRATES

JUICES

Most Beneficial:	1 Portion =		Yin	Neutral	Yang	Yin/Yang Score
	Raw	Cooked				
Black Cherry + *	1/3 cup		X			-3
Pineapple *	1/4 cup		X			-3
Water w/ Lemon	N/A		N/A			N/A

Neutral:	1 Portion =		Yin	Neutral	Yang	Yin/Yang Score
	Raw	Cooked				
Apricot	1/4 cup		X			-3
Boysenberry	1/4 cup		X			-3
Carrot *	1/3 cup		X			-1
Celery +	3/4 cup		X			-1
Cranberry *	1/4 cup		X			-3
Cucumber	3/4 cup		X			-1
Grape *	1/4 cup		X			-3
Grapefruit + *	1/3 cup		X			-3
Guava	1/3 cup		X			-3
Orange ⊕	1/3 cup		X			-3
Papaya *	1/4 cup		X			-3
Pomegranate	1/3 cup		X			-3
Prune + *	1/5 cup		X			-3
Tomato + *	1 cup		X			-1
Vegetable * ■	3/4 cup		X			-2
V-8 Juice *	3/4 cup		X			-2

Least Beneficial:	1 Portion =		Yin	Neutral	Yang	Yin/Yang Score
	Raw	Cooked				
Apple + *	1/3 cup		X			-3
Apple Cider + *	1/3 cup		X			-3
Cabbage	1 cup		X			-2
Orange (Regular) *	1/3 cup		X			-3

+ Organic Is Preferable   * Highly Glycemic   ⊕ Acid Neutralized   ■ Acceptable Fruits & Vegetables Only

CARBOHYDRATES

PASTAS AND FLOURS

Most Beneficial:	1 Portion =		Yin	Neutral	Yang	Yin/Yang Score
None						

Neutral:	1 Portion =		Yin	Neutral	Yang	Yin/Yang Score
	Raw	Cooked				
Barley Flour	2/3 oz.			X		0
Buckwheat	1/2 oz.			X		0
Kamut	1/2 oz.			X		0
Kasha	1/2 oz.			X		0
Artichoke Pasta (Jerusalem)		1/4 cup		X		0
Quinoa Flour	1/2 oz.			X		0
Rice, Basmati *		1/5 cup		X		0
Rice, Brown *		1/5 cup		X		0
Rice Flour, Brown *	1/2 oz.			X		0
Rice, Wild *		1/5 cup		X		0
Rye Flour (100%) + *	3/4 oz.			X		0
Soy Flour	1/2 oz.			X		0
Spelt Flour	2/3 oz.			X		0
Spelt Noodles	1/4 cup			X		0

Least Beneficial:	1 Portion =		Yin	Neutral	Yang	Yin/Yang Score
	Raw	Cooked				
Bulgar Wheat Flour	1/2 oz.			X		0
Couscous Flour	1/2 oz.			X		0
Durum Wheat Flour	1/2 oz.			X		0
Gluten Flour	1 oz.			X		0
Graham Flour	1/2 oz.			X		-2
Oat Flour	1/2 oz.			X		0
Rice, White		1/5 cup		X		0
Rice Flour, White	1/2 oz.			X		0
Soba Noodles		1/4 cup		X		0
Semolina Pasta		1/4 cup		X		0
Spinach Pasta		1/4 cup		X		0
Sprouted Wheat Flour	1 1/2 oz.			X		0
White Flour	3/4 oz.			X		0
Whole Wheat Flour	1 oz.			X		0

+ Organic Is Preferable   * Highly Glycemic   ⊕ Acid Neutralized   ■ Acceptable Fruits & Vegetables Only

CARBOHYDRATES

VEGETABLES

Most Beneficial:	1 Portion =		Yin	Neutral	Yang	Yin/Yang Score
	Raw	Cooked				
Artichokes +	Small		X			-1
Jerusalem Artichokes	Small		X			-1
Barley, Green	N/A	N/A	X			-2
Beet Greens	5 1/2 cups		X			-2
Blue Green Algae	N/A	N/A	X			-1
Broccoli +	2 cups		X			-1
Choy Sum +	2 cups		X			-1
Chicory Greens	1 cup		X			-2
Chicory Roots	1 cup		X			-1
Collard Greens +	1 cup		X			-2
Dandelion Greens +	1 2/3 cups		X			-2
Escarole +	7 1/2 cups		X			-2
Garlic	10 cloves		X			-1
Horseradish (Pods)	2 cups				X	+1
Kale +	1 cup		X			-2
Kelp	4 oz.		X			-2
Kohlrabi +	1 cup		X			-2
Leeks +	1 cup		X			-1
Okra +		1 cup	X			-1
Parsley +	5 cups		X			-2
Parsnips *	1/3 cup		X			-1
Pepper, Red (chopped) +	1 cup		X			-1
Pumpkins (mashed)		3/4 cup	X			-1
Purslane +	6 1/2 cups	1 2/3 cups	X			-2
Romaine Lettuce +	6 cups		X			-2
Red Chard		1 cup	X			-2
Red Onions	1 cup		X			-1
Seaweed		3 1/2 oz.	X			-2
Spanish Onions	1 cup		X			-1
Spinach +	4 cups		X			-2
Spirulina	1 1/2 oz.		X			-2
Sweet Potato +		1/3 potato	X			-1
Swiss Chard +		1 cup	X			-2
Turnips (mashed) +		1 cup	X			-1
Turnip Greens		1 1/2 cups	X			-2
Yellow Onions	1 cup		X			-1

+ Organic Is Preferable   * Highly Glycemic   ⊕ Acid Neutralized   ■ Acceptable Fruits & Vegetables Only

Neutral:	1 Portion =		Yin	Neutral	Yang	Yin/Yang Score
	Raw	Cooked				
Arugula	11 1/4 cups		X			-2
Asparagus		12 spears	X			-1
Bamboo Shoots	3 3/4 cups	1 cup	X			-1
Beets		1/2 cup	X			-1
Bok Choy +		3 cups	X			-2
Carrots	3 1/2 oz.	1/2 cup	X			-1
Celery	2 cups		X			-1
Cilantro (Coriander)		2 1/2 cups	X			-2
Cucumber (Whole) +	1		X			-1
Cucumber (Sliced) +	1 cup		X			-1
Daikon Radish	2 1/2 cups		X			-1
Dill Weed +	15 cups		X			-1
Endive	7 1/2 cups		X			-2
Hominy (grits)		1/3 cup	X			-1
Hummus	1/4 cup		X			-1
Lettuce, Bibb (5" head)	2 head		X			-2
Lettuce, Boston (5" head)	2 head		X			-2
Lettuce, Iceberg (6" head) +	1 head		X			-2
Lettuce, Mesclun +	1 head		X			-2
Abalone Mushrooms	3 cups	1 cup	X			-1
Mushrooms, Enoki	3 cups	1 cup	X			-1
Mushrooms, Portobello	3 cups	1 cup	X			-1
Mushrooms, Oyster	3 cups	1 cup	X			-1
Mushrooms, Tree	3 cups	1 cup	X			-1
Onions, Green (Scallions)	1 cup	1/2 cup	X			-1
Peppers, Chili (Chopped)	2/3 cup		X			-1
Peppers, Green (Chopped)	2 1/4 cups		X			-1
Peppers, Jalapeno (Chopped)	3 oz.		X			-1
Peppers, Poblano (Chopped) +	3 oz.		X			-2
Peppers, Serrano (Chopped) +	2/3 cup		X			-1
Peppers, Yellow (Chopped)	2 1/4 cups		X			-1
Radicchio	7 oz.		X			-1
Radishes +	4 cups		X			-1
Rapini	2 cups		X			-1
Red Algae	N/A	N/A	X			-1
Rutabaga +	3/4 cup	1/2 cup	X			-1
Shallots	2 oz.		X			-1
Sprouts, Mung	3 cups		X			-1
Sprouts, Radish	3 cups		X			-1
Squash, Acorn +		1/2 cup	X			-1

+ Organic Is Preferable   * Highly Glycemic   ⊕ Acid Neutralized   ■ Acceptable Fruits & Vegetables Only

Neutral: (continued)	1 Portion =		Yin	Neutral	Yang	Yin/Yang Score
	Raw	Cooked				
Squash, Butternut +		1/2 cup	X			-1
Squash, Yellow +		1 1/4 cups	X			-1
Taro	1/3 cup	1/5 cup	X			-1
Tomatillo	1 cup		X			-1
Tomato +	2		X			-1
Water Chestnuts	1/3 cup		X			-1
Watercress	22 1/2 cups		X			-2
Yams		1/3 cup	X			-1
Zucchini		1 1/2 cups	X			-1

Least Beneficial:	1 Portion =		Yin	Neutral	Yang	Yin/Yang Score
	Raw	Cooked				
Cabbage, Chinese	3 cups	1 1/3 cups	X			-2
Cabbage, Red	3 cups	1 1/3 cups	X			-2
Cabbage, White	3 cups	1 1/3 cups	X			-2
Corn, White		1/4 cups	X			-1
Corn, Yellow		1/4 cups	X			-1
Cauliflower		2 cups	X			-1
Eggplant +		1 1/2 cups	X			-1
Fiddlehead Ferns	10 cups		X			-2
Mushrooms, Domestic	3 cups	1 cup	X			-1
Mushrooms, Shitake	3 cups	1 cup	X			-2
Mustard Greens	3 1/4 cups	3 cups	X			-1
Potatoes, Red +		1/3 cup	X			-1
Potatoes, Sweet		1/3 cup	X			-1
Potatoes, White		1/3 cup	X			-1
Sauerkraut	1 cup		X			-2
Sprouts, Alfalfa	11 cups		X			-1
Sprouts, Brussels	1 1/4 cups		X			-1

FATS

NUTS AND SEEDS

Most Beneficial:	1 Portion =		Yin	Neutral	Yang	Yin/Yang Score
	Raw	Cooked				
Flax Seed	3/4 tsp.		X			-1
Hemp Seeds	3/4 tsp.		X			-1
Pumpkin Seeds	3/4 tsp.		X			-1
Walnuts	1/2 tsp.		X			-2

+ Organic Is Preferable   * Highly Glycemic   ⊕ Acid Neutralized   ■ Acceptable Fruits & Vegetables Only

Neutral:	1 Portion =		Yin	Neutral	Yang	Yin/Yang Score
	Raw	Cooked				
Almonds	1 tsp.		X			-2
Almond Butter	1/2 tsp.		X			-2
Chestnuts	3/4 oz.		X			-2
Filbert Nuts	1/2 tsp.		X			-2
Hickory Nuts	1/2 tsp.		X			-2
Macadamia	1 large		X			-2
Pecans	1/2 tsp.		X			-2
Pignola (Pine Seeds)	1 tsp.		X			-1
Sesame Butter (Tahini)	1/3 tbsp.		X			-1
Sesame Seeds	1 tsp.		X			-1
Sunflower Butter	3/4 tsp.		X			-1
Sunflower Seeds	3/4 tsp.		X			-1
Watermelon Seeds	3/4 tsp.		X			-1

Least Beneficial:	1 Portion =		Yin	Neutral	Yang	Yin/Yang Score
	Raw	Cooked				
Brazil	1/2 nut		X			-2
Cashews	2 nuts		X			-2
Cashew Butter	2/3 tsp.		X			-2
Lychee Nut (1C)	2 oz.		X			-3
Peanuts	6 nuts		X			-2
Peanut Butter	1/2 tsp.		X			-2
Pistachios	2/3 tsp.		X			-2
Poppy Seeds	1 1/4 tsp.		X			-1
Radish Seeds	1 tsp.		X			-1

FATS

OILS AND OTHER FATS

Most Beneficial:	1 Portion =		Yin	Neutral	Yang	Yin/Yang Score
	Raw	Cooked				
Borage Oil	1/3 tsp.		X			-2
Black Currant Oil	1/3 tsp.		X			-2
Hemp Seed Oil	1/3 tsp.		X			-2
Flaxseed Oil (Linseed)	1/3 tsp.		X			-2
Olive Oil	1/3 tsp.		X			-2
Salmon Oil	1/3 tsp.		X			-2

+ Organic Is Preferable   * Highly Glycemic   Acid Neutralized   ■ Acceptable Fruits & Vegetables Only

Neutral:	1 Portion =		Yin	Neutral	Yang	Yin/Yang Score
	Raw	Cooked				
Butter	1/3 tsp.		X			-1
Canola Oil	1/3 tsp.		X			-2
Cod Liver Oil	1/3 tsp.		X			-2
Ghee	1/3 tsp.		X			-1
Olives (Green)	3		X			-2
Sesame Seed Oil	1/3 tsp.		X			-2
Tahini	1/2 tsp.		X			-2

Least Beneficial:	1 Portion =		Yin	Neutral	Yang	Yin/Yang Score
	Raw	Cooked				
Avocado	1 tbsp.		X			-2
Coconut Oil	1/3 tsp.		X			-2
Corn Oil	1/3 tsp.		X			-2
Cottonseed Oil	1/3 tsp.		X			-2
Cream (half & half)	1 tbsp.		X			-1
Cream Cheese	1 tsp.		X			-1
Hydrogenated Oil	1/3 tsp.		X			-2
Lard	1/3 tsp.		X			-2
Olives (Black)	3		X			-2
Olives (Greek)	3		X			-2
Olives (Spanish)	3		X			-2
Palm Oil	1/3 tsp.		X			-2
Peanut Oil	1/3 tsp.		X			-2
Safflower Oil	1/3 tsp.		X			-2
Shortening, vegetable	1/3 tsp.		X			-2
Sour Cream	1/2 tbsp		X			-1
Sour Cream, Light	1 tbsp		X			-1

MISCELLANEOUS

BEVERAGES

Most Beneficial:	1 Portion =		Yin	Neutral	Yang	Yin/Yang Score
	Raw	Cooked				
Club Soda	N/A			X		<
Green Tea (Decaffeinated)	N/A			X		<
Purified Water	N/A			X		<
Seltzer Water	N/A			X		<

+ Organic Is Preferable   * Highly Glycemic   ⊕ Acid Neutralized   ■ Acceptable Fruits & Vegetables Only

Neutral:	1 Portion =		Yin	Neutral	Yang	Yin/Yang Score
	Raw	Cooked				
Beer (Light)	4 oz.			X		0
Beer (Regular)	4 oz.			X		0
Cappuccino, Decaf ⊕	N/A				X	<
Champagne	4 oz		X			-3
Coffee, Decaf ⊕	N/A		X			<
Green Tea	N/A			X		<
Sparkling Water	N/A			X		<
Sports Drink (Natural)	1/3 cup				X	-3
Tea, Black, Decaf ⊕	N/A				X	<
Tea, Black, Regular ⊕	N/A				X	<
Wine, Red	4 oz.		X			-3
Wine, White	4 oz.		X			-3

Least Beneficial:	1 Portion =		Yin	Neutral	Yang	Yin/Yang Score
	Raw	Cooked				
Cappuccino, Decaf	N/A				X	<
Cappuccino, Regular	N/A				X	<
Coffee, Decaf	N/A				X	<
Coffee, Regular	N/A				X	<
Latte'	1 cup		X			-2
Liquors, Distilled	1 oz.			X		0
Soda, Diet	2 1/2 oz.		X			-3
Sodas (other)	2 1/2 oz.		X			-3
Sports Drink (Artificial)	1/3 cup		X			-3
Tea, Black, Decaffeinated	N/A				X	<
Tea, Black, Regular	N/A				X	<

MISCELLANEOUS

CONDIMENTS

Most Beneficial:	1 Portion =	Yin	Neutral	Yang	Yin/Yang Score
None					

Neutral:	1 Portion =		Yin	Neutral	Yang	Yin/Yang Score
	Raw	Cooked				
Apple Butter *	2 tsp.		X			-3
Braggs Amino Acids	N/A				X	<
Jam * ■	2 tsp.		X			-3
Jelly * ■	2 tsp.		X			-3
Mayonnaise (Vegetarian)	1 tsp.		X			-2
Mustard	N/A				X	<
Salad Dressing	N/A		X			<
Soy Sauce	N/A				X	<
Tamarind	N/A				X	<
Worcestershire Sauce	N/A				X	<

Least Beneficial:	1 Portion =		Yin	Neutral	Yang	Yin/Yang Score
	Raw	Cooked				
Barbecue Sauce	2 tbsp.		X			-3
Candy Bar	1/4 bar		X			-3
Cocktail Sauce	2 tbsp.		X			-3
Dill Pickles	9		X			-1
Ketchup	2 tbsp.		X			-2
Kosher Pickles	9 oz.		X			-1
Maple Syrup	2 tsp		X			-3
Mayonnaise (Dairy)	1 tsp		X			-1
Plum Sauce	1 1/2 tbsp.		X			-3
Sweet Pickles	1 1/2		X			-1
Sour Pickles	9		X			-1
Relish	4 tsp.		X			-2
Teriyaki Sauce	1 tbsp.		X			-3

MISCELLANEOUS

SPICES

Most Beneficial:	1 Portion =		Yin	Neutral	Yang	Yin/Yang Score
	Raw	Cooked				
Carob	1 oz.		X			-3
Curry	N/A				X	<
Dulse	N/A		X			<
Garlic	N/A				X	<
Ginger	N/A				X	<
Kelp	N/A		X			<
Parsley	N/A				X	<
Pepper, Cayenne	N/A				X	<
Turmeric (Tuber)	N/A		X			<
Turmeric (Rhizome)	N/A				X	<

Neutral:	1 Portion =		Yin	Neutral	Yang	Yin/Yang Score
	Raw	Cooked				
Agar	N/A		X			<
Allspice	N/A				X	<
Almond Extract	N/A		X			<
Anise	N/A		X			<
Arrowroot Starch	1 tsp.		X			-1
Barley, Malt	3 tsp.		X			-2
Basil	N/A		X			<
Bay Leaf	N/A		X			<
Bergamot	N/A		X			<
Black Strap Molasses	1/2 tsp.		X			-3

+ Organic Is Preferable   * Highly Glycemic   ⊕ Acid Neutralized   ■ Acceptable Fruits & Vegetables Only

Neutral: (continued)	1 Portion =		Yin	Neutral	Yang	Yin/Yang Score
	Raw	Cooked				
Brewer's Yeast	N/A		X			<
Brown Rice Syrup	3 tsp.		X			-3
Caraway Seeds	N/A		X			<
Cardamom	N/A				X	<
Chervil	N/A				X	<
Chives	N/A		X			<
Chocolate	1 oz.		X			-3
Cloves	N/A				X	<
Coriander	N/A				X	<
Cream of Tartar	N/A		X			<
Cumin	N/A				X	<
Dill	N/A		X			<
Fennel	N/A		X			<
Gelatin	N/A			X		<
Honey	1/2 tbsp.		X			-3
Horseradish	N/A				X	<
Marjoram	N/A		X			<
Mint	N/A		X			<
Miso	N/A			X		<
Mustard	N/A				X	<
Paprika	N/A				X	<
Peppercorn	N/A				X	<
Red Pepper	N/A				X	<
Peppermint	N/A		X			<
Pimento	N/A				X	<
Rice Syrup	3 tsp.		X			-3
Rosemary	N/A		X			<
Saffron	N/A			X		<
Sage	N/A				X	<
Salt	N/A		X			<
Savory	N/A				X	<
Spearmint	N/A		X			<
Stevia	N/A		X			<
Sucanat	2 tsp.		X			-3
Tapioca	N/A		X			<
Tarragon	N/A		X			<
Thyme	N/A			X		<
Wintergreen	N/A		X			‹

+ Organic Is Preferable   * Highly Glycemic   ⊕ Acid Neutralized   ■ Acceptable Fruits & Vegetables Only

Least Beneficial:	1 Portion =		Yin	Neutral	Yang	Yin/Yang Score
	Raw	Cooked				
Capers	N/A				X	<
Cinnamon	N/A				X	<
Cornstarch	1 tsp.		X			-1
Corn Syrup *	2 tsp.		X			-3
Nutmeg	N/A				X	<
Pancake Syrup *	2 tsp.		X			-3
Pepper, Ground Black	N/A				X	<
Pepper, White	N/A				X	<
Sugar, Brown *	2 tsp.		X			-3
Sugar, Confectionery *	1 tbsp.		X			-3
Sugar, White *	2 tsp.		X			-3
Vanilla	N/A		X			<
Vinegar, Apple Cider	N/A				X	<
Vinegar, Balsamic	N/A				X	<
Vinegar, Red Wine	N/A				X	<
Vinegar, White	N/A				X	<

MISCELLANEOUS

TEAS and/or HERBS

Most Beneficial:	1 Portion =		Yin	Neutral	Yang	Yin/Yang Score
	Raw	Cooked				
Cayenne	N/A				X	<
Chickweed	N/A		X			<
Dandelion	N/A		X			<
Deglycyrrhizinated licorice	N/A			X		<
Fenugreek	N/A				X	<
Ginger	N/A				X	<
Green Tea	N/A			X		<
Hops	N/A			X		<
Linden	N/A		X			<
Milk Thistle	N/A		X			<
Mulberry	N/A		X			<
Parsley	N/A				X	<
Peppermint	N/A		X			<
Rosehip	N/A			X		<
Sage	N/A				X	<
Sarsaparilla	N/A			X		<
Slippery Elm	N/A			X		<

+ Organic Is Preferable   * Highly Glycemic   ⊕ Acid Neutralized   ■ Acceptable Fruits & Vegetables Only

Neutral:	1 Portion =		Yin	Neutral	Yang	Yin/Yang Score
	Raw	Cooked				
Catnip	N/A		X			<
Chamomile	N/A			X		<
Dong Quai	N/A				X	<
Elder	N/A				X	<
Ginseng, American	N/A		X			<
Hawthorne	N/A				X	<
Horehound	N/A		X			<
Licorice Root	N/A			X		<
Mullein	N/A		X			<
Raspberry Leaf	N/A			X		<
Skullcap	N/A		X			<
Spearmint	N/A		X			<
Thyme	N/A			X		<
Valerian	N/A				X	<
Vervain	N/A		X			<
White Birch	N/A		X			<
White Oak Bark	N/A		X			<
Yarrow	N/A			X		<

Least Beneficial:	1 Portion =		Yin	Neutral	Yang	Yin/Yang Score
	Raw	Cooked				
Alfalfa	N/A			X		<
Aloe Vera	N/A		X			<
Burdock	N/A		X			<
Cascara sagrada	N/A		X			<
Colt's Foot	N/A		X			<
Corn silk	N/A		X			<
Echinacea	N/A		X			<
Gentian	N/A		X			<
Ginseng, Siberian	N/A				X	<
Goldenseal	N/A		X			<
Red Clover	N/A		X			<
Rhubarb	N/A			X		<
St. John's Wort	N/A		X			<
Senna	N/A		X			<
Shepherd's Purse	N/A			X		<
Strawberry Leaf	N/A		X			<
Yellowdock	N/A		X			<

+ Organic Is Preferable   * Highly Glycemic   ⊕ Acid Neutralized   ■ Acceptable Fruits & Vegetables Only

Blood Type O Recipes

INSTRUCTIONS FOR USE:

The following pages provide five recipes specific for this particular blood type: breakfast, lunch, dinner, dessert and one snack. Each recipe takes into account the correct foods for this specific blood type, the proper ratio of proteins, carbohydrates and fats (Macrobalance™ Portions) and an acceptable Yin Yang energetic score. In compliance with the 4th piece of the New Millennium Diet puzzle, it is recommended that organic foods be used as much as possible. Each meal (breakfast, lunch and dinner) offers the user three, four, five or six Portion amounts.

The recipe consists of two parts. Part one, a shopping list that provides the correct amount of ingredients necessary according to the 4 different Portion sizes. The shopping list also shows the amount in which the various Portion sizes contribute towards the total Yin Yang score.

Part two is the Preparation section and provides simple to follow instructions in preparing the recipe.

It is very simple to use the recipes, it is done in three easy steps:
1. **Determine the correct amount of Portions needed (Chapter 7).**
2. **In the recipe, refer to the Grocery List, select the correct Portion column and obtain the ingredients in the amounts listed.**
3. **Prepare the recipe according to the Preparation instructions in Part two.**

It's that simple to enjoy a complete Macrobalanced™ meal. Bon appetit!

Breakfast: Italian Scramble
Blood Type O

Shopping List

	Portion Size			
	3	4	5	6
Ingredients:	**Amount of Ingredient**			
Proteins:				
Whole Egg(s)	2 eggs	3 eggs	4 eggs	5 eggs
Mozzarella Cheese	1 oz	1 oz	1 1/4 oz	1 1/3 oz
Carbohydrates:				
Bell Peppers (chopped)	3/4 cup	1 1/5 cup	1 1/2 cup	1 2/3 cup
Zucchini (chopped)	1 1/3 cup	1 2/3 cup	2 1/4 cup	2 2/3 cup
Onions (chopped)	3/5 cup	4/5 cup	1 cup	1 1/5 cup
Tomato (chopped)	1/2 cup	3/4 cup	1 cup	1 1/4 cup
Fats and Oils:				
Olive Oil	1 tsp	1 1/3 tsp	1 2/3 tsp	2 tsp
Spices:				
Sea Salt	pinch	pinch	pinch	pinch
Oregano (dried)	pinch	pinch	pinch	pinch
Turmeric	pinch	pinch	pinch	pinch
Basil (dried)	pinch	pinch	pinch	pinch
Marjoram	pinch	pinch	pinch	pinch
Yin (-)/Yang(+) (excess)	-2	-2	-1	-1

Preparation:

In a saute pan, cook the vegetables in the olive oil until soft. Once cooked, add the tomatoes and the five herbs and spices. Simmer for 4 to 6 minutes. Add the eggs and grated mozzarella to the vegetable mixture. Scramble until eggs have solidified. Serve immediately while warm.

Lunch: Tex Mex Chili
Blood Type O

Shopping List

Ingredients:	Portion Size			
	3	4	5	6
	Amount of Ingredient			
Proteins:				
Lean Ground Beef	3 oz	4 oz	5 oz	6 oz
Mozzarella Cheese	1 oz	1 1/3 oz	1 2/3 oz	2 oz
Carbohydrates:				
Red Beans (canned)	3/8 cup	1/2 cup	5/8 cup	3/4 cup
Onions (diced)	3/8 cup	1/3 cup	5/8 cup	3/4 cup
Celery (diced)	3/8 cup	1/2 cup	5/8 cup	3/4 cup
Tomato (canned)	3/5 cup	4/5 cup	1 cup	1 1/5 cup
Tomato (puree)	1/8 cup	1/6 cup	1/5 cup	1/4 cup
Fats and Oils:				
Canola Oil	2/3 tsp	2/3 tsp	2/3 tsp	2/3 tsp
Sunflower Seeds	3/4 tsp	1 tsp	2 1/4 tsp	3 tsp
Spices:				
Garlic (minced)	1/2 cl	2/3 cl	1 cl	1 1/4 cl
Basil (dried)	3/8 tsp	1/2 tsp	1/2 tsp	3/4 tsp
Tabasco Sauce	1 1/2 tsp	1 1/2 tsp	3/4 tsp	3/4 tsp
Sea Salt	pinch	pinch	pinch	pinch
Yin (-)/Yang(+) (excess)	-2	-2	-3	-3

Preparation:

Heat the oil, saute onions, beef, beans and celery in a saucepan until lightly cooked. Add water, tomato puree, diced tomatoes, herbs, spices and cook until thoroughly heated. Add mozzarella cheese and sunflower seeds as topping. Serve warm.

Snack: Tomato Mozzarella
Blood Type O

Shopping List

	Portion Size		
	1	2	3
Ingredients:	**Amount of Ingredient**		
Proteins:			
Mozzarella Cheese	1 oz	3 oz	3 oz
Carbohydrates:			
Tomato	1 medium	2 medium	2 1/2 medium
Fats and Oils:			
Sunflower Seeds	1 tsp	2 tsp	3 tsp
Spices:			
Sea Salt	pinch	pinch	pinch
Yin (-)/Yang(+) (excess)	0	1	1

Preparation:
Slice tomatoes and mozzarella. Sprinkle sunflower seeds on top.
Lightly season with sea salt.

Dinner: Mandarin Shrimp and Beef
Blood Type O

Shopping List

Ingredients:	Portion Size			
	3	4	5	6
	Amount of Ingredient			
Proteins:				
Shrimp (large)	1 1/2 oz	2 oz	2 1/2 oz	3 oz
Beef (cubed)	2 oz	2 2/3 oz	3 1/3 oz	4 oz
Carbohydrates:				
Bell Peppers (green)	1 cup	1 1/4 cup	1 1/2 cup	2 cup
Snow Peas	3/4 cup	1 cup	1 1/4 cup	1 1/2 cup
Bean Sprouts	1 1/8 cup	1 1/2 cup	1 7/8 cup	2 1/4 cup
Green Onion (chopped)	3/4 cup	1 cup	1 1/4 cup	1 1/2 cup
Tomato (chopped)	3/8 cup	1/2 cup	5/8 cup	3/4 cup
Fats and Oils:				
Olive Oil	1/4 tsp	1/3 tsp	1/2 tsp	3/4 tsp
Butter	1/2 tsp	2/3 tsp	5/8 tsp	1 tsp
Spices:				
Ginger	1 1/2 tsp	2 tsp	2 1/3 tsp	3 tsp
Apple Cider Vinegar	1 1/2 tbsp	2 tbsp	2 1/2 tbsp	3 tbsp
Hot Sauce	3/4 tsp	1 tsp	1 1/4 tsp	1 1/2 tsp
White Wine	1/4 tsp	1/4 tsp	1/4 tsp	1/4 tsp
Yin (-)/Yang(+) (excess)	-2	-3	-2	-3

Preparation:

In a saucepan add the sprouts, snow peas and bell peppers to 1 cup of water and cook until tender. In a separate saucepan place the oil, butter, shrimp, beef and green onions and cook for 5 to 10 minutes until done. Add the beef/shrimp mixture, tomatoes, wine, hot sauce, small amount of water and ginger. Continue to cook another 5 to 6 minutes. Add the vegetables to the beef and shrimp mixture. Stir and serve.

Dessert: Frozen Pineapple Cream
Blood Type O

Shopping List

Ingredients:	Portion Size		
	1	2	3
	Amount of Ingredient		
Proteins:			
Egg Whites	1/4 egg	1/2 egg	3/4 egg
Unflavored Gelatin	1/4 env.	1/2 env.	3/4 env.
Soy Yogurt (plain)	1/4 cup	1/2 cup	3/4 cup
Carbohydrates:			
Pineapple	1/4 cup	1/2 cup	3/4 cup
Arrowroot Powder**	1 1/3 tsp	2 tsp	2 1/4 tsp
Fats and Oils:			
Sunflower Seeds (chopped)	2/3 tsp	1 1/3 tsp	2 tsp
Spices:			
Ginger	1/6 tsp	1/5 tsp	1/3 tsp
Orange Extract	1/4 tsp	1/3 tsp	1/3 tsp
Yin (-)/Yang(+) (excess)	-2	-2	-4

Preparation:

In a saucepan, place the pineapple, gelatin, arrowroot,** ginger, orange extract and yogurt. Heat until warmed thoroughly. Set aside until cool. Place the egg whites in a mixing bowl and whip until firm. Add the egg mixture and sunflower seeds to the cooled fruit mixture. Stir the mixture, place into freezer until frozen. Serve cold.

**Arrowroot Powder should be well-mixed with 3 to 5 teaspoons of cold water before adding to the other ingredients.

Chapter 9

Blood Type A: Agrarian

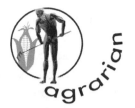

Health and Dietary Characteristics

- 25% Protein
  50% Carbohydrate
  25% Fat
- The First True Vegan
- Sensitive Digestive Tract
- Adaptive Immune System
- Strong Adaptive Potential to
  Environmental Pressures
- Agricultural-Based Diet for Maximum
  Physical and Mental Health

Personality Characteristics

- Handles Stress Well
- Noncompetitive and Relaxed
- Adaptable to Any Situation
- Creative
- Sensitive

BLOOD TYPE A—CHARACTERISTICS

PERSONALITY CHARACTERISTICS

Type A individuals compose approximately 40% of the world population. They are suited for a more civilized environment and better equipped to deal with the stressors produced in our industrialized age, such as pollution and congestion. They appear more able to handle societal stresses found in an organized living situation in comparison to other blood types. Blood Type A people do well in a more relaxed, noncompetitive environment, where they are able to foster the creative and sensitive aspects of their being. However, they can be very adaptive to changing circumstances. This is why they were able to make it through the agricultural revolution and tolerated it so well. A types, in fact, can adapt to any type of situation, even if that means stepping up and taking a leadership role.

PHYSIOLOGY AND DIETARY CHARACTERISTICS

Type A stands for agrarian. Agrarian, according to the American Heritage Dictionary, refers to someone concerned with land, its ownership, cultivation, or tenure. This definition explains why Type A people have adapted to foods that are produced from the land, such as fruits, vegetables, and grains as opposed to meat-based food sources. As a matter of fact, red meat is actually considered a poison for blood Type A. Also, many refined and processed foods, which are increasingly becoming the staple of the American diet, react poorly with the sensitive immune system that blood Type A possesses.

It is vital to eat foods in as natural a state as possible. Organic and locally produced foods contain more nutrients and health-giving properties than commercial foods. Many of my patients who have been big meat eaters find this concept to be a bit difficult to live with at first, but within a short period of time after incorporating this type of dietary plan, they often report that they have never felt better. In addition, as their immune system improves, they develop greater resistance to infective agents such as viruses, bacteria, and parasites.

Most A types have a genetic predisposition for cancer, diabetes, heart disease, and immune system–related conditions, including chronic fatigue syndrome. Following this diet reduces the risk of developing these illnesses.

Weight Management

The blood Type A diet has a tremendous impact on the potential for weight and fat loss. Results can occur very rapidly. By following the program, you will quickly learn what your body already knows. You will find that you are simply tapping into the innate intelligence that already exists.

You will find, for instance, that persistent problems with fat and water retention are often resolved by eliminating meat, especially red meat, from your diet. The blood Type A individual has a metabolic system that functions better with higher carbohydrates, especially carbohydrates that come from vegetables, grains, and soy-based foods. Their system is not designed for the standard macronutrient ratio of 30% protein, 40% carbohydrates, and 30% fat. Instead, it is geared for a combination of 25% protein, 50% carbohydrates, and 25% fat. This modification is based on hundreds of Type A individuals who experienced poor results attempting to follow the zone protocol of 40:30:30. Initially, they did well with that combination, but then failed to make progress and often gained weight back. The reason for this is that the higher protein amount in the zone approach can cause water weight loss initially, but over time promotes weight and fat storage. This is because of the higher insulin secretion produced by the body to deal with the larger amount of protein.

Thirty percent protein, recommended in the zone diet, is considered to be too high for an A blood type. Reducing protein by just 5%, down to 25%, can have a significant impact. This is due to the fact that blood Type A individuals have a very sensitive immunological and metabolic system. The subtle downsizing of protein causes dramatic results in their physiology.

Type As do poorly with protein derived from red meat sources. They have a lower stomach acid level compared to blood Type O individuals. Reduced stomach acid makes it more difficult for the digestive tract to effectively break down protein into amino acids. The strain can cause sluggishness in the system, leading to poor digestion, gas, bloating and fatigue.

Dairy-based foods are also problematic. Poor digestibility promotes increased insulin stimulation and fat storage. Milk products also contain lectins which can damage the intestinal lining and impair absorption and assimilation. The result again is gas, bloating, and indigestion.

There are a specific number of grains that A types can eat without problems. Wheat is acceptable because of their agrarian background; however, only in moderate amounts. If eaten excessively, wheat may cause acidity and metabolic imbalance, especially in the bloodstream and in the muscle tissues.

It is important for all types, and particularly individuals with blood Type A, to try to eat foods with low toxicity. Organic is best. The reason is obvious, but in the case of A types who are extra sensitive, this practice helps to protect their immune system and enhance their body's ability to detoxify and eliminate poisons.

Foods Encouraging Fat Gain:

Red meat, dairy products, kidney beans, lima beans, excessive wheat consumption.

Foods Encouraging Fat Loss:

Vegetable oils, soy-based foods, an assortment of vegetables (except for the ones highlighted as least beneficial vegetables) and pineapples.

Exercise

Blood Type A individuals react strongly to stress and because of that their immune systems can become weakened more readily. For this reason, they need to choose their type of exercise carefully. Exercise is a form of stress on the body. A types do not want to overdo it.

Among the best exercises for this blood type is Qigong or tai chi, which emphasizes slow or stationary movement patterns. These disciplines were developed by the Chinese 2,000–3,000 years ago as a way of building the internal qi (pronounced chee), the life force flowing through the body, which regulates the acupuncture channels. Such activities help to calm the nervous system, keeping open the flow of energy to stabilize the physiology.

In addition, moderate exercises such as bicycling, swimming, or light jogging can be performed. They are preferred over more strenuous activities. Marathons and triathlons should be performed with caution. They put a tremendous amount of stress on the more delicate Type A nervous system.

Typically, 30–60 minutes of exercise is sufficient. Meditation is also excellent for many blood Type A individuals. It helps to focus the thought process and calm the nerves, allowing the body to regenerate and heal. Yoga, especially Hatha yoga, is effective for toning muscles, joints and ligaments, as well as the cardiovascular system. If you integrate aerobic or weight-lifting type activities, follow up with some type of meditation or yoga stretching moves to help balance the neuro-muscular system.

If blood Type A individuals, or any blood type for that matter, participate in any type of seriously strenuous activities, I recommend taking large amounts of a nutrient known as MSM (methylsulfonylmethane). MSM is excellent for preventing the typical muscle soreness that is associated with intense physical workouts or peak performance activities. I also recommend small amounts of calming herbs such as valerian root or kava kava after intense workouts. In addition, arnica, a popular homeopathic remedy, should always be kept on hand in case of sprains or strains. It is amazingly effective to prevent the normal swelling that occurs after trauma. St. John's wort is also useful to keep the mind on an even keel.

DIETARY SPECIFICS

PROTEINS

MEAT AND POULTRY

Meats, in general, have a negative effect on blood Type A's physiological functions because of their high lectin content. Most red meats should be avoided. Poultry and fish can be eaten in limited quantity. However, if you philosophically or otherwise choose to avoid meat altogether, then follow your beliefs.

Living in a meat-eating culture — such as in America and many Western countries — often makes it difficult to follow a vegetarian diet. It's worth the effort; it can substantially reduce your risk of developing cancer, heart disease, diabetes, and immune system illnesses. The closer you are able to follow it, the higher the probability that you will not develop these types of conditions over your lifetime.

Poultry, in limited quantity, is considered neutral for most A types. However, it is the highest rated Yang food, so if you choose to eat poultry, balance it out with the appropriate amounts of Yin-containing foods, such as fruits, leafy vegetables and nuts. If fish is a more preferable meat choice for you, do not eat it with fruit. Fruit is such a high Yin food that it will totally unbalance the Yin-Yang state of the meal.

Regarding the Rh factor, Type A negative individuals can include partridge, pheasant, and quail among their neutral foods.

A types should definitely avoid any type of processed meats. They often contain nitrates, chemical additives that are considered carcinogens, which may contribute to the development of stomach cancer.

It is also recommended to avoid antacids. The Type A stomach environment is more alkaline than most of the other blood types. Antacids further reduce the stomach acid level, making it more difficult to digest even a limited amount of meat. If indigestion occurs, it is advisable to use ginger root or a digestive enzyme instead. If digestion still remains a problem, then a betain hydrochloride supplement may help to activate the digestive enzymes in your stomach.

PROTEINS

SEAFOOD

Seafood is tolerated to a moderate degree, certainly much better than meat. Sole and flounder are high in bad lectins. Avoid these fish, especially if you suffer from any intestinal condition. The lectins can cause or aggravate inflammation within the bowel lining.

In addition, there is a snail that's known as *Helix pomatia*, which actually contains a very important lectin that has been shown to neutralize mutated Type A cells, such as those found in many types of cancer. This is especially important for women who have breast cancer, because it can help to neutralize these types of cancerous tissues.

Type A negative individuals can eat anchovies, spiney lobster, and scallops. A positive individuals should not.

In the seafood listings, at the end of this chapter, you will notice that many fish you might think are acceptable have been grouped into the least beneficial category. This is because many fish are contaminated with environmental toxins.

PROTEINS

DAIRY

Avoid milk products because of the high amount of lactose, the milk sugar in dairy products. Type A individuals, however, can consume a small amount of fermented dairy products because the fermenting process removes a large amount of the lactose. If possible, purchase organic dairy products such as organic yogurt, eggs, and sour cream. You are even better off utilizing milk replacements such as rice, almond, soy and oat milk. I regard soy milk as the best substitute. It contains high concentrations of isoflavones, natural substances found in soy with anticancer and antioxidant properties. Goat's milk is another natural replacement for cow's milk. It has a much lower level of lectins and antigens.

A types are generally allergic to cow's milk because of lactose, which contains D-galactosamine, the sugar molecule that makes up the blood Type B antigen. Blood Type A individuals will reject anything with blood Type B antigens. Consequently, blood Type A's reject cow's milk that contains this particular sugar.

A types have a tendency to produce large amounts of mucus. Milk and dairy lead to increased mucus secretion because of its Yin nature, which is phlegm producing. Type A people with asthma, allergies, or other allergic conditions, including children with recurrent ear infections, experience significant relief by eliminating dairy.

CARBOHYDRATES

BEANS AND LEGUMES

Soy beans are a form of carbohydrate but are also high in protein. They are, in fact, the only bean or legume considered as a protein source for A types. The other beans listed in the highly beneficial or neutral section are considered solely as carbohydrates. Many vegetarians combine rice and beans to make a balanced protein source. It is important to understand, however, that the amount of protein in these foods is minor relative to their carbohydrate content.

If you plan on following a strict vegetarian approach, tofu (soybean curd) will supply a large source of your protein needs in the New Millennium Diet. If available, make sure the tofu you buy is organic without additives. Preservatives are used in some of the more commercially available tofu products. If at all possible, buy your tofu at a health food store.

Avoid kidney, lima, navy, and garbanzo beans. They contain lectins that can increase insulin production, throwing you out of balance. Excess insulin is associated with diabetes and fat gain.

Regarding the Rh factor, garbanzo beans are OK for A negatives, but not for A positives.

CARBOHYDRATES

GRAINS AND CEREALS

A types can tolerate a wide variety of cereals and grains because their bodies have adapted to these types of food over the last 20,000 years. Within the general category, certain types of grains and cereals are more favorable than others. Wheat is still the biggest concern because it contains lectins that may be offensive to some people. It is a good idea to determine your wheat tolerance level, that is, how much you can eat on a regular basis. Wheat, of course, is used in many products, including breads, cakes and cookies. If you are suffering with candidiasis or any type of allergic condition, you should consider reducing your wheat consumption to two to three times per week, or perhaps cut it out altogether.

CARBOHYDRATES

BREADS

Your preference should be sprouted breads. Be alert to the wheat content. I recommend Essene or Ezekiel bread as the most beneficial. The sprouting process reduces much of the gluten and lectin content, making them acceptable for A types. In general, breads, cereals and grains have a higher glycemic index, which means that their carbohydrate content becomes converted into sugar more rapidly. But as long as you are following the 25:50:25 dietary approach, higher glycemic foods can be tolerated to a greater degree. Soy flours may have a slightly unpleasant taste but if mixed with other types of flours that are blood type acceptable, they are tolerated and can be used in the making of pancakes or muffins.

CARBOHYDRATES

PASTAS AND FLOURS

Most of the traditional pastas should be avoided because they contain semolina flour. Acceptable grains for pastas include spelt, kamut, quinoa, buckwheat, and rice.

CARBOHYDRATES

VEGETABLES

Vegetables are a mainstay for Type A. All vegetables are Yin foods. It is important they be slightly steamed or cooked in order to reduce the amount of Yin energy. If you follow a full vegan approach this is particularly important. Try to aim for an overall Yin-Yang score as close to neutral as possible; you won't be able to eat enough Yang foods to balance out the large amount of Yin in the diet. Cooking the food reduces the Yin potential, thus helping to achieve an energetic balance. This doesn't mean that raw foods should be avoided. Just be aware of the Yin-Yang balance. If you frequently eat poultry, introduce more raw vegetables into your diet to balance out the excessive Yang tendencies found in the poultry.

Do not eat foods listed as least beneficial. They can negatively affect the digestive function. Foods such as olives, peppers, potatoes, sweet potatoes, yams, tomatoes, and cabbage should all be avoided.

It is best to buy organically grown vegetables, especially at a time when more and more genetically engineered foods are appearing in the produce marketplace. Many commercially available vegetables have been genetically modified with insect genes, fish genes, and even human genes in order to alter the growth pattern or resistance to certain types of pests. Many scientists question the safety of these foods, which are not specially labeled. Organic food has not been genetically engineered. Therefore you can feel safe that your family will not be consuming altered foods.

Candida patients should avoid raw foods because such foods can negatively impact the spleen and pancreas function, leading to an overgrowth of fungus.

CARBOHYDRATES

FRUITS

Fruits are very dense carbohydrates. You only need a small quantity to provide a full New Millennium carbohydrate portion. Fruits are the most Yin of all foods. They are given a score of -3 in our Yin-Yang scale. If you eat poultry, you can easily balance the meal with fruit. This does not apply for people who are suffering with candidiasis, who should avoid fruit.

There are a large number of highly beneficial fruits that A types can consume. Grapefruit, pineapples, apricots, plums, and lemons are fine, but avoid mangoes and papayas. Even though these tropical fruits contain beneficial levels of digestive enzymes, the lectins may potentially disrupt the A individual's more sensitive digestive system. Many melons contain high levels of molds, so avoid melons except for those that are in the neutral or most beneficial lists.

Bad news for banana lovers! They are not for A types. They have elevated lectin levels and a high glycemic rating.

CARBOHYDRATES

JUICES

Black cherry juice is a highly beneficial juice. However, it can cause staining of the teeth if they are porous, a result of not getting enough calcium in the diet (see calcium under supplements below). Adequate calcium strengthens and hardens the enamel surface.

I recommend drinking at least one glass of water per day mixed with 10–15 drops of lemon juice. This helps to detoxify the system and to eliminate excess phlegm and toxic accumulations within the body.

FATS

NUTS AND SEEDS

Fat makes up 25% of your New Millennium Diet. Nuts and seeds are considered excellent sources of fat in the program. They contain high levels of beneficial monounsaturated oil.

Peanuts, however, are a no-no. While they have been touted in the past as being highly beneficial for A types, they are the most toxic food in the entire American diet, according to an FDA study. The average peanut contains dozens of chemicals as well as aflatoxin, a toxic substance produced by a mold that infests almost every peanut produced in the world. Even if peanuts contain lectins with anticancer properties, which has been reported in the medical literature, the number of seriously toxic compounds outweighs any such benefits. If you have candida, you must avoid peanuts even if they are organic.

I like to use macadamia nuts or sunflower seeds to fill out my fat requirement in meals, especially when I am eating out. Using nuts and seeds in this manner is easy. Usually one small macadamia nut or a half of a large nut is equivalent to one fat Portion. For example, if you were to have a three-Portion meal, then you would eat at least three small macadamia nuts to meet your fat requirement.

In regard to the Rh factor, A negative types can consume pistachios. A positives should still avoid them.

FATS

OILS

Monounsaturated fats, such as olive oil, are the best fats for your blood type. Sufficient fat is critical in order to balance out the high level of carbohydrates consumed. Fat slows down the entry of carbohydrates into the bloodstream, so that there isn't a tidal wave of insulin. Remember: Excess insulin leads to fat storage.

MISCELLANEOUS

BEVERAGES

Coffee is beneficial for many of you. It increases stomach acid and improves digestion. Don't get carried away, though. Not more than one to two cups a day. Coffee has the potential to damage the adrenal glands because it increases the production of adrenaline. Decaf is preferred.

If you enjoy red wine, choose organic red. They contain natural sulfites, not synthetic compounds. Green tea is an excellent beverage, replete with natural substances shown to have anticancer and antioxidant properties.

MISCELLANEOUS

CONDIMENTS

Avoid any condiment containing tomato or vinegar, including ketchup, pickles, and Worcestershire sauces. Vinegar is a fermented substance that is not well suited to A types. It can irritate their stomach lining and can cause imbalances. Also try to avoid condiments with dairy. Mustard is the most beneficial condiment for your blood type.

MISCELLANEOUS

SPICES

Sorry to pass along this bit of bad news, but most of you should avoid sugar and chocolates. If you can't help yourself, please limit your indulgence. These foods put a strain on your adrenal gland and that can weaken the whole physiology. They are refined foods and, as stated earlier, most A types do not fare well on such food. If you need to sweeten things up, use brown rice syrups instead of the more refined sugars. It's a good substitute and will not cause the imbalances generated by processed sugars. Stevia is another excellent sugar substitute. It's actually an herb from South America that has recently been given approval by the FDA.

Kelp is an excellent salt or spice substitute. It contains iodine, an important mineral for proper thyroid gland function. Type A individuals have a tendency toward low thyroid gland function.

MISCELLANEOUS

SUPPLEMENTS

B Complex Vitamins

Vitamin B's, especially B_{12}, are particularly lacking in the vegan type of diet which blood Type As should be following. B_{12} in particular is vital for the proper functioning of many neurological and energy-generating systems in the body. It's a good idea to take some additional B_{12} if you're following a strict vegetarian diet.

There are excellent B_{12} supplements that are delivered sublingually, that is, they are absorbed under the tongue directly into the bloodstream, bypassing the digestive tract. This is a good way to obtain extra B_{12}. I would avoid niacin supplements (vitamin B_3) because it can put stress on your liver and in excess could cause liver damage.

Vitamin C

Vitamin C, especially the nonacidic (buffered) type which has been bound to a mineral, such as sodium ascorbate or calcium ascorbate, is the preferred form of this important vitamin. Ascorbic acid, the acidic form of vitamin C, can be irritating to the sensitive digestive tract of most A types. Buffered vitamin C also has a higher bio-availability, meaning more of it is absorbed into the body. Take between 1,500–3,000 milligrams per day.

Vitamin C has powerful immune-enhancing characteristics. It also has the ability to bind up toxins in the bloodstream, and escort them out of the body through the urine, one of the few vitamins known to have this property. I am a firm believer in the detoxification power of vitamin C. I often recommend intravenous drips of vitamin C at my clinic for patients to accelerate the detoxification process. However, you can help your body significantly detoxify itself from accumulated toxins merely by following the New Millennium Diet.

Vitamin E

Vitamin E is another excellent supplement to fortify your diet. I prefer the tocotrienol version of the vitamin. It has 60 times more antioxidant power than regular vitamin E. I recommend doses in the range of 400–800 IU per day for regular vitamin E, and 150 IU for the tocotrenol variety.

Calcium

Calcium is a vital mineral for all people. It is particularly so for A types who shouldn't eat much dairy. Dairy, of course, is a major source of dietary calcium. The best and most bio-available form of calcium as a supplement is microcrystalline hydroxyapatite. Take a daily dose ranging from 1,000–1,200 milligrams. You should be able to locate microcrystalline hydroxyapatite at your health food store. If you can't find it, use calcium lactate. Avoid calcium carbonate, which requires a high level of stomach acid and is not suited for the blood Type A digestive tracts.

Iron

Iron supplements are beneficial because your diet lacks common foods rich in iron. Women should be particularly alert to this need because of the iron lost in the blood during menses. I recommend any form of natural iron supplement.

The homeopathic remedy Ferrum metallicum can be very effective for improving cases of anemia. Use the 6C potency and take it three times per day. Many health food stores carry homeopathic remedies.

Herbs

Stimulating herbs are useful to boost immune system function. Examples are echinacea, astragalus, ginseng, and licorice root. They nourish the thymus gland and bone marrow, important centers in the body for production of white blood cells and other immuno-logical factors.

Other important herbs are chamomile and valerian. These are proven antistress herbs that act as natural tranquilizers. Often they can replace medications prescribed for in-somnia. Of course, consult with your doctor prior to use.

Another wonderful herb is milk thistle. It has a special affinity for the liver, helping this pivotal organ to rid itself of toxins and repair damaged tissue. It's one of the few substances known to be protective against mushroom poisoning. It has saved numerous lives from toxic effects of poisonous mushrooms.

Stay away from antacids. Use ginger instead, or deglycyrrhizinated licorice (DGL), or pearl coix for indigestion needs.

Noni Juice

Noni juice is an excellent herb derived from the morinda citrofolia plant of the South Pacific. It has been shown to improve high blood sugar levels in diabetes and accellerate wound healing.

Enzymes

Digestive enzymes, especially plant-based products derived from aspergillus, a type of fungus, are excellent supplements for boosting the digestive ability of A types who may have weak digestion. Another type of supplement called probiotics is helpful in main-taining good digestive function. Probiotics supplements usually contain billions of ben-eficial bacterial strains, such as acidophilus and bifidus, that are involved in numerous important activities in the gut. Beneficial bacteria are often destroyed by antibiotics.

Blood Type A Food Chart

25% Protein—50% Carbohydrate—25% Fat

Proper Food Ratio

The proper macronutrient ratio for blood Type A is 25% protein, 50% carbohydrate and 25% fat. One Portion of protein equals 5.75 grams, one Portion of carbohydrates equals 11.5 grams and one Portion of fat equals 2.5 grams. You will only use this information if you want to use a food not listed in the food groups. Otherwise, all food listings are designated in their appropriate Portion requirements.

Classification of Foods

Three (3) food classifications are used in the New Millennium Diet Plan. They are most beneficial, neutral and least beneficial foods. These classifications are based on blood type compatibility, glycemic index, toxicity levels and other food characteristics.

These factors have been carefully analyzed and weighed against each other to determine their appropriate designation within the food classifications. For example, peanuts and peanut butter have been considered as a *favorable food* by other diet plans. In this diet plan, they have been rated as *least beneficial,* due to the fact that they contain over 180 chemical residues. Similar reclassification of foods have been made on this basis.

It is important that you realize this distinction in your meal planning to achieve maximum results.

Most Beneficial Foods

These foods demonstrate optimum blood type compatibility and contain the lowest level of toxic chemical residues. They should be selected as your first choice in diet planning.

Neutral Foods

These foods are neutral in their blood type compatibility, but may contain slightly higher levels of toxic chemical residues. They should be selected as your second choice in diet planning.

Least Beneficial Foods

These foods demonstrate the least blood type compatibility and may contain the highest levels of toxic chemical residues. They should be considered as the last choice in diet planning and be consumed only on a very limited basis if at all.

Rh Factor—Type A Positive and Type A Negative

The Type A positive and Type A negative diets are very similar except for certain foods that are in bold type in the least beneficial section of the different food classifications. Type A negatives can consider the bold type foods in the chart as neutral foods unless you have a known allergic reaction to the food. However, Type A positives must look at those bold foods as least beneficial. This system applies to all blood types. This is the only pertinent difference between Type A negatives and Type A positives.

FOOD GROUPS USED IN THE CHART

PROTEINS
- MEAT • POULTRY • EXOTICS
- SEAFOOD
- DAIRY PRODUCTS

CARBOHYDRATES
- BEANS and LEGUMES
- GRAINS and CEREALS
- BREADS
- PASTAS and FLOURS
- VEGETABLES
- FRUITS
- JUICES

FATS
- NUTS and SEEDS
- OILS and other Fats

MISCELLANEOUS
- BEVERAGES
- CONDIMENTS
- SPICES • TEAS • HERBS

FOOD CHART LEGEND

+ Organic Is Preferable

* Highly Glycemic

⊕ Acid Neutralized

■ Acceptable Fruits & Vegetables Only

< This food possibly has a Yin or Yang energy, but for our diet planning is considered negligible

1P 1 Protein Portion

1C 1 Carbohydrate Portion

1F 1 Fat Portion

*1P/1C/1F This food contains 1 Portion of protein, 1 Portion of carbohydrate and 1 Portion of Fat in the serving size listed

* Note: The number before the letter will always signify the amount of Protein-Carbohydrates-Fat Portions in the serving size listed.

PROTEINS

MEAT • POULTRY • EXOTICS

Most Beneficial:	1 Portion =		Yin	Neutral	Yang	Yin/Yang Score
None						

Neutral:	1 Portion =		Yin	Neutral	Yang	Yin/Yang Score
	Raw	Cooked				
Alligator		1 1/4 oz.			X	+2
Chicken (Breast, deli, ground)		1 1/4 oz.			X	+3
Chicken (Breast, skinless)		3/4 oz.			X	+3
Chicken, (dark, skinless)		3/4 oz.			X	+3
Chicken (hot dog)		3/4 link			X	+3
Cornish Hens		3/4 oz.			X	+3
Ostrich		1 1/4 oz.			X	+3
Soy Burger		1/3 patty			X	+1
Soy (hot dog)		3/4 link			X	+1
Soy Sausage		1 2/3 link			X	+1
Soy Sausage Patty		3/4 patty				+1
Tempeh (1P/1C)		1 1/4 oz.	X		X	+1/-1
Tofu (firm or extra firm)		2 1/2 oz.			X	+2
Tofu (soft or regular) (1P/1C)		2 1/2 oz.	X		X	+1/-1
Turkey		3/4 oz.			X	+3
Turkey (bacon)		2 1/2 strips			X	+3
Turkey (breast, skinless)		3/4 oz.			X	+3
Turkey (breast, deli, ground)		1 1/4 oz.			X	+3
Turkey (hot dog)		3/4 link			X	+3

+ Organic Is Preferable   * Highly Glycemic   ⊕ Acid Neutralized   ■ Acceptable Fruits & Vegetables Only

CHAPTER 9
BLOOD TYPE A: AGRARIAN

Least Beneficial:	1 Portion =		Yin	Neutral	Yang	Yin/Yang Score
	Raw	Cooked				
Bacon		2 1/2 strips			X	+1
Beef, Ground 10–15%		1 1/4 oz.			X	+2
Beef (hot dog)		3/4 link			X	+2
Beef, Lean		3/4 oz.			X	+2
Buffalo		3/4 oz.			X	+2
Canadian Bacon		3/4 oz.			X	+1
Duck		1 1/4 oz.			X	+3
Goose		3/4 oz.			X	+3
Ham, Lean		3/4 oz.			X	+1
Ham, Deli		1 1/4 oz.			X	+1
Heart, Beef		3/4 oz.			X	+2
Kidney, Beef		3/4 oz.			X	+2
Kielbasa		1 2/3 oz.			X	+2
Lamb		3/4 oz.			X	+2
Liver, Beef		3/4 oz.			X	+2
Mutton		3/4 oz.			X	+2
Partridge		1 1/4 oz.			X	+3
Pepperoni		3/4 oz.			X	+2
Pheasant		1 1/4 oz.			X	+3
Pork		3/4 oz.			X	+1
Pork (hot dog)		3/4 link			X	+1
Pork Chop		3/4 oz.			X	+1
Pork Sausage		1 2/3 links			X	+1
Quail		1 1/4 oz.			X	+3
Rabbit		3/4 oz.			X	+2
Rattlesnake		1 1/4 oz.			X	+2
Salami		3/4 oz.			X	+2
Tripe (beef)		1 1/4 oz.			X	+2
Veal		3/4 oz.			X	+2
Venison (domestic)		3/4 oz.			X	+2
Venison (imported)		3/4 oz.			X	+2

PROTEIN

DAIRY PRODUCTS
(Protein-rich dairy sources unless otherwise noted)

Most Beneficial:	1 Portion =		Yin	Neutral	Yang	Yin/Yang Score
	Raw	Cooked				
Cheese (soy)	3/4 oz.				X	+2
Milk (soy) (1C)	1 cup		X			-1
Yogurt, Soy (plain) (1P/1/2C)	1/3 cup		X		X	+1/-1

+ Organic Is Preferable   * Highly Glycemic   ⊕ Acid Neutralized   ■ Acceptable Fruits & Vegetables Only

Neutral:	1 Portion =		Yin	Neutral	Yang	Yin/Yang Score
	Raw	Cooked				
Cheese (almond)	3/4 oz.				X	+2
Cheese (goat)	3/4 oz.				X	+2
Eggs	1 small				X	+3
Egg white	2 small				X	+3
Farmer	3/4 oz.				X	+2
Feta	3/4 oz.				X	+2
Ice Cream, Soy (1C) *	1 cup		X			-3
Ice Cream, Rice (1C) *	1 cup		X			-3
Kefir (1P/1/2C/1F)	3/4 cup		X		X	+1/-1/-1
Milk, Almond (1C) *	1 cup		X			-2
Milk, Goat (1P/1/2C/1F)	3/4 cup		X		X	+1/-1/-1
Milk, Oat (1C) *	1 cup		X			-2
Milk, Rice (1C) *	1 cup		X			-2
Mozzarella	3/4 oz.				X	+2
Ricotta	2 oz.				X	+2
String Cheese	3/4 oz.				X	+2
Yogurt, Plain, (lowfat) (1P/1/2C)	1/3 cup		X		X	+1/-1
Yogurt, Frozen (1C) *	1/3 cup		X			-3
Yogurt, Goat (plain) (1C/1/2C/3F) *	1/3 cup		X		X	+1/-1/-1
Yogurt with fruit (1C) + ■	1/3 cup		X			-3

Least Beneficial:	1 Portion =		Yin	Neutral	Yang	Yin/Yang Score
	Raw	Cooked				
American Cheese	3/4 oz.				X	+2
Blue Cheese	3/4 oz.				X	+2
Brie	3/4 oz.				X	+2
Buttermilk (1P/1/2C/3F)	3/4 cup		X		X	+1/-1/-1
Camembert	3/4 oz.				X	+2
Casein	3/4 oz.				X	+2
Cheddar	3/4 oz.				X	+2
Colby	3/4 oz.				X	+2
Cottage Cheese	3/4 oz.				X	+2
Egg (substitute)	1/5 cup				X	+2
Edam	3/4 oz.				X	+2
Emmenthal	3/4 oz.				X	+2
Gouda	3/4 oz.				X	+2
Gruyere	3/4 oz.				X	+2
Ice Cream (1C) *	1/3 cup		X			-3
Jarlsberg	3/4 oz.				X	+2
Milk (evaporated)	1/3 cup		X			-1
Milk, Ice (1C) *	1/3 cup		X			-3
Milk (Lowfat) (1C) (1P/1/2C)	3/4 cup		X		X	+1/-1
Milk Shake (1C) *	1/3 cup		X			-3
Milk (skim) (1P/1/2C)	3/4 oz.		X		X	'+1/-1
Milk (whole) (1P/1/2C/3F)	3/4 cup		X		X	+1/-1/-1

Least Beneficial: (cont.)	1 Portion =		Yin	Neutral	Yang	Yin/Yang Score
	Raw	Cooked				
Monterey Jack	3/4 oz.				X	+2
Muenster	3/4 oz.				X	+2
Parmesan	3/4 oz.				X	+2
Provolone	3/4 oz.				X	+2
Neufchatel	3/4 oz.				X	+2
Sherbet	1/3 cup		X			-3
Swiss Cheese	3/4 oz.				X	+2
Whey	1/4 oz.				X	+2

PROTEINS

SEAFOOD

Most Beneficial:	1 Portion =		Yin	Neutral	Yang	Yin/Yang Score
	Raw	Cooked				
Abalone		1 1/4 oz.			X	+1
Arctic Char		1 1/4 oz.			X	+1
Bream		1 1/4 oz.			X	+1
Butterfish (imported)		1 1/4 oz.			X	+1
Cod (imported)		1 1/4 oz.			X	+1
Grouper		1 1/4 oz.			X	+1
Marlin		1 1/4 oz.			X	+1
Menpachi		1 1/4 oz.			X	+1
Milkfish		1 1/4 oz.			X	+1
Monkfish		1 1/4 oz.			X	+1
Palani		1 1/4 oz.			X	+1
Pickerel		1 1/4 oz.			X	+1
Pollock		1 1/4 oz.			X	+1
Red Snapper		1 1/4 oz.			X	+1
Salmon (Pacific)		1 1/4 oz.			X	+1
Sardine		3/4 oz.			X	+1
Sea Bass (imported)		3/4 oz.			X	+1
Silver Perch		1 1/4 oz.			X	+1
Snail		1 1/4 oz.			X	+1
Talapia		1 1/4 oz.			X	+1
Trout (imported)		3/4 oz.			X	+1
Trout, Sea		3/4 oz.			X	+1
Wahoo		1 1/4 oz.			X	+1

+ Organic Is Preferable   * Highly Glycemic   ⊕ Acid Neutralized   ■ Acceptable Fruits & Vegetables Only

Neutral:	1 Portion =		Yin	Neutral	Yang	Yin/Yang Score
	Raw	Cooked				
Albacore (tuna)		3/4 oz.			X	+1
Angle Shark		1 1/4 oz.			X	+1
Belt Fish		1 1/4 oz.			X	+1
Bonito		1 1/4 oz.			X	+1
Mackerel		1 1/4 oz.			X	+1
Mahi Mahi		1 1/4 oz.			X	+1
Mud Fish		1 1/4 oz.			X	+1
Mullet (imported)		1 1/4 oz.			X	+1
Ocean Perch		1 1/4 oz.			X	+1
Orange Roughy		1 1/4 oz.			X	+1
Porgy		1 1/4 oz.			X	+1
Ribbonfish		1 1/4 oz.			X	+1
Sand Dabs		1 1/4 oz.			X	+1
Sailfish		1 1/4 oz.			X	+1
Sea Urchin (roe)		3/4 oz.			X	+1
Shark, Thresher		1 1/4 oz.			X	+1
Smelt		1 1/4 oz.			X	+1
Snapper		1 1/4 oz.			X	+1
Spot		1 1/4 oz.			X	+1
Tarpon		1 1/4 oz.			X	+1
Tuna (canned)		3/4 oz.			X	+1
Tuna (steak)		3/4 oz.			X	+1
Whitefish		1 1/4 oz.			X	+1
White Perch		1 1/4 oz.			X	+1
Whiting		1 1/4 oz.			X	+1
Yellow Perch		1 1/4 oz.			X	+1
Yellowtail		3/4 oz.			X	+1

Least Beneficial:	1 Portion =		Yin	Neutral	Yang	Yin/Yang Score
	Raw	Cooked				
Anchovy		3/4oz.			X	+1
Barracuda		1 1/4 oz.			X	+1
Beluga		1 1/4 oz.			X	+1
Black Cod		1 1/4 oz.			X	+1
Bluefish		1 1/4oz.			X	+1
Bluegill Bass		3/4oz.			X	+1
Buffalo Fish		1 1/4 oz.			X	+1
Carp		1 1/4 oz.			X	+1
Catfish		1 1/4 oz.			X	+1
Caviar	1 1/4 oz.				X	+1
Clam		1 1/4 oz.			X	+1

+ Organic Is Preferable   * Highly Glycemic   ⊕ Acid Neutralized   ■ Acceptable Fruits & Vegetables Only

Least Beneficial:	1 Portion =		Yin	Neutral	Yang	Yin/Yang Score
	Raw	Cooked				
Cod (domestic)		1 1/4 oz.			X	+1
Coho Salmon (Great Lakes)		1 1/4 oz.			X	+1
Conch		1 1/4 oz.			X	+1
Crab		1 1/4 oz.			X	+1
Crayfish		1 1/4 oz.			X	+1
Croaker		1 1/4 oz.			X	+1
Eel		1 1/4 oz.			X	+1
Flounder		1 1/4 oz.			X	+1
Frog		1 1/4 oz.			X	+1
Gray sole		1 1/4 oz.			X	+1
Haddock		1 1/4 oz.			X	+1
Hake		1 1/4 oz.			X	+1
Halibut		1 1/4 oz.			X	+1
Herring (fresh)		1 1/4 oz.			X	+1
Herring (pickled)		1 1/4 oz.			X	+1
Lobster		3/4oz.			X	+1
Lobster (spiny)		3/4oz.			X	+1
Lox (smoked salmon)		1 1/4 oz.			X	+1
Mullet (domestic)		1 1/4 oz.			X	+1
Mussels		1 1/4 oz.			X	+1
Octopus		1 1/4 oz.			X	+1
Oysters		1 1/4 oz.			X	+1
Pike		1 1/4 oz.			X	+1
Scallops		1 1/4 oz.			X	+1
Sea Bass (domestic)		3/4oz.			X	+1
Shad		1 1/4 oz.			X	+1
Shark		1 1/4 oz.			X	+1
Sheephead		1 1/4 oz.			X	+1
Shrimp		1 1/4 oz.			X	+1
Sole		1 1/4 oz.			X	+1
Squid (calamari)		2 oz.			X	+1
Striped Bass		3/4oz.			X	+1
Sturgeon		1 1/4 oz.			X	+1
Swordfish		1 1/4 oz.			X	+1
Tilefish		1 1/4 oz.			X	+1
Trout, Rainbow		3/4oz.			X	+1
Turtle		1 1/4 oz.			X	+1
Walleye		1 1/4 oz.			X	+1
Weakfish		1 1/4 oz.			X	+1
White Bass		3/4oz.			X	+1
Yellow Perch		1 1/4 oz.			X	+1

+ Organic Is Preferable   * Highly Glycemic   ⊕ Acid Neutralized   ■ Acceptable Fruits & Vegetables Only

CARBOHYDRATES

BEANS AND LEGUMES

Most Beneficial:	1 Portion =		Yin	Neutral	Yang	Yin/Yang Score
	Raw	Cooked				
Aduke Beans		1/5 cup	X			-1
Adzuki Beans		1/5 cup	X			-1
Bean Sprouts	12 1/2 cups		X			-1
Black Beans		1/2 cup	X			-1
Black-eyed Peas		1/2 cup	X			-1
Broad Beans		2/3 cup	X			-1
Cannellini Beans		1/2 cup	X			-1
Green Beans		1 1/4 cup	X			-1
Jicama Beans		2/3 cup	X			-1
Mung Beans		1/2 cup	X			-1
Pinto Beans +		1/2 cup	X			-1
Red Soy Beans		1/2 cup	X			-1
Domestic Lentils	1/2 cup	1/3 cup	X			-1
Green Lentils	1/2 cup	1/3 cup	X			-1
Red Lentils	1/2 cup	1/3 cup	X			-1

Neutral:	1 Portion =		Yin	Neutral	Yang	Yin/Yang Score
	Raw	Cooked				
Fava Beans		1/2 cup	X			-1
Green Peas		1/2 cup	X			-1
Northern Beans		1/2 cup	X			-1
Red Soy Beans		1/2 cup	X			-1
Snap Beans		1/2 cup	X			-1
String Beans		1 1/4 cups	X			-1
White Beans		1/2 cup	X			-1
Pea Pods		1/2 cup	X			-1
Snow Peas		1/2 cup	X			-1

Least Beneficial:	1 Portion =		Yin	Neutral	Yang	Yin/Yang Score
	Raw	Cooked				
Copper Beans		1/2 cup	X			-1
Garbanzo Beans		1/3 cup	X			-1
Kidney Beans		1/2 cup	X			-1
Lima Beans		1/3 cup	X			-1
Navy Beans		1/3 cup	X			-1
Refried Beans		1/3 cup	X			-1
Red Beans		1/2 cup	X			-1
Tamarind Beans		1/2 cup	X			-1

+ Organic Is Preferable   * Highly Glycemic   ⊕ Acid Neutralized   ■ Acceptable Fruits & Vegetables Only

CARBOHYDRATES

BREADS

Most Beneficial:	1 Portion =		Yin	Neutral	Yang	Yin/Yang Score
	Raw	Cooked				
Essene Bread	2 1/2 oz.			X		0
Ezekiel Bread	1 slice			X		0
Soya Flour Bread	1 1/4 slice			X		0
Sprouted Wheat Bread	2/3 slice			X		0

Neutral:	1 Portion =		Yin	Neutral	Yang	Yin/Yang Score
	Raw	Cooked				
Bagels, Wheat	1/3 bagel			X		0
Brown Rice Bread	2/3 slice			X		0
Brown Rice Cakes	1 1/4 cakes			X		0
Corn Muffins	1/3			X		0
Fin Crisp	2 1/2 pieces			X		0
Gluten-Free Bread	2/3 slice			X		0
Ideal Flat Bread	2 1/2 pieces			X		0
Kamut Bread	1 1/4 slice			X		0
Millet Bread	2/3 slice			X		0
Oat Bran Muffins	1/2 muffin			X		0
100% Rye Bread +	1 slice			X		0
Spelt Bread	2/3 slice			X		0
Wasa Bread	1 1/4 slice			X		0

Least Beneficial:	1 Portion =		Yin	Neutral	Yang	Yin/Yang Score
	Raw	Cooked				
Bread Sticks (hard)	1 1/4 stick			X		0
Bread Sticks (soft)	2/3 stick			X		0
Cake	1/2 piece		X			-2
Doughnut	1/2		X			-2
Durum Wheat	2/3 slice			X		0
English Muffins	1/3 muffin			X		0
Graham Crackers	1 3/4 crackers		X			-2
High Protein Bread	2/3 slice			X		0
Matzos (wheat)	1/2 board			X		0
Melba Toast	2/3 slice			X		0
Multi-Grain Bread	2/3 slice			X		0
Pancakes (wheat) 4"	2/3			X		0
Pita Bread	1/3 pocket			X		0
Pumpernickel.	3/4 slice			X		0
Rice Cakes, white	1 1/4			X		0
Rice Crackers	7 Crackers			X		0
Rye Crisps	4 pieces			X		0

+ Organic Is Preferable   * Highly Glycemic   ⊕ Acid Neutralized   ■ Acceptable Fruits & Vegetables Only

Least Beneficial: (continued)	1 Portion =		Yin	Neutral	Yang	Yin/Yang Score
	Raw	Cooked				
Saltine Crackers	4			X		0
Vita, Rye	4 pieces			X		0
Waffle, Wheat	2/3			X		0
Wheat Bran Muffins	1/3			X		0
Whole Wheat Bread	2/3 slice			X		0

CARBOHYDRATES

FRUITS

Most Beneficial:	1 Portion =		Yin	Neutral	Yang	Yin/Yang Score
	Raw	Cooked				
Apricots +	3 3/4		X			-3
Blackberries +	1 cup		X			-3
Blueberries +	2/3 cup		X			-3
Boysenberries	2/3 cup		X			-3
Cherries +	10		X			-3
Cranberries +	1 cup		X			-3
Figs, Fresh *	1 1/4 piece		X			-3
Grapefruit	2/3		X			-3
Lemons	1 1/4		X			-3
Pineapple (cubed)	2/3 cup		X			-3
Plums, Dark +	1 1/4		X			-3
Plums, Green +	1 1/4		X			-3
Plums, Red +	1 1/4		X			-3

Neutral:	1 Portion =		Yin	Neutral	Yang	Yin/Yang Score
	Raw	Cooked				
Apples +	2/3		X			-3
Currants, Black	1 cup		X			-3
Currants, Red	1 cup		X			-3
Currants, White	1 cup		X			-3
Dates +	2 1/2		X			-3
Elderberries	2/3 cup		X			-3
Feiojas (Medium) +	2 1/2		X			-3
Figs, Dried *	1 1/4 piece		X			-3
Gooseberries	1 1/4 cup		X			-3
Grapes, Black +	2/3 cup		X			-3
Grapes, Concord +	2/3 cup		X			-3
Grapes, Green +	2/3 cup		X			-3
Grapes, Red +	2/3 cup		X			-3
Guava	2/3 cup		X			-3
Kiwi	1 1/4		X			-3

+ Organic Is Preferable　　* Highly Glycemic　　⊕ Acid Neutralized　　■ Acceptable Fruits & Vegetables Only

Neutral: (continued)	1 Portion =		Yin	Neutral	Yang	Yin/Yang Score
	Raw	Cooked				
Kumquat	3 3/4		X			-3
Limes	1 1/4		X			-3
Loganberries	1 cup		X			-3
Melons, Canang	3/4 cup		X			-3
Melons, Casaba +	3/4 cup		X			-3
Melons, Christmas	3/4 cup		X			-3
Melons, Crenshaw +	3/4 cup		X			-3
Melons, Musk	3/4 cup		X			-3
Melons, Spanish	3/4 cup		X			-3
Watermelons	1 cup		X			-3
Nectarines (medium)+	2/3		X			-3
Peaches, (medium) +	1 1/4		X			-3
Peaches (canned) +	2/3 cup		X			-3
Pears (medium) +	2/3		X			-3
Pears (canned) +	2/3 cup		X			-3
Persimmons (medium)+	1 1/4		X			-3
Pomegranates (medium)	1/2		X			-3
Prickly Pears	1/2		X			-3
Prunes +	2 1/2		X			-3
Raisins (organic only)	1 1/4 tbsp		X			-3
Raspberries	1 1/4 cup		X			-3
Star Fruit (medium)	1 1/2		X			-3
Strawberries +	1 1/4 cup		X			-3

Least Beneficial:	1 Portion =		Yin	Neutral	Yang	Yin/Yang Score
	Raw	Cooked				
Bananas	1/2		X			-3
Cactus	1/2 cup		X			-3
Coconut	6 2/3 oz.		X			-3
Mangoes	2/3 cup		X			-3
Melon, Bitter	1/2		X			-3
Melon, Cantaloupe +	1/2		X			-3
Melon, Honeydew +	1/2		X			-3
Oranges	3/4		X			-3
Papaya	1 1/4 cup		X			-3
Plantains	1 2/3 oz.		X			-3
Raisins (commercial)	1 1/4 tbsp		X			-3
Rhubarb (diced)	3 cups		X			-3
Tangerines	1 2/3		X			-3

+ Organic Is Preferable   * Highly Glycemic   ⊕ Acid Neutralized   ■ Acceptable Fruits & Vegetables Only

CARBOHYDRATES

GRAINS & CEREALS

Most Beneficial:	1 Portion =		Yin	Neutral	Yang	Yin/Yang Score
	Raw	Cooked				
Amaranth	2/3 oz.			X		0
Buckwheat	2/3 oz.			X		0
Kasha	2/3 oz.			X		0
Rice Bran	1/2 cup			X		0

Neutral:	1 Portion =		Yin	Neutral	Yang	Yin/Yang Score
	Raw	Cooked				
Barley	2/3 tbsp.			X		0
Brown Rice (puffed) *	1/2 oz.			X		0
Cornflakes *	1/2 oz.			X		0
Cornmeal *	2/3 oz.			X		0
Cream of Brown Rice *		1/2 cup		X		0
Grits	2/3 oz.	1/2 cup		X		0
Kamut (flakes)	2/3 oz.			X		0
Millet *	2/3 oz.			X		0
Oat Bran	1/2 oz.			X		0
Oatmeal (slow cooking)	2/3 oz.	1/2 cup		X		0
Spelt (flakes)	2/3 oz.			X		0

Least Beneficial:	1 Portion =		Yin	Neutral	Yang	Yin/Yang Score
	Raw	Cooked				
Cream of Wheat *	2/3 oz.	1/2 cup		X		0
Cream of White Rice *	2/3 oz.	1/2 cup		X		0
Familia	2/3 oz.	1/2 cup		X		0
Farina	2/3 oz.	1/2 cup		X		0
Granola	2/3 oz.			X		0
Grape Nuts	2/3 oz.			X		0
Rice, White (puffed)	1/2 oz.			X		0
Seven Grains *	3/4 oz.			X		0
Shredded Wheat *	2/3 oz.			X		0
Wheat Bran	2/3 oz.			X		0
Wheat Germ	1 1/4 oz			X		0

+ Organic Is Preferable   * Highly Glycemic   ⊕ Acid Neutralized   ■ Acceptable Fruits & Vegetables Only

CARBOHYDRATES

JUICES

Most Beneficial:	1 Portion =		Yin	Neutral	Yang	Yin/Yang Score
	Raw	Cooked				
Apricot	1/3 cup		X			-3
Black Cherry + *	1/2 cup		X			-3
Carrot *	1/2 cup		X			-1
Celery +	1 cup		X			-1
Grapefruit + *	1/2 cup		X			-3
Pineapple *	1/3 cup		X			-3
Water w/ Lemon	N/A			X		N/A

Neutral:	1 Portion =		Yin	Neutral	Yang	Yin/Yang Score
	Raw	Cooked				
Apple + *	1/2 cup		X			-3
Apple Cider + *	1/2 cup		X			-3
Boysenberry	1/3 cup		X			-3
Cabbage	1/4 cup		X			-2
Cranberry *	1/3 cup		X			-3
Cucumber	1 cup		X			-1
Grape *	1/3 cup		X			-3
Orange ⊕	1/2 cup		X			-3
Pomegranate	1/2 cup		X			-3
Prune + *	1/4 cup		X			-3
Vegetable ■	1 1/4 cup		X			-2

Least Beneficial:	1 Portion =		Yin	Neutral	Yang	Yin/Yang Score
	Raw	Cooked				
Orange (regular) *	1/2 cup		X			-3
Guava	1/2 cup		X			-3
Papaya *	1/3 cup		X			-3
Tomato	1 1/4 cups		X			-1
V-8 Juice	1 cup		X			-2

+ Organic Is Preferable   * Highly Glycemic   ⊕ Acid Neutralized   ■ Acceptable Fruits & Vegetables Only

CARBOHYDRATES

PASTAS AND FLOURS

Most Beneficial:	1 Portion =		Yin	Neutral	Yang	Yin/Yang Score
	Raw	Cooked				
Artichoke Pasta (Jerusalem)		1/3 cup		X		0
Buckwheat Flour	2/3 oz.			X		0
Kamut Flour	2/3 oz.			X		0
Kasha	2/3 oz.			X		0
Oat Flour	2/3oz.			X		0
Rice Flour, Brown *	2/3 oz.			X		0
Rye Flour	1 oz.			X		0
Soba Noodles		1/3 cup		X		0
Soy Flour	2/3 oz.			X		0

Neutral:	1 Portion =		Yin	Neutral	Yang	Yin/Yang Score
	Raw	Cooked				
Couscous	2/3 oz.			X		0
Barley Flour	3/4 oz.			X		0
Bulgur Wheat Flour	2/3 oz.			X		0
Durum Wheat Flour	2/3 oz.			X		0
Gluten Flour	1 1/4 oz.			X		0
Quinoa Flour	2/3 oz.			X		0
Rice, Basmati *		1/4 cup		X		0
Rice, Brown *		1/4 cup		X		0
Rice, Wild *		1/4 cup		X		0
Spelt Flour	3/4 oz.			X		0
Spelt Noodles		1/3 cup		X		0
Sprouted Wheat Flour	2 oz.			X		0

Least Beneficial:	1 Portion =		Yin	Neutral	Yang	Yin/Yang Score
	Raw	Cooked				
Graham Flour *	2/3 oz.			X		-2
Rice, White *		1/4 cup		X		0
Semolina Pasta		1/3 cup		X		0
Spinach Pasta		1/3 cup		X		0
White Flour *	1 oz.			X		0
White Rice Flour *	2/3 oz.			X		0
Whole Wheat Flour *	1 1/4 oz.			X		0

+ Organic Is Preferable   * Highly Glycemic   ⊕ Acid Neutralized   ■ Acceptable Fruits & Vegetables Only

CARBOHYDRATES

VEGETABLES

Most Beneficial:	1 Portion =		Yin	Neutral	Yang	Yin/Yang Score
	Raw	Cooked				
Artichokes, Domestic+	Medium		X			-1
Artichokes, Jerusalem +	Medium		X			-1
Barley Greens	N/A	N/A	X			-2
Beet Greens	7cups		X			-2
Blue Green Algae	N/A	N/A	X			-2
Broccoli +	2 1/2 cups		X			-1
Carrots	4 1/2 oz.	2/3 cup	X			-1
Chicory Greens	1 1/4 cups		X			-2
Chicory Roots	1 1/4 cups		X			-2
Collard Greens +	1 1/4 cups		X			-2
Dandelion Greens +	2 cups		X			-2
Dill Weed +	18 3/4 cups		X			-1
Escarole +	9 1/2 cups		X			-2
Garlic	12 1/2 cloves		X			-1
Horseradish (pods)	2 1/2 cups		X			-1
Kale +	1 1/4 cups		X			-2
Kelp	5 oz.		X			-2
Kohlrabi +	1 1/4 cups		X			-2
Leeks +	1 1/4 cups		X			-1
Lettuce, Romaine +	9 cups		X			-2
Okra +		1 1/4 cups	X			-1
Onions, Red	1 1/4 cups		X			-1
Onions, Spanish	1 1/4 cups		X			-1
Onions, Yellow	1 1/4 cups		X			-1
Parsley +	6 1/4 cups		X			-2
Parsnips *	1/2 cup		X			-1
Pumpkins (mashed)		1 cup	X			-1
Red Algae	N/A	N/A	X			-1
Red Chard		1 1/4 cup	X			-2
Spinach +	5 cups		X			-2
Spirulina	2 oz.		X			-2
Sprouts, Alfalfa	13 3/4 cups		X			-1
Swiss Chard +		1 1/4 cup	X			-2
Taro	1/2 cup	1/4 cup	X			-1
Turnip Greens +		2 cups	X			-2
Turnips (mashed) +		1 1/4 cup	X			-1
Watercress	28 cups		X			-1

+ Organic Is Preferable　　* Highly Glycemic　　⊕ Acid Neutralized　　■ Acceptable Fruits & Vegetables Only

Neutral:	1 Portion =		Yin	Neutral	Yang	Yin/Yang Score
	Raw	Cooked				
Arugula	14 cups		X			-1
Asparagus		15 spears	X			-1
Bamboo Shoots	4 3/4 cups	1 1/4 cup	X			-2
Beets		2/3 cups	X			-1
Bok Choy +		3 3/4 cups	X			-1
Cauliflower		2 1/2 cups	X			-1
Celery +	2 1/2 cups		X			-2
Choy Sum +	2 1/2 cups		X			-1
Cilantro (coriander)		3 cups	X			-1
Corn, White		1/3 cup	X			-1
Corn, Yellow		1/3 cup	X			-1
Cucumber (whole) +	1 1/4		X			-1
Cucumber (sliced)	1 1/4 cups		X			-1
Daikon Radish	3 cups		X			-1
Endive	9 cups		X			-2
Hominy (Grits)		1/2 cup	X			-1
Lettuce, Bibb (5" head)	2 1/2 head		X			-2
Lettuce, Boston (5" head)	2 1/2 head		X			-2
Lettuce, Iceberg (6" head) +	1 1/4 head		X			-2
Lettuce, Mesclun +	1 1/4 head		X			-2
Mushrooms, Abalone	3 3/4 cups	1 1/4 cup	X			-1
Mushrooms, Enoki	3 3/4 cups	1 1/4 cup	X			-1
Mushrooms, Portobello,	3 3/4 cups	1 1/4 cup	X			-1
Mushrooms, Oyster	3 3/4 cups	1 1/4 cup	X			-1
Mushrooms, Tree	3 3/4 cups	1 1/4 cup	X			-1
Mustard Greens	4 cups	3 3/4 cups	X			-2
Onions, Green (scallions)	1 1/4 cup	2/3 cup	X			-1
Peppers, Chili	3/4 cup		X			-1
Peppers, Poblano +	3 3/4 oz.		X			-1
Radicchio	8 3/4 oz		X			-1
Radishes +	5 cups		X			-2
Rapini	2 1/2 cups		X			-1
Rutabaga +	3/4 cup	1/2 cup	X			-1
Seaweed		4 1/2 oz.	X			-2
Shallots	2 1/2 oz.		X			-1
Sprouts, Brussels	1 1/2 cups		X			-1
Sprouts, Mung	3 3/4 cups		X			-1
Sprouts, Radish	3 3/4 cups		X			-1
Squash, Acorn +		2/3 cup	X			-1
Squash, Butternut +		2/3 cup	X			-1
Squash, Yellow +		1 1/2 cups	X			-1
Water Chestnuts	1/2 cup		X			-1
Zucchini		2 cups	X			-1

+ Organic Is Preferable   * Highly Glycemic   ⊕ Acid Neutralized   ■ Acceptable Fruits & Vegetables Only

Least Beneficial:	1 Portion =		Yin	Neutral	Yang	Yin/Yang Score
	Raw	Cooked				
Cabbage, Chinese	3 3/4 cups	1 2/3 cups	X			-2
Cabbage, Red	3 3/4 cups	1 2/3 cups	X			-2
Cabbage, White	3 3/4 cups	1 2/3 cups	X			-2
Eggplant +	2 cups		X			-1
Fiddlehead Ferns	12 1/2 cups		X			-2
Hummus	1/3 cup		X			-1
Mushrooms, Domestic	3 3/4 cups	1 1/4 cup	X			-1
Mushrooms, Shitake	3 3/4 cups	1 1/4 cup	X			-1
Peppers, Green (chopped)	2 3/4 cups		X			-1
Peppers, Jalapeno (chopped)	3 3/4 oz.		X			-1
Peppers, Red (chopped)	2 3/4 cups		X			-1
Peppers, Serrano (chopped) +	3/4 cup		X			-1
Peppers, Yellow (chopped)	2 3/4 cups		X			-1
Potatoes, Red +	1/2 cup		X			-1
Potatoes, Sweet	1/2 cup		X			-1
Potatoes, White	1/2 cup		X			-1
Purslane +	8 cups	2 cups	X			-2
Sauerkraut	1 1/4 cup		X			-2
Tomatillo	1 1/4 cup		X			-1
Tomato +	2 1/2		X			-1
Yams (medium)		2/3	X			-1

FATS

NUTS AND SEEDS

Most Beneficial:	1 Portion =		Yin	Neutral	Yang	Yin/Yang Score
	Raw	Cooked				
Flax Seeds	2/3 tsp.		X			-1
Hemp Seeds	2/3 tsp.		X			-1
Pumpkin Seeds	2/3 tsp.		X			-1

Neutral:	1 Portion =		Yin	Neutral	Yang	Yin/Yang Score
	Raw	Cooked				
Almond Butter	1/3 tsp.		X			-2
Almond Nuts	3/4 tsp.		X			-2
Chestnuts	2/3 oz.		X			-2
Filbert Nuts	1/3 tsp.		X			-2
Hickory Nuts	1/3 tsp.		X			-2
Lychee Nuts (1C)	2 1/2 oz.		X			-3
Macadamia Nuts	1 small		X			-2
Pignolia (pine seeds)	3/4 tsp.		X			-1
Poppy seeds	1 tsp.		X			-1

+ Organic Is Preferable   * Highly Glycemic   ⊕ Acid Neutralized   ■ Acceptable Fruits & Vegetables Only

Neutral:	1 Portion =		Yin	Neutral	Yang	Yin/Yang Score
	Raw	Cooked				
Sesame Seeds	1/4 tsp.		X			-1
Sesame Butter (Tahini)	1/4 tbsp.		X			-1
Sunflower Butter	2/3 tsp.		X			-1
Sunflower Seeds	2/3 tsp.		X			-1
Walnuts	1/3 tsp.		X			-2
Watermelon Seeds	2/3 tsp.		X			-1

Least Beneficial:	1 Portion =		Yin	Neutral	Yang	Yin/Yang Score
	Raw	Cooked				
Brazil	1/3 nut		X			-2
Cashews	1 1/2 nuts		X			-2
Cashew Butter	1/2 tsp.		X			-2
Peanuts	5 nuts		X			-2
Peanut Butter	1/3 tsp.		X			-2
Pistachios	1/2 tsp.		X			-2
Radish Seeds	3/4 tsp.		X			-1

FATS

OILS AND OTHER FATS

Most Beneficial:	1 Portion =		Yin	Neutral	Yang	Yin/Yang Score
	Raw	Cooked				
Black Currant Oil	1/4 tsp.		X			-2
Hemp Seed Oil	1/4 tsp.		X			-2
Flax Seed Oil (Linseed)	1/4 tsp.		X			-2
Olive Oil	1/4 tsp.		X			-2

Neutral:	1 Portion =		Yin	Neutral	Yang	Yin/Yang Score
	Raw	Cooked				
Avocado	3/4 tbsp		X			-2
Borage Oil	1/4 tsp.		X			-2
Canola Oil	1/4 tsp.		X			-2
Cod Liver Oil	1/4 tsp.		X			-2
Olives (green)	2 1/2		X			-2
Salmon Oil	1/4 tsp.		X			-2
Tahini	1/3 tsp		X			-2

+ Organic Is Preferable   * Highly Glycemic   ⊕ Acid Neutralized   ■ Acceptable Fruits & Vegetables Only

Least Beneficial:	1 Portion =		Yin	Neutral	Yang	Yin/Yang Score
	Raw	Cooked				
Butter	1/4 tsp.		X			-1
Coconut Oil	1/4 tsp.		X			-2
Corn Oil	1/4 tsp.		X			-2
Cottonseed Oil	1/4 tsp.		X			-2
Cream (half & half)	3/4 tbsp.		X			-1
Cream Cheese	3/4 tsp.		X			-1
Ghee	1/4 tsp.		X			-1
Hydrogenated Oil	1/4 tsp.		X			-2
Lard	1/4 tsp.		X			-2
Olives (black)	2 1/2		X			-2
Olives (green)	2 1/2		X			-2
Olives (Spanish	2 1/2		X			-2
Palm Oil	1/4 tsp.		X			-2
Peanut Oil	1/4 tsp.		X			-2
Safflower Oil	1/4 tsp.		X			-2
Sesame Seed Oil	1/4 tsp.		X			-2
Sour Cream	1/3 tbsp.		X			-1
Sour Cream, Light	3/4 tbsp.		X			-1
Vegetable Shortening	1/4 tsp.		X			-2

MISCELLANEOUS

BEVERAGES

Most Beneficial:	1 Portion =		Yin	Neutral	Yang	Yin/Yang Score
	Raw	Cooked				
Coffee, Decaf	N/A				X	<
Coffee, Regular	N/A				X	<
Green Tea	N/A			X		<
Green Tea (decaffeinated)	N/A			X		<
Wine, Red	5 oz.		X			-3
Purified Water	N/A			X		<

Neutral:	1 Portion =		Yin	Neutral	Yang	Yin/Yang Score
	Raw	Cooked				
Cappuccino, Decaf	N/A				X	<
Champagne	5 oz.		X			-3
Sports Drink (natural)	1/2 cup		X			-3
Sparkling Water	N/A					<
Wine, White	5 oz.		X			-3

+ Organic Is Preferable   * Highly Glycemic   ⊕ Acid Neutralized   ■ Acceptable Fruits & Vegetables Only

Least Beneficial:	1 Portion =		Yin	Neutral	Yang	Yin/Yang Score
	Raw	**Cooked**				
Beer (light)	5 oz.			X		0
Beer (regular)	5 oz.			X		0
Cappuccino (regular)	N/A				X	<
Club Soda	N/A			X		<
Latte'	1 cup		X			-2
Liquors, Distilled	1 1/4 oz.			X		0
Seltzer Water	N/A			X		<
Soda, Diet	3 oz.		X			-3
Sodas (other)	3 oz.		X			-3
Sport Drink (artificial)	1/2 cup		X			-3
Tea, Black, Decaffeinated	N/A				X	<
Tea, Black (regular)	N/A				X	<

MISCELLANEOUS

CONDIMENTS

Most Beneficial:	1 Portion =		Yin	Neutral	Yang	Yin/Yang Score
	Raw	**Cooked**				
"Bragg's" Amino Acids	N/A				X	<
Mustard	N/A				X	<
Soy Sauce	N/A				X	<
Tamarind	N/A				X	<

Neutral:	1 Portion =		Yin	Neutral	Yang	Yin/Yang Score
	Raw	**Cooked**				
Apple Butter	2 1/2 tsp.		X			-3
Fruit Jams ■	2 1/2 tsp.		X			-3
Fruit Jellies ■	2 1/2 tsp.		X			-3
Dill Pickles	11 1/2		X			-1
Kosher Pickles	11 1/2		X			-1
Mayonnaise (vegetarian) (1F)	3/4 tsp.			X		-1
Salad Dressing	N/A		X			<
Sour Pickles	11 1/2		X			-1
Sweet Pickles	2		X			-1

+ Organic Is Preferable   * Highly Glycemic   ⊕ Acid Neutralized   ■ Acceptable Fruits & Vegetables Only

Least Beneficial:	1 Portion =		Yin	Neutral	Yang	Yin/Yang Score
	Raw	Cooked				
Candy Bar	1/3 Bar		X			-3
Barbecue Sauce	2 1/2 tbsp.		X			-3
Cocktail Sauce	2 1/2 tbsp.		X			-3
Ketchup	2 1/2 tbsp.		X			-2
Maple Syrup	2 1/2 tsp.		X			-3
Mayonnaise, (dairy)	3/4 tsp.		X			-1
Plum Sauce	2 tbsp.		X			-3
Relish	5 tsp.		X			-2
Teriyaki Sauce	1 1/4 tbsp.		X			-3
Worcestershire Sauce	N/A		X			<

MISCELLANEOUS

SPICES

Most Beneficial:	1 Portion =		Yin	Neutral	Yang	Yin/Yang Score
	Raw	Cooked				
Barley Malt	3 3/4 tsp.		X			-2
Black Strap Molasses	2/3 tsp.		X			-3
Carob	1 1/4 oz		X			-3
Cinnamon	N/A				X	<
Curry	N/A				X	<
Dill	N/A		X			<
Dulse	N/A		X			<
Garlic	N/A				X	<
Ginger	N/A				X	<
Kelp	N/A		X			<
Miso	N/A			X		<
Parsley	N/A				X	<
Turmeric (tuber)	N/A		X			<
Turmeric (rhizone)	N/A				X	<

Neutral:	1 Portion =		Yin	Neutral	Yang	Yin/Yang Score
	Raw	Cooked				
Agar	N/A		X			<
Allspice	N/A				X	<
Almond Extract	N/A		X			<
Anise	N/A		X			<
Arrowroot Starch	1 1/4 tsp.		X			-1
Basil	N/A		X			<
Bay Leaf	N/A		X			<

+ Organic Is Preferable   * Highly Glycemic   ⊕ Acid Neutralized   ■ Acceptable Fruits & Vegetables Only

Neutral: (continued)	1 Portion =		Yin	Neutral	Yang	Yin/Yang Score
	Raw	Cooked				
Bergamot	N/A		X			<
Brewer's Yeast	N/A		X			<
Brown Rice Syrup	3 3/4 tsp.		X			-3
Caraway Seeds	N/A		X			<
Cardamom	N/A				X	<
Chervil	N/A				X	<
Chives	N/A		X			<
Chocolate *	1 1/4 oz.		X			-3
Cloves	N/A				X	<
Coriander	N/A				X	<
Cornstarch	1 1/4 tsp.		X			-1
Cream of Tartar	N/A		X			<
Cumin	N/A				X	<
Fennel	N/A		X			<
Honey *	2/3 tbsp.		X			-3
Horseradish	N/A				X	<
Marjoram	N/A		X			<
Mint	N/A		X			<
Mustard	N/A				X	<
Nutmeg	N/A				X	<
Paprika	N/A				X	<
Peppermint	N/A		X			<
Pimento	N/A				X	<
Rice Syrup *	3 3/4 tsp.		X			-3
Rosemary	N/A		X			<
Saffron	N/A			X		<
Sage	N/A				X	<
Salt	N/A		X			<
Savory	N/A				X	<
Spearmint	N/A		X			<
Stevia	N/A		X			<
Sucanat	2 1/2 tsp.		X			-3
Tapioca	N/A		X			<
Tarragon	N/A		X			<
Thyme	N/A			X		<
Vanilla	N/A		X			<

+ Organic Is Preferable   * Highly Glycemic   ⊕ Acid Neutralized   ■ Acceptable Fruits & Vegetables Only

Least Beneficial:	1 Portion =		Yin	Neutral	Yang	Yin/Yang Score
	Raw	Cooked				
Capers	N/A				X	<
Corn Syrup *	2 1/2 tsp.		X			-3
Gelatin	N/A			X		<
Pancake Syrup *	2 1/2 tsp.		X			-3
Pepper Cayenne	N/A				X	<
Pepper, Ground Black	N/A				X	<
Pepper, Red	N/A				X	<
Pepper, White	N/A				X	<
Peppercorn	N/A				X	<
Sugar, Brown *	2 1/2 tsp.		X			-3
Sugar, Confectionery *	1 1/4 tbsp.		X			-3
Sugar, White *	2 1/2 tsp.		X			-3
Vinegar, Apple Cider	N/A				X	<
Vinegar, Balsamic	N/A				X	<
Vinegar, Red Wine	N/A				X	<
Vinegar, White	N/A				X	<
Wintergreen	N/A		X			<

MISCELLANEOUS

TEAS and/or HERBS

Most Beneficial:	1 Portion =		Yin	Neutral	Yang	Yin/Yang Score
	Raw	Cooked				
Alfalfa	N/A			X		<
Aloe Vera	N/A		X			<
Burdock	N/A		X			<
Chamomile	N/A			X		<
Dandelion	N/A		X			<
Deglycerrhizinated licorice	N/A			X		<
Echinacea	N/A		X			<
Fenugreek	N/A				X	<
Ginger	N/A				X	<
Ginseng, American	N/A		X			<
Green Tea	N/A			X		<
Hawthorne	N/A				X	<
Milk Thistle	N/A		X			<
Rosehip	N/A			X		<
St. John's Wort	N/A		X			<
Slippery Elm	N/A			X		<
Valerian	N/A				X	<

+ Organic Is Preferable   * Highly Glycemic   ⊕ Acid Neutralized   ■ Acceptable Fruits & Vegetables Only

Neutral:	1 Portion =		Yin	Neutral	Yang	Yin/Yang Score
	Raw	Cooked				
Chickweed	N/A		X			<
Colt's Foot	N/A		X			<
Dong Quai	N/A				X	<
Elder	N/A				X	<
Gentian	N/A		X			<
Goldenseal	N/A		X			<
Hops	N/A			X		<
Horehound	N/A		X			<
Licorice Root	N/A			X		<
Linden	N/A		X			<
Mulberry	N/A		X			<
Mullein	N/A		X			<
Parsley	N/A				X	<
Peppermint	N/A		X			<
Raspberry Leaf	N/A			X		<
Sage	N/A				X	<
Sarsaparilla	N/A			X		<
Senna	N/A		X			<
Shepherd's Purse	N/A			X		<
Skullcap	N/A		X			<
Spearmint	N/A		X			<
Strawberry Leaf	N/A		X			<
Thyme	N/A			X		<
Vervain	N/A		X			<
White Birch	N/A		X			<
White Oak Bark	N/A		X			<
Yarrow	N/A			X		<
Yellowdock	N/A		X			<

Least Beneficial:	1 Portion =		Yin	Neutral	Yang	Yin/Yang Score
	Raw	Cooked				
Catnip	N/A		X			<
Cayenne	N/A				X	<
Cascara sagrada	N/A		X			<
Corn silk	N/A		X			<
Ginseng, Siberian	N/A				X	<
Red Clover	N/A		X			<
Rhubarb	N/A			X		<

+ Organic Is Preferable   * Highly Glycemic   ⊕ Acid Neutralized   ■ Acceptable Fruits & Vegetables Only

Blood Type A Recipes

INSTRUCTIONS FOR USE:

The following pages provide five recipes specific for this particular blood type: breakfast, lunch, dinner, dessert and one snack. Each recipe takes into account the correct foods for this specific blood type, the proper ratio of proteins, carbohydrates and fats (Macrobalance™ Portions) and an acceptable Yin Yang energetic score. In compliance with the 4th piece of the New Millennium Diet puzzle, it is recommended that organic foods be used as much as possible. Each meal (breakfast, lunch and dinner) offers the user three, four, five or six Portion amounts.

The recipe consists of two parts. Part one, a shopping list that provides the correct amount of ingredients necessary according to the 4 different Portion sizes. The shopping list also shows the amount in which the various Portion sizes contribute towards the total Yin Yang score.

Part two is the Preparation section and provides simple to follow instructions in preparing the recipe.

It is very simple to use the recipes, it is done in three easy steps:
1. **Determine the correct amount of Portions needed (Chapter 7).**
2. **In the recipe, refer to the Grocery List, select the correct Portion column and obtain the ingredients in the amounts listed.**
3. **Prepare the recipe according to the Preparation instructions in Part two.**

It's that simple to enjoy a complete Macrobalanced™ meal. Bon appetit!

Breakfast: Italian Scramble
Blood Type A

Shopping List

Ingredients:	Portion Size			
	3	4	5	6
	Amount of Ingredient			
Proteins:				
Whole Egg(s)	2 eggs	3 eggs	4 eggs	5 eggs
Mozzarella Cheese	1 oz	1 oz	1 1/4 oz	1 1/3 oz
Carbohydrates:				
Portabello Mushrooms	3/4 cup	1 1/5 cup	1 1/2 cup	1 2/3 cup
Zucchini (chopped)	1 1/3 cup	1 2/3 cup	2 1/4 cup	2 2/3 cup
Onions (chopped)	3/5 cup	4/5 cup	1 cup	1 1/5 cup
Apples (sliced)	1/2 cup	3/4 cup	1 cup	1 1/4 cup
Fats and Oils:				
Olive Oil	1 tsp	1 1/3 tsp	1 2/3 tsp	2 tsp
Sunflower Seed Butter	2/3 tsp	1 tsp	1 1/8 tsp	1 1/3 tsp
Spices:				
Sea Salt	pinch	pinch	pinch	pinch
Oregano (dried)	pinch	pinch	pinch	pinch
Turmeric	pinch	pinch	pinch	pinch
Basil (dried)	pinch	pinch	pinch	pinch
Marjoram	pinch	pinch	pinch	pinch
Yin (-)/Yang(+) (excess)	-2	-3	-4	-3

Preparation:

In a saute pan, cook the vegetables in the olive oil until soft. Once cooked, add the five spices, eggs, sunflower butter and grated mozzarella to the vegetable mixture. Scramble until eggs have solidified. Cook the apple slices in a separate pan lightly sprayed with olive oil. Serve immediately while warm.

Lunch: Chicken Black Bean Stew
Blood Type A

Shopping List

	Portion Size			
	3	4	5	6
Ingredients:	**Amount of Ingredient**			
Proteins:				
Chicken	2 1/2 oz	3 1/3 oz	4 1/4 oz	5 oz
Carbohydrates:				
Black Beans (cooked)	1/2 cup	2/3 cup	3/4 cup	1 cup
Onions (chopped)	1/4 cup	1/3 cup	1/2 cup	3/5 cup
Zucchini (chopped)	1/3 cup	1/2 cup	3/4 cup	2/3 cup
Green Beans (chopped)	1/2 cup	2/3 cup	5/6 cup	1 cup
Apples (sliced)	1/2 cup	2/3 cup	5/6 cup	1 cup
Fats and Oils:				
Canola Oil	1 tsp	1 1/3 tsp	1 2/3 tsp	2 tsp
Spices:				
Vegetarian Broth	1/4 cup	1/3 cup	3/4 cup	3/4 cup
Parsley	3/4 tsp	1 tsp	1 1/4 tsp	1 1/2 tsp
Sea Salt	pinch	pinch	pinch	pinch
Cinnamon	pinch	pinch	pinch	pinch
Yin (-)/Yang(+) (excess)	-2	-2	-3	-3

Preparation:

In a lightly olive oil sprayed saucepan, heat the zucchini, onions, parsley and sea salt with the vegearian broth. Cook until vegetables are tender. Separately cook the chicken in the canola oil until tender and then mix with vegetable stew. Simmer for another 4 to 6 minutes, then serve. Cook the sliced apples in a saucepan, lightly sprayed with olive oil, until tender. Sprinkle with cinnamon, serve as a dessert.

Snack: Cucumber, Carrot and Mozzarella
Blood Type A

Shopping List

	Portion Size		
	1	2	3
Ingredients:	**Amount of Ingredient**		
Proteins:			
Mozzarella Cheese	3/4 oz	1 1/2 oz	2 1/4 oz
Carbohydrates:			
Cucumbers	1/2 cup	1 cup	1 1/2 cup
Carrots	1/2 cup	1 cup	1 1/2 cup
Fats and Oils:			
Sunflower butter	3/4 tsp	1 1/2 tsp	2 1/4 tsp
Spices:			
Sea Salt	pinch	pinch	pinch
Yin (-)/Yang(+) (excess)	-1	0	1

Preparation:
Cut the mozzarella and vegetables into desired portions. Use sunflower butter as a spread. Sprinkle with sea salt.

Dinner: Dill Salmon and Asparagus
Blood Type A

Shopping List

Ingredients:	Portion Size			
	3	4	5	6
	Amount of Ingredient			
Proteins:				
Salmon	3 3/4 oz	5 oz	6 1/5 oz	7 1/2 oz
Carbohydrates:				
Onions (chopped)	1 cup	1 1/3 cup	1 2/3 cup	2 cup
Asparagus (chopped)	1 1/2 cups	2 cups	2 1/2 cups	3 cups
Yellow Corn	1/8 cup	1/6 cup	1/5 cup	1/4 cup
Chickpeas (canned)	1/4 cup	1/3 cup	2/5 cup	1/2 cup
Fats and Oils:				
Olive Oil	3/4 tsp	1 tsp	1 1/4 tsp	1 1/2 tsp
Spices:				
Dill (dried)	pinch	pinch	pinch	pinch
Garlic Powder	pinch	pinch	pinch	pinch
Chives (fresh)	pinch	pinch	pinch	pinch
Sea Salt	pinch	pinch	pinch	pinch
Hot Sauce	dash	dash	dash	dash
Yin (-)/Yang(+) (excess)	-3	-4	-5	-5

Preparation:

Lightly spray bottom of baking pan with olive oil spray. Place onions, yellow corn, asparagus and chickpeas on the bottom of the pan. Place the salmon fillet over the vegetables, add olive oil. Sprinkle the fish with garlic powder and dill. Add 1 cup of water and dash of hot sauce, cover and bake 35 to 40 minutes at 350°. Remove liquid, sprinkle on chives and sea salt. Serve hot.

Dessert: Frozen Cherry Cream
Blood Type A

Shopping List

	Portion Size		
	1	2	3
Ingredients:	**Amount of Ingredient**		
Proteins:			
Egg Whites	1 egg	2 eggs	3 eggs
Soy Yogurt (plain)	1/2 cup	1 cup	1 1/2 cup
Carbohydrates:			
Cherries	1/4 cup	1/2 cup	3/4 cup
Arrowroot Powder**	1 1/3 tsp	2 tsp	2 1/4 tsp
Fats and Oils:			
Almonds (finely chopped)	2/3 tsp	1 1/3 tsp	2 tsp
Spices:			
Ginger	1/8 tsp	1/5 tsp	1/3 tsp
Orange Extract	1/4 tsp	1/3 tsp	1/3 tsp
Yin (-)/Yang(+) (excess)	0	-1	0

Preparation:

In a saucepan, place the cherries, ginger, orange extract, yogurt and arrowroot powder**. Heat until warmed thoroughly. Set aside until cool. Place the egg whites in a mixing bowl and whip until firm. Add the egg whites and almonds to the cooled fruit mixture. Stir the mixture, place into freezer until frozen. Serve cold.

**Arrowroot Powder should be well-mixed with 3 to 5 teaspoons of cold water before adding to the other ingredients.

Chapter 10

Blood Type B: Balance

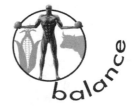

Health and Dietary Characteristics

- 30% Carbohydrate
  40% Protein
  30% Fat
- Hardy Immune System
- Strong Digestive Tract
- Widest Variety of Food Choices
- Dairy Tolerant

Personality Characteristics

- Creative Thinkers
- Must Maintain Balance with Mental, Emotional and Physical State
- Adaptive and Flexible Individuals
- Balance of Aggressive and Intuitive Natures

BLOOD TYPE B—CHARACTERISTICS

PERSONALITY CHARACTERISTICS

Type B personalities epitomize the essence of balance in their healthy, natural state. They are very adaptive and flexible individuals who have learned to change rapidly to new and unusual environments, geography, and cultures. They have some of the aggressive nature of O types and the intuitiveness of A types, which helps them create a balanced state when dealing with unusual circumstances. They do very well in business and entrepreneurial endeavors. Many B types are of Asian descent. The Asian tradition is known for its emphasis on achieving mental, emotional, and spiritual balance. Going back to these concepts is the key to unlocking the inherent potential for vital energy and good health. B types make up approximately 9% of the world population.

PHYSIOLOGY AND DIETARY CHARACTERISTICS

Type B individuals must balance the differing characteristics of their blood type for optimum health. The 30% protein, 40% carbohydrate, 30% macronutrient ratio is recommended. The New Millennium Diet for Type B individuals accommodates a meat and dairy tradition, giving them problem-free access to many sources of proteins.

Blood Type B is the culmination of many evolutionary tendencies. They have the ability to eat an agrarian diet as well as be hunter in style. Type B's, in fact, have the widest choices in foods because of their ability to tolerate both dairy products and meat.

There is one major no-no, chicken. Chicken contains a powerful lectin that can damage Type B immune systems. The Type B immune system is hardy and has more resistance to infective agents than A or AB types. Fortunately they have less susceptibility to many of the most common diseases of the industrial world, such as heart disease, cancer, and diabetes. B types most commonly suffer from autoimmune disorders — multiple sclerosis, lupus, rheumatoid arthritis, and chronic fatigue. Following the broad B type diet improves one's ability to resist genetic predispositions towards these types of diseases.

Weight Management

In order to enhance fat loss, it is important to avoid high-lectin foods. For Type B that means corn, buckwheat, chicken, wheat, lentils, and peanuts. Be sure to follow the New Millennium macronutrient ratios of 30% protein, 40% carbohydrate, and 30% fat. Avoid wheat-containing products because of the high amount of gluten and lectins found in these foods. Gluten and lectins interfere with digestion, and can even damage glandular and organ tissue, preventing proper function. This often leads to metabolic imbalance.

Foods Encouraging Fat Gain

Chicken, corn, lentils, peanuts, sesame seeds, buckwheat and wheat.

Foods Encouraging Fat Loss

High chlorophyll-containing vegetables, meat and dairy products.

Exercise

B types require a more balanced approach to exercise. You do not need the heavy physical exertion required by O types. However, a moderate level of physical exertion is recommended. Activities such as tennis, racquetball, or aerobics are well suited for Type Bs. Moderate weight training for at least 30–60 minutes a day, 4–5 times a week, maintains good bone mass and is especially useful for women who are at risk of osteoporosis.

DIETARY SPECIFICS

PROTEINS

MEATS AND POULTRY

Chicken is a major problem food for blood type B. It contains a special lectin in its muscle tissue that aggressively agglutinates the blood. This can lead to numerous types of hematological and immune system disorders. It is also a good idea to limit consumption of red meat and instead choose other types of game, including lamb, mutton, rabbit, and venison.

Game is the best meat source. Turkey and pheasant are acceptable poultry alternatives. Neither contain the bad lectins that are found in chicken. Eggs do not contain the lectins that are found in the adult chicken muscle tissue. So eggs are OK.

PROTEINS

SEAFOOD

Seafood is an excellent source of protein for Type Bs. Salmon and cod are particularly rich in the beneficial omega-3 essential fatty acids that can play an important role in balancing hormonal disturbances. Avoid shellfish, including mussels, shrimp, lobster, and crab. They contain lectins that are similar to the lectins found in chicken, and are harmful for most B types.

PROTEINS

DAIRY

Your blood type is the only one that permits consumption of dairy in large quantities. The sugar antigen found in Type B blood is D-galactosamine, the same sugar found in most milks. This means that the sugar in milk, lactose, does not agglutinate in Type Bs the way it does in O or A types. From an evolutionary perspective, Type B blood emerged from the herdsman tradition where milk and game was a mainstay of the diet.

Type B individuals of Asian ancestry do very well on dairy products. Their systems respond superbly to dairy. However, there may be some difficulty adapting to dairy in the beginning, especially if there is no history of dairy consumption in a person's lineage. To facilitate the introduction of dairy into the diet it is useful to use a lactase-based enzyme product. You can find such products in health food stores. Cultured or soured dairy products, such as yogurt and kefir, are very beneficial. Once tolerance to these foods has been developed, milk, ice cream, and cheeses can be more easily introduced.

B types of African descent are usually lactose intolerant; however, there are relatively few such individuals. Soy and rice milk products are acceptable for most B types. However, whole milk products are preferable.

CARBOHYDRATES

BEANS AND LEGUMES

One of the most important ways to keep insulin levels in check, outside of using the 30-40-30 macronutrient approach, is to avoid excessive consumption of beans and legumes. In particular, stay away from lentils, pinto beans, black-eyed peas, garbanzo beans, and azuki beans. These foods contain high levels of lectins that can interfere with the insulin-glucagon axis. Insulin causes fat to be stored and prevents its utilization for energy.

Asians typically consume large amounts of legumes. Reducing the amount of legumes eaten will definitely improve the health of a Type B Asian. Legumes and beans rank as a -1, meaning they are mildly Yin.

Black-eyed peas are tolerated and considered a neutral food by B negatives. Type B positives should avoid them.

CARBOHYDRATES

GRAINS AND CEREALS

Type B's should reduce the amount of wheat eaten. Wheat lectins actually act as an artificial insulin molecule, causing increased insulin receptor cell stimulation, even without the presence of insulin. This is why excessive wheat consumption does lead to excess fat reserves and fat storage, while preventing the utilization of fat as a fuel source.

Type B's should also avoid rye, kasha, and buckwheat. They contain lectins in a level that has the potential to damage the vascular lining, leading to increased blood disorders, including strokes. In place of wheat and other high-lectin cereals, grain choices should be spelt, oatmeal and rice. Most grains rank high on the glycemic index. By reducing their consumption Type B's will experience greater fat loss.

CARBOHYDRATES

BREADS

Essene or Ezekiel bread, which are sprouted wheat breads, are best. The sprouting process eliminates the bad lectins commonly found in wheat. These breads are processed at lower temperatures, which allows the enzymes and important nutrients to remain stable and available for assimilation. Avoid rye bread. Its lectin content causes disturbances in the blood.

CARBOHYDRATES

PASTAS AND FLOURS

Be careful; most pastas have a very high glycemic index, which can lead to insulin disturbances. If the macronutrient ratios are properly balanced, they will minimize this insulin response; however, it is a good idea to limit pasta. B types should also limit the use of rye flour.

CARBOHYDRATES

VEGETABLES

Your biggest vegetable no-no is the tomato. Tomatoes contain panhemaglutinins, lectins that agglutinate, especially blood Types A and B. O and AB types react much less to these lectins.

The tomato aside, there is a wide range of vegetables choices for Type B's compared to other blood types. They can eat potatoes, yams, and even cabbage, whereas most of the other types must avoid them. Green leafy vegetables are important providers of nutrition. Eat ample amounts. Limit intake of olives. They contain molds that may disturb the immune system of Type B individuals.

CARBOHYDRATES

FRUITS

Avoid coconuts, persimmons, and pomegranates. The lectin content is detrimental. However, there are plenty of good choices among the acidic fruits. Type Bs have an ability to readily buffer the acid content.

Fruits have a very high Yin score of -3. They should be eaten in moderation and balanced with appropriate high Yang foods.

CARBOHYDRATES

JUICES

B types are fairly unique in their ability to tolerate cabbage, a food with a very powerful fat- and fluid-reducing potential. It offers a sure-fire way to lose weight or detoxify. Cabbage juice is a particularly effective way to accomplish either one, and can be blended with any number of other beneficial vegetable juices. Cabbage juice is an excellent choice for a fasting program. Juice fresh cabbage, preferably organic, and drink two to three quarts a day, up to three days in a row. Cabbage juice can also be used as a meal replacement, even though it does not fit the macronutrient ratio concept. However, in this respect it is being used in a medicinal way for detoxification, helping the body to rid itself of assorted poisons that have accumulated in the cells over time. These toxins must be eliminated in order to attain higher levels of health and to reduce the risk of cancer and degenerative diseases. Avoid tomato juice, even in Bloody Marys, unless on vacation and you just want to indulge. It should not become a habit.

FATS

NUTS AND SEEDS

There are only certain nuts that are acceptable. Macadamia is one. One large macadamia nut is equivalent to one fat Portion in the New Millennium Diet. Avoid peanuts, pistachios, pumpkin seeds, filberts, and pine nuts. They contain lectins that are detrimental to Type B individuals.

FATS

OILS

Olive oil is the most beneficial oil. It is a monounsaturated fat, promoting healthy digestion, especially when used in combination with the New Millennium–based ratios of 30% protein, 40% carbohydrate, and 30% fat. Avoid cottonseed, peanut, and sesame oil. They all contain lectins that can be potentially harmful to the digestive and immunological systems of Type B individuals.

MISCELLANEOUS

BEVERAGES

Stay away from distilled liquors. They can put a major stress on the liver. Red wine and beer are OK in limited amounts. These drinks tend to increase fat accumulation because of their high glycemic rating. In balance with proteins and fats they are tolerable.

Most sodas, even natural sodas, should be avoided. Green tea is a good choice. It contains compounds found to have anticancer properties, notably against stomach cancer. A number of studies have shown that green tea has a protective effect for individuals with a family or cultural history of stomach cancer.

MISCELLANEOUS

CONDIMENTS

Avoid condiments with tomato. That means ketchup and tomato sauces. Tomato-based condiments lead to fat gain even if they are a low-calorie product. Organic jams and jellies are preferable over the commercially available varieties. Salad dressings, especially those that contain milk products, are acceptable.

MISCELLANEOUS

SPICES

Keep in mind that most individuals have either an excess Yin or Yang state. This means they are a bit too hot or a bit too cool, in terms of their body's energetic balance. Most of the highly beneficial spices for blood type B are warming herbs, which suggests that B types tend to be a little on the Yin side. This generalization, of course, does not apply to all. An individual determination requires consulting a practitioner knowledgeable in Chinese medicine.

You should definitely avoid black and white peppers because of the lectins they contain. Many natural sweeteners may be problematic. These include barley malt and corn syrup. Such ingredients may cause intestinal irritation. Cayenne pepper is an excellent herb for strengthening and tonifying the digestive tract and organs. It helps to prevent poor circulation by moving the blood. It can be used regularly.

MISCELLANEOUS

TEAS AND HERBS

There are only a few teas that are truly not recommended for B types. Fenugreek should not be used by pregnant women to stimulate breast milk production. It reacts poorly in the B type system. Aloe vera should be limited or avoided altogether. Ginseng can over-stimulate the kidneys if used in excess .

Rose hip tea is an excellent source of vitamin C. It helps to enhance immune system function, increasing the body's defense against viral and bacterial agents. Ginger is very useful for settling the stomach. In addition, it is a good antiparasitic herb and tea, and should be used when eating game or sushi. It helps destroy bacteria that are present in improperly cooked meats. Use ginger either in the form of ginger root or ginger tea as an excellent digestive and antimicrobe remedy.

MISCELLANEOUS

SUPPLEMENTS

Multivitamins

It is important for B types to take a multiple vitamin that is blood type–specific, even if much of the diet contains foods reportedly high in vitamins and minerals. Our modern-day farming techniques reduce the amount of nutrients present in the soil, which in turn reduces the amount present in our foods. In addition, the time involved in transporting food from the grower to the grocery further lowers the nutrient content.

In our high-tech, high-pollution age, we need to use nutrients as a protective means to ensure that our bodies are able to function to their maximum potential. Research has repeatedly shown that nutritional supplements provide an excellent form of nutritional insurance against many of the degenerative diseases that have reached epidemic proportions throughout our industrialized world.

Minerals

The consumption of high calcium-containing dairy products generally ensures an adequate level of this important mineral. However, magnesium is another story, and is often in short supply. Magnesium is a critical mineral not only for strong bones but also for hundreds of enzyme reactions in the body. Magnesium deficiency aggravates stress reactions. This is one very important mineral.

Magnesium is found in green leafy vegetables, which is recommended for B blood types. For added insurance, supplement with magnesium glycinate, the most bio-available form of the mineral. Take it at bedtime. It is better absorbed then and also contributes to relaxation of the muscles and nervous system, and promotes deeper, sounder sleep. I recommend 500 to 1,000 milligrams of magnesium at bedtime. Go slow with magnesium. If too much is taken it will act as a laxative. If Type Bs do not eat the dairy products recommended in this book, then they will need to step up their calcium. In that case, take a combination calcium-magnesium supplement. The preferable form of calcium is microcrystalline hydroxyapatite. This combination also should be taken at bedtime.

Herbs

Ginkgo biloba is an excellent brain fortifier that helps improve memory and mental acuity. It is widely used throughout Europe and the United States for patients with dementia, Alzheimer's disease, and Parkinson's. Numerous studies have validated its benefits.

Licorice, or DGL as it is commonly called, is another useful herb for B types. It has powerful antiviral and healing qualities, as well as antiulcer and antiindigestion properties. It can be used freely in place of antacids and other types of stomach acid blockers such as Prilosec. Before stopping any medication, consult a physician. DGL is available at health food stores in a de-glycyrrhizinated form. This means that the glycerin content has been reduced, the portion that has negative effects on human physiology. Licorice with glycerin can lead to elevated blood pressure and fluid retention. It is advisable to use licorice under the supervision of a physician who is educated in herbology.

Lecithin

Lecithin is a nutrient that helps to regulate the immune system. When taken in adequate quantity, it can also thin the blood.

Noni Juice

Noni juice, which comes from the tropical morinda citrofolia plant, is excellent for B blood type individuals. It contains a substance known as prexeronine, which is converted into xeronine in the body. This ingredient is very effective for lowering blood pressure and improving symptoms of diabetes and arthritis.

Vegetarian Enzymes

Digestive enzymes are an important aid for B types who may want to change from a vegetarian diet to a more meat- and dairy-based diet as recommended by the New Millennium program. Vegetarian enzymes, made from the *Aspergillus* species of fungus, are the most effective. Study the label of the enzyme product to be sure it is an *Aspergillus* product and not an animal-based enzyme. The latter type may have a suppressive effect on the pancreas. Usually two capsules 15–20 minutes before a meal can help reduce some of the negative side effects associated with the transition to meat. Within two to four weeks after introducing red meat and dairy into the diet, the body should be able to adapt to the change and increase its own production of digestive enzymes necessary for the breakdown of these foods.

Bromelain, a pineapple enzyme, is also very effective in helping to break down proteins. As a supplement, it can be taken 15–20 minutes prior to eating a meat-based meal. The recommended dosage is 500–1,000 milligrams. Bromelain is also an excellent anti-inflammatory agent and can be used in place of Advil or Tylenol for many inflammatory conditions. If it is used for this purpose, it should be taken an hour before or after meals, so that it does not have a digestive effect. In this way, it is absorbed in its pre-enzyme form that allows it to go to work as an anti-inflammatory. Doses in the range of 2,000–6,000 milligrams between meals are often effective for acute situations where any type of ligament, tendon or muscular injury has occurred.

Blood Type B Food Chart

30% Protein—40% Carbohydrate—30% Fat

Proper Food Ratio

The proper macronutrient ratio for blood Type B is 30% protein, 40% carbohydrate and 30% fat. One Portion of protein equals 7 grams, one Portion of carbohydrates equals 9 grams and one Portion of fat equals 3 grams. You will only use this information if you want to use a food not listed in the food groups. Otherwise, all food listings are designated in their appropriate Portion requirements.

Classification of Foods

Three (3) food classifications are used in the New Millennium Diet Plan. They are most beneficial, neutral and least beneficial foods. These classifications are based on blood type compatibility, glycemic index, toxicity levels and other food characteristics.

These factors have been carefully analyzed and weighed against each other to determine their appropriate designation within the food classifications. For example, raisins have been considered as a *favorable food* by other diet plans. In this diet plan, they have been rated as *least beneficial*, due to the fact that they contain over 113 chemical residues. Similar reclassification of foods have been made on this basis.

It is important that you realize this distinction in your meal planning to achieve maximum results.

Most Beneficial Foods

These foods demonstrate optimum blood type compatibility and contain the lowest level of toxic chemical residues. They should be selected as your first choice in diet planning.

Neutral Foods

These foods are neutral in their blood type compatibility, but may contain slightly higher levels of toxic chemical residues. They should be selected as your second choice in diet planning.

Least Beneficial Foods

These foods demonstrate the least beneficial blood type compatibility and may contain the highest levels of toxic chemical residues. They should be considered as the last choice in diet planning and be consumed only on a very limited basis if at all.

Rh Factor—Type B Positive and Type B Negative

There are no known differences between Type B positives and Type B negatives.

FOOD GROUPS USED IN THE CHART

PROTEINS
- MEAT · POULTRY · EXOTICS
- SEAFOOD
- DAIRY PRODUCTS

CARBOHYDRATES
- BEANS and LEGUMES
- GRAINS and CEREALS
- BREADS
- PASTAS and FLOURS
- VEGETABLES
- FRUITS
- JUICES

FATS
- NUTS and SEEDS
- OILS and other Fats

MISCELLANEOUS
- BEVERAGES
- CONDIMENTS
- SPICES · TEAS · HERBS

FOOD CHART LEGEND

+ Organic Is Preferable
* Highly Glycemic
⊕ Acid Neutralized
■ Acceptable Fruits & Vegetables Only
< This food possibly has a Yin or Yang energy, but for our diet planning is considered negligible

1P 1 Protein Portion
1C 1 Carbohydrate Portion
1F 1 Fat Portion
*1P/1C/1F This food contains 1 Portion of protein, 1 Portion of carbohydrate and 1 Portion of Fat in the serving size listed

* Note: The number before the letter will always signify the amount of Protein-Carbohydrates-Fat Portions in the serving size listed.

PROTEINS

MEAT • POULTRY • EXOTICS

Most Beneficial:	1 Portion =		Yin	Neutral	Yang	Yin/Yang Score
	Raw	Cooked				
Lamb		1 oz.			X	+2
Mutton		1 oz.			X	+2
Venison (Domestic)		1 oz.			X	+2

Neutral:	1 Portion =		Yin	Neutral	Yang	Yin/Yang Score
	Raw	Cooked				
Alligator		1 1/2 oz.			X	+2
Beef (lean cuts) +		1 oz.			X	+2
Beef, Ground (10–15% fat) +		1 1/2 oz.			X	+2
Buffalo		1 oz.			X	+2
Heart (beef) +		1 oz.			X	+2
Pheasant		1 1/2 oz.			X	+3
Ostrich		1 1/2 oz.			X	+3
Rabbit		1 oz.			X	+2
Soy Burger		1/2 patty			X	+1
Soy (hot dog)		1 link			X	+1
Soy Sausage		2 links			X	+1
Soy Sausage Patty		1 patty			X	+1
Tofu (soft or regular)(1P/1C)		3 oz.	X		X	+1/-1
Tofu (firm or extra firm)		3 oz.			X	+2
Tripe		1 1/2 oz.			X	+2
Turkey		1 oz.			X	+3
Turkey (breast, deli, ground)		1 1/2 oz.			X	+3
Turkey (hot dog)		1 link			X	+3
Turkey (bacon) 3 strips		3 strips			X	+3
Turkey (breast, skinless)		1 oz			X	+3
Veal +		1 oz.			X	+2

Least Beneficial:	1 Portion =		Yin	Neutral	Yang	Yin/Yang Score
	Raw	Cooked				
Bacon		3 strips			X	+1
Bacon (Canadian)		1 oz.			X	+1
Beef (hot dog)		1 link			X	+2
Chicken (breast, deli) +		1 1/2 oz.			X	+3
Chicken (breast, skinless) +		1 oz.			X	+3
Chicken (dark, skinless) +		1 oz.			X	+3
Chicken (hot dogs)		1 link			X	+3
Cornish Hens		1 oz.			X	+3
Duck		1 1/2 oz.			X	+3
Goose		1 1/2 oz.			X	+3
Ham (deli)		1 1/2 oz.			X	+1
Ham (lean)		1 oz.			X	+1
Kielbasa		2 oz.			X	+2
Kidney (beef)		1 oz.			X	+2
Liver (beef)		1 oz.			X	+2
Partridge		1 1/2 oz.			X	+3
Pepperoni		1 oz.			X	+2
Pork		1 oz.			X	+1
Pork (chop)		1 oz.			X	+1
Pork (hot dog)		1 Link			X	+1
Pork (sausage)		2 Links			X	+1
Quail		1 1/2 oz.			X	+3
Rattlesnake		1 1/2 oz.			X	+2
Salami		1 oz.			X	+2
Tempeh (1P/1C)		1 1/2 oz.	X		X	+1/-1
Venison (imported)		1 1/2 oz.			X	+2

PROTEIN

DAIRY PRODUCTS

(Protein rich dairy sources unless otherwise noted)

Most Beneficial:	1 Portion =		Yin	Neutral	Yang	Yin/Yang Score
	Raw	Cooked				
Eggs	1 large				X	+3
Egg White	2 large				X	+3
Feta	1 oz.				X	+2
Cheese (goat)	1 oz.				X	+2
Cottage Cheese (low fat)	2 oz.				X	+2
Farmer	1 oz.				X	+2
Kefir (1P/1C)	1 cup		X		X	+1/-1
Milk, Goat (1P/1C/2F)	1 cup		X		X	+1/-1/-1
Milk, Low fat (1P/1C) +	1 cup		X		X	+1/-1
Milk, Oat (1C)	3/4 cup		X			-2
Yogurt, Goat, Plain (1P/1C/2F)	1/2 cup		X		X	+1/-1/-1

Most Beneficial:	1 Portion =		Yin	Neutral	Yang	Yin/Yang Score
	Raw	Cooked				
Mozzarella	1 oz.				X	+2
Ricotta, skim	2 1/2 oz.				X	+2
Skim Milk (1P/1C)	1 cup		X		X	+1/-1
Yogurt, Plain (lowfat) (1P/1C) +	1/2 cup		X		X	+1/-1

Neutral:	1 Portion =		Yin	Neutral	Yang	Yin/Yang Score
	Raw	Cooked				
Brie	1 oz.				X	+2
Buttermilk (1P/1C/2F)	1 cup		X		X	+1/-1/-1
Camembert	1 oz.				X	+2
Casein	1 oz.				X	+2
Cheese (almond)	1 oz.				X	+2
Cheese (soy)	1 oz.				X	+2
Colby	1 oz.				X	+2
Edam	1 oz.				X	+2
Emmenthal	1 oz.				X	+2
Gouda	1 oz.				X	+2
Gruyere	1 oz.				X	+2
Ice Cream (soy)	1 cup		X			-3
Ice Cream (rice)	1 cup		X			-3
Jarlsberg	1 oz.				X	+2
Milk, Almond (1C)	3/4 cup		X			-2
Milk, Rice (1C)	3/4 cup		X			-2
Milk, Soy (1C)	3/4 cup		X			-2
Milk, Whole (1P/1C/1F) +	1 cup		X		X	+1/-1/-1
Muenster	1 oz.				X	+2
Parmesan	1 oz.				X	+2
Provolone	1 oz.				X	+2
Neufchatel	1 oz.				X	+2
Monterey Jack	1 oz.				X	+2
Swiss	1 oz.				X	+2
Whey	1/3 oz.				X	+2
Yogurt, Frozen (1C)*	1/3 cup		X			-3
Yogurt, Soy (plain) (1P/1C)	1/2 cup		X		X	+1/-1
Yogurt with fruit (1C) +■	1/4 cup		X			-3

Least Beneficial:	1 Portion =		Yin	Neutral	Yang	Yin/Yang Score
	Raw	Cooked				
American Cheese	1 oz.				X	+2
Blue Cheese	1 oz.				X	+2
Cheddar	1 oz.				X	+2
Egg (substitute)	1/4 cup				X	+2
Ice Cream (1C)	1/4 cup		X			-3
Ice Milk (1C) *	1/4 cup		X			-3
Milk, Evaporated	1/4 cup		X			-1
Milk shake (1C) *	1/4 cup		X			-3
Sherbet	1/4 cup		X			-3
String Cheese	1 oz.				X	+2

+ Organic Is Preferable * Highly Glycemic ⊕ Acid Neutralized ■ Acceptable Fruits & Vegetables Only

PROTEINS

SEAFOOD

Most Beneficial:	1 Portion =		Yin	Neutral	Yang	Yin/Yang Score
	Raw	Cooked				
Arctic char		1 1/2 oz.			X	+1
Belt fish		1 1/2 oz.			X	+1
Butterfish (imported)		1 1/2 oz.			X	+1
Cod (imported)		1 1/2 oz.			X	+1
Flounder		1 1/2 oz.			X	+1
Gray sole		1 1/2 oz.			X	+1
Grouper		1 1/2 oz.			X	+1
Haddock		1 1/2 oz.			X	+1
Hake		1 1/2 oz.			X	+1
Halibut		1 1/2 oz.			X	+1
Lobster (spiny)		1 oz.			X	+1
Mahi Mahi		1 1/2 oz.			X	+1
Monkfish		1 1/2 oz.			X	+1
Mullet (imported)		1 1/2 oz.			X	+1
Ocean Perch		1 1/2 oz.			X	+1
Pickerel		1 1/2 oz.			X	+1
Porgy		1 1/2 oz.			X	+1
Salmon (Pacific)		1 1/2 oz.			X	+1
Sand Dabs		1 1/2 oz.			X	+1
Sardine		1 oz.			X	+1
Shad		1 1/2 oz.			X	+1
Sole		1 1/2 oz.			X	+1
Talapia		1 1/2 oz.			X	+1
Trout, Sea		1 oz.			X	+1
Whiting		1 1/2 oz.			X	+1

Neutral:	1 Portion =		Yin	Neutral	Yang	Yin/Yang Score
	Raw	Cooked				
Abalone		1 1/2 oz.			X	+1
Albacore (Tuna)		1 oz.			X	+1
Bonito		1 1/2 oz.			X	+1
Mackerel		1 1/2 oz.			X	+1
Marlin		1 1/2 oz.			X	+1
Orange Roughy		1 1/2 oz.			X	+1
Pollock		1 1/2 oz.			X	+1
Ribbonfish		1 1/2 oz.			X	+1
Sailfish		1 1/2 oz.			X	+1

+ Organic Is Preferable   * Highly Glycemic   ⊕ Acid Neutralized   ■ Acceptable Fruits & Vegetables Only

Neutral:	1 Portion =		Yin	Neutral	Yang	Yin/Yang Score
	Raw	Cooked				
Scallop		1 1/2 oz.			X	+1
Sea Bass (imported)		1 oz.			X	+1
Sea Urchin		1 oz.			X	+1
Silver Perch		1 1/2 oz.			X	+1
Smelt		1 1/2 oz.			X	+1
Snapper		1 1/2 oz.			X	+1
Snapper (red)		1 1/2 oz.			X	+1
Spot Fish		1 1/2 oz.			X	+1
Squid (calamari)		2 1/2 oz.			X	+1
Tarpon		1 1/2 oz.			X	+1
Thresher Shark		1 1/2 oz.			X	+1
Tilefish		1 1/2 oz.			X	+1
Trout (imported)		1 oz.			X	+1
Tuna (canned)		1 oz.			X	+1
Tuna (steak)		1 oz.			X	+1
Wahoo		1 1/2 oz.			X	+1
Whitefish		1 1/2 oz.			X	+1
White Perch		1 1/2 oz.			X	+1

Least Beneficial:	1 Portion =		Yin	Neutral	Yang	Yin/Yang Score
	Raw	Cooked				
Anchovies		1 oz.			X	+1
Angle Shark		1 1/2 oz.			X	+1
Barracuda		1 1/2 oz.			X	+1
Beluga		1 1/2 oz.			X	+1
Black Cod		1 1/2 oz.			X	+1
Bluefish		1 1/2 oz.			X	+1
Bluegill Bass		1 oz.			X	+1
Bream		1 1/2 oz.			X	+1
Buffalo Fish		1 1/2 oz.			X	+1
Carp		1 1/2 oz.			X	+1
Catfish		1 1/2 oz.			X	+1
Caviar	1 1/2 oz.				X	+1
Clam		1 1/2 oz.			X	+1
Cod (domestic)		1 1/2 oz.			X	+1
Coho Salmon (Great Lks.)		1 1/2 oz.			X	+1
Conch		1 1/2 oz.			X	+1
Crab		1 1/2 oz.			X	+1
Crayfish		1 oz.			X	+1
Croaker		1 1/2 oz.			X	+1
Eel		1 1/2 oz.			X	+1
Frog		1 1/2 oz.			X	+1

+ Organic Is Preferable   * Highly Glycemic   ⊕ Acid Neutralized   ■ Acceptable Fruits & Vegetables Only

Least Beneficial:	1 Portion =		Yin	Neutral	Yang	Yin/Yang Score
	Raw	Cooked				
Herring		1 1/2 oz.			X	+1
Herring (pickled)		1 1/2 oz.			X	+1
Lobster		1 oz.			X	+1
Lox (smoked salmon)		1 1/2 oz.			X	+1
Menpachi		1 1/2 oz.			X	+1
Milkfish		1 1/2 oz.			X	+1
Mud Fish		1 1/2 oz.			X	+1
Mullett (domestic)		1 1/2 oz			X	+1
Mussels		1 1/2 oz.			X	+1
Octopus		1 1/2 oz.			X	+1
Oysters		1 1/2 oz.			X	+1
Palani		1 1/2 oz.			X	+1
Pike		1 1/2 oz.			X	+1
Sea Bass (domestic)		1 oz.			X	+1
Sea Herring		1 oz.			X	+1
Shark		1 1/2 oz.			X	+1
Sheephead		1 1/2 oz.			X	+1
Shrimp		1 1/2 oz.			X	+1
Snail		1 1/2 oz.			X	+1
Striped Bass		1 oz.			X	+1
Sturgeon		1 1/2 oz.			X	+1
Swordfish		1 1/2 oz.			X	+1
Trout (domestic)		1 oz.			X	+1
Turtle		1 1/2 oz.			X	+1
Walleye		1 1/2 oz.			X	+1
Weakfish		1 1/2 oz.			X	+1
White Bass		1 oz.			X	+1
Yellow Perch		1 1/2 oz.			X	+1
Yellowtail Tuna		1 1/2 oz.			X	+1

CARBOHYDRATES

BEANS and LEGUMES

Most Beneficial:	1 Portion =		Yin	Neutral	Yang	Yin/Yang Score
	Raw	Cooked				
Cannellini Beans		1/3 cup	X			-1
Kidney Beans		1/3 cup	X			-1
Lima Beans *		1/4 cup	X			-1
Navy Beans		1/4 cup	X			-1

+ Organic Is Preferable   * Highly Glycemic   ⊕ Acid Neutralized   ■ Acceptable Fruits & Vegetables Only

Neutral:	1 Portion =		Yin	Neutral	Yang	Yin/Yang Score
	Raw	Cooked				
Broad Beans		1/2 cup	X			-1
Fava Beans		1/3 cup	X			-1
Green Beans		1 cup	X			-1
Green Peas		1/3 cup	X			-1
Jicama Beans		1/2 cup	X			-1
Mung Beans		1/3 cup	X			-1
Northern Beans		1/3 cup	X			-1
Pea Pods		1/3 cup	X			-1
Snow Peas		1/3 cup	X			-1
Red Beans		1/3 cup	X			-1
Red Soy Beans		1/3 cup	X			-1
Snap Beans		1/3 cup	X			-1
String Beans		1 cup	X			-1
Tamarind Beans		1/3 cup	X			-1
White Beans		1/3 cup	X			-1

Least Beneficial:	1 Portion =		Yin	Neutral	Yang	Yin/Yang Score
	Raw	Cooked				
Aduke Beans		1/6 cup	X			-1
Adzuki Beans		1/6 cup	X			-1
Bean Sprouts		10 cups	X			-1
Black Beans		1/3 cup	X			-1
Black-eyed Peas		1/3 cup	X			-1
Copper Beans		1/3 cup	X			-1
Garbanzo Beans		1/4 cup	X			-1
Pinto Beans +		1/3 cup	X			-1
Refried Beans		1/4 cup	X			-1
Domestic Lentils	1/3 cup	1/4 cup	X			-1
Green Lentils	1/3 cup	1/4 cup	X			-1
Red Lentils	1/3 cup	1/4 cup	X			-1

CARBOHYDRATES

BREADS

Most Beneficial:	1 Portion =		Yin	Neutral	Yang	Yin/Yang Score
	Raw	Cooked				
Essene Bread		2 oz.		X		0
Ezekiel Bread		3/4 slice		X		0
Spelt Bread		1/2 slice		X		0
Wasa		1 slice		X		0

+ Organic Is Preferable   * Highly Glycemic   ⊕ Acid Neutralized   ■ Acceptable Fruits & Vegetables Only

Neutral:	1 Portion =		Yin	Neutral	Yang	Yin/Yang Score
	Raw	Cooked				
Brown Rice Bread *		1/2 slice		X		0
Brown Rice Cakes		1 cake		X		0
Fin Crisp		1 slice		X		0
Gluten-Free Bread		1/2 slice		X		0
High Protein Bread		1/2 slice		X		0
Ideal Flat Bread		2 piece		X		0
Millet Bread *		1/2 slice		X		0
Oat Bran Muffins		1/3 muffin		X		0
Pumpernickel		2/3 slice		X		0
Soya Flour Bread		1 slice		X		0
Sprouted Wheat Bread		1/2 slice		X		0

Least Beneficial:	1 Portion =		Yin	Neutral	Yang	Yin/Yang Score
	Raw	Cooked				
Bagels, Wheat		1/4 bagel		X		0
Bread Sticks (hard)		1 stick		X		0
Bread Sticks (soft)		1/2 stick		X		0
Cake		1/3 piece	X			-2
Corn Muffins		1/4 muffin		X		0
Doughnut		1/3	X			-2
Durum Wheat		1/2 slice		X		0
English Muffins		1/4 muffin		X		0
Graham Crackers		1 1/3 crackers	X			-2
Kamut		1 slice		X		0
Matzo, Wheat		1/3 Board		X		0
Melba toast		1/2 slice		X		0
Multi-Grain Bread		1/2 slice		X		0
Pancakes (wheat) 4"		1/2		X		0
Pita Bread (pocket)		1/4 pocket		X		0
Rice Cakes (white)		1 cake		X		0
Rice Crackers		6 crackers		X		0
Rye Bread (100%)		3/4 slice		X		0
Rye Crisp		3 pieces		X		0
Saltine Crackers		3		X		0
Vita Rye		3 pieces		X		0
Waffle (wheat)		1/2		X		0
Wheat Bran Muffins		1/2 muffin		X		0
Whole Wheat Bread		1/2 slice		X		0

+ Organic Is Preferable   * Highly Glycemic   ⊕ Acid Neutralized   ■ Acceptable Fruits & Vegetables Only

CARBOHYDRATES

FRUITS

Most Beneficial:	1 Portion =		Yin	Neutral	Yang	Yin/Yang Score
	Raw	Cooked				
Cherries +	8		X			-3
Feiojas (medium) +	2		X			-3
Grapes, Black +	1/2 cup		X			-3
Grapes, Concord +	1/2 cup		X			-3
Grapes, Green +	1/2 cup		X			-3
Grapes, Red +	1/2 cup		X			-3
Plums, Dark +	1		X			-3
Plums, Green +	1		X			-3
Plums, Red +	1		X			-3
Pineapple	1/2 cup		X			-3
Raspberries	1 cup		X			-3

Neutral:	1 Portion =		Yin	Neutral	Yang	Yin/Yang Score
	Raw	Cooked				
Apples +	1/2		X			-3
Apricots +	3		X			-3
Bananas	1/3		X			-3
Blackberries	3/4 cup		X			-3
Blueberries +	1/2 cup		X			-3
Boysenberries	1/2 cup		X			-3
Cactus	1/3 cup		X			-3
Cranberries +	3/4 cup		X			-3
Currants, Black	3/4 cup		X			-3
Currants, Red	3/4 cup		X			-3
Currants, White	3/4 cup		X			-3
Dates +	2		X			-3
Elderberries	1/2 cup		X			-3
Figs (dried) *	1 piece		X			-3
Figs (fresh) *	1 piece		X			-3
Gooseberries	1 cup		X			-3
Grapefruit	1/2		X			-3
Guava	1/2 cup		X			-3
Kiwi	1		X			-3
Kumquat	3		X			-3
Lemons	1		X			-3
Limes	1		X			-3
Loganberries	3/4 cup		X			-3
Mangoes	1/3 cup		X			-3

+ Organic Is Preferable   * Highly Glycemic   ⊕ Acid Neutralized   ■ Acceptable Fruits & Vegetables Only

Neutral:	1 Portion =		Yin	Neutral	Yang	Yin/Yang Score
	Raw	Cooked				
Melons, Bitter	1/4		X			-3
Melons, Cantaloupe +	1/4		X			-3
Melons, Canang	2/3 cup		X			-3
Melons, Casaba +	2/3 cup		X			-3
Melons, Crenshaw +	2/3 cup		X			-3
Melons, Christmas	2/3 cup		X			-3
Melons, Honeydew +	1/4		X			-3
Melons, Musk	2/3 cup		X			-3
Melons, Spanish	2/3 cup		X			-3
Watermelons	3/4 cup		X			-3
Nectarines (medium)+	1/2		X			-3
Oranges	1/2		X			-3
Papaya	3/4 cup		X			-3
Peaches, (medium) +	1		X			-3
Peaches (canned) +	1/2 cup		X			-3
Pears (medium) +	1/2		X			-3
Pears (canned) +	1/2 cup		X			-3
Plantains	1 oz.		X			-3
Prunes +	2		X			-3
Raisins (organic only) + *	1 tbsp.		X			-3
Strawberries +	1 cup		X			-3
Tangerines	1		X			-3

Least Beneficial:	1 Portion =		Yin	Neutral	Yang	Yin/Yang Score
	Raw	Cooked				
Coconut	5 1/3 oz.		X			-3
Pears, Prickly	3/4		X			-3
Persimmons (medium) +	1/3		X			-3
Pomegranates (medium) +	1/3		X			-3
Raisins (commercial)	1 tbsp.		X			-3
Rhubarb	2 1/2 cups		X			-3
Star Fruit (Medium)	1 1/3		X			-3

CARBOHYDRATES

GRAINS and CEREALS

Most Beneficial:	1 Portion =		Yin	Neutral	Yang	Yin/Yang Score
	Raw	Cooked				
Oat Bran	1/3 oz.			X		0
Oatmeal (slow cooking)	1/2 oz.	1/3 cup		X		0
Rice Bran	1/2 oz.			X		0
Spelt (Flakes)	1/2 oz.			X		0

+ Organic Is Preferable   * Highly Glycemic   ⊕ Acid Neutralized   ■ Acceptable Fruits & Vegetables Only

Neutral:	1 Portion =		Yin	Neutral	Yang	Yin/Yang Score
	Raw	Cooked				
Cream of Brown Rice*		1/3 cup		X		0
Familia	1/2 oz.	1/3 cup		X		0
Farina	1/2 oz.	1/3 cup		X		0
Granola	1/2 oz.			X		0
Grapenuts	1/2 oz.			X		0
Grits	1/2 oz.	1/3 cup		X		0
Millet *	1/2 oz.			X		0
Rice, Brown (puffed)	1/3 cup			X		0

Least Beneficial:	1 Portion =		Yin	Neutral	Yang	Yin/Yang Score
	Raw	Cooked				
Amaranth (flakes)	1/2 oz.			X		0
Barley (dry flakes)	1/2 tbsp.			X		0
Buckwheat (dry)	1/2 oz.			X		0
Cornflakes *	1/3 cup			X		0
Cornmeal *	1/2 oz.			X		0
Cream of Wheat *	1/2 oz.	1/3 cup		X		0
Cream of White Rice *	1/2 oz.	1/3 cup		X		0
Kamut (flakes)	1/2 oz.			X		0
Kasha	1/2 oz.			X		0
Rice, White (puffed)	1/5 cup			X		0
Rye	1/2 oz			X		0
Seven Grain *	2/3 oz.			X		0
Shredded Wheat *	1/2 oz.			X		0
Wheat Bran	1/2 oz.			X		0
Wheat Germ	1 oz.			X		0

CARBOHYDRATES

JUICES

Most Beneficial:	1 Portion =		Yin	Neutral	Yang	Yin/Yang Score
	Raw	Cooked				
Cabbage	1 cup		X			-2
Celery +	3/4 cup		X			-1
Grape *	1/4 cup		X			-3
Pineapple *	1/4 cup		X			-3
Water w/ Lemon	N/A			X		N/A

+ Organic Is Preferable   * Highly Glycemic   ⊕ Acid Neutralized   ■ Acceptable Fruits & Vegetables Only

Neutral:	1 Portion =		Yin	Neutral	Yang	Yin/Yang Score
	Raw	**Cooked**				
Apple + *	1/3 cup		X			-3
Apple Cider + *	1/3 cup		X			-3
Apricot	1/4 cup		X			-3
Black Cherry + *	1/3 cup		X			-3
Boysenberry	1/4 cup		X			-3
Carrot *	1/3 cup		X			-1
Cranberry *	1/4 cup		X			-3
Cucumber	3/4 cup		X			-1
Grapefruit + *	1/3 cup		X			-3
Orange *	1/3 cup		X			-3
Papaya *	1/4 cup		X			-3
Prune + *	1/5 cup		X			-3
Vegetable * ■	3/4 cup		X			-2

Least Beneficial:	1 Portion =		Yin	Neutral	Yang	Yin/Yang Score
	Raw	**Cooked**				
V-8 Juice *	3/4 cup		X			-2
Pomegranate Juice	1/3 cup		X			-3
Tomato + *	1 cup		X			-1

CARBOHYDRATES

PASTAS and FLOURS

Most Beneficial:	1 Portion =		Yin	Neutral	Yang	Yin/Yang Score
	Raw	**Cooked**				
Oat Flour	1/2 oz.			X		0

Neutral:	1 Portion =		Yin	Neutral	Yang	Yin/Yang Score
	Raw	**Cooked**				
Quinoa Flour	1/2 oz.			X		0
Rice, Basmati *		1/5 cup		X		0
Rice, Brown *		1/5 cup		X		0
Rice Flour, Brown *	1/2 oz.			X		0
Semolina Pasta		1/4 cup		X		0
Soya Flour	1/2 oz			X		0
Spelt Flour	2/3 oz.			X		0
Spelt Noodles	1/4 cup			X		0
Spinach Pasta		1/4 cup		X		0
Sprouted Wheat Flour	1 1/2 oz.			X		0

+ Organic Is Preferable   * Highly Glycemic   ⊕ Acid Neutralized   ■ Acceptable Fruits & Vegetables Only

Least Beneficial:	1 Portion =		Yin	Neutral	Yang	Yin/Yang Score
	Raw	Cooked				
Artichoke Pasta		1/4 cup		X		0
Barley Flour	2/3 oz.			X		0
Buckwheat	1/2 oz.			X		0
Bulgar Wheat Flour	1/2 oz.			X		0
Couscous Flour	1/2 oz.			X		0
Durum Wheat Flour	1/2 oz.			X		0
Gluten Flour	1/2 oz.			X		0
Graham Flour	1/2 oz.			X		-2
Kamut	1/2 oz			X		0
Kasha	1/2 oz.			X		0
Rice Flour + *	4/5 oz.			X		0
Rice, White		1/5 cup		X		0
Rice Flour, White	1/2 oz			X		0
Rice, Wild *		1/5 cup		X		0
Rye Flour (100%) + *	4/5 oz.			X		0
Soba Noodles		1/4 cup		X		0
White Flour	3/4 oz.			X		0
Whole Wheat Flour	1 oz.			X		0

CARBOHYDRATES

VEGETABLES

Most Beneficial:	1 Portion =		Yin	Neutral	Yang	Yin/Yang Score
	Raw	Cooked				
Beet Greens	5 1/2 cups		X			-2
Beets		1/2 cup	X			-1
Broccoli	2 cups		X			-1
Cabbage, Chinese	3 cups	1 1/3 cups	X			-2
Cabbage, Red	3 cups	1 1/3 cups	X			-2
Cabbage, White	3 cups	1 1/3 cups	X			-2
Carrots *	3 1/2 oz.	1/2 cup	X			-1
Cauliflower		2 cups	X			-1
Choy Sum +	2 cups		X			-1
Cilantro (coriander)		2 1/2 cups	X			-2
Collard Greens +	2 1/2 cups		X			-2
Eggplant +		1 1/2 cups	X			-1
Kale +	1 cup		X			-2
Kelp	4 oz.		X			-2
Mushrooms, Shitake	3 cups	1 cup	X			-1
Mustard Greens	3 1/4 cups	3 cups	X			-2
Parsley +	5 cups		X			-2
Parsnips *	1/3 cup		X			-1
Peppers, Green (chopped)	2 1/4 cups		X			-1
Peppers, Jalapeno (chopped)	3 oz.		X			-1

+ Organic Is Preferable   * Highly Glycemic   ⊕ Acid Neutralized   ■ Acceptable Fruits & Vegetables Only

Most Beneficial: (continued)	1 Portion =		Yin	Neutral	Yang	Yin/Yang Score
	Raw	Cooked				
Peppers, Red (chopped) +	1 cup		X			-1
Peppers, Pablano (chopped) +	3 oz.		X			-1
Peppers, Serrano (chopped) +	2/3 cup		X			-1
Peppers, Yellow (chopped)	2 1/4 cups		X			-1
Potato, Sweet +		1/3 potato	X			-1
Red Chard		1 cup	X			-2
Spirulina	1 1/2 oz.		X			-2
Sprouts, Brussels	1 1/4 cups		X			-1
Tomatillo	1/3		X			-1
Yams		1/3	X			-1

Neutral:	1 Portion =		Yin	Neutral	Yang	Yin/Yang Score
	Raw	Cooked				
Arugula	11 1/4 cups		X			-2
Asparagus		12 spears	X			-1
Bamboo Shoots	3 3/4 cup	1 cup	X			-1
Barley Greens	N/A		X			-2
Blue Green Algae	N/A		X			-1
Bok Choy +		3 cup	X			-2
Celery +	2 cups		X			-1
Chicory Greens	1 cup		X			-1
Chicory Roots	2/3 cup		X			-1
Cilantro (coriander)		2 1/2 cup	X			-2
Cucumber, whole	1		X			-1
Cucumber, sliced	1 cup		X			-1
Daikon Radish	2 1/2 cups		X			-1
Dandelion Greens +	1 2/3 cups		X			-2
Dill Weed +	15 cups		X			-1
Endive	7 1/2 cups		X			-2
Escarole +	7 1/2 cups		X			-2
Garlic	10 cloves		X			-1
Hominy (grits)	1/3 cup		X			-1
Horseradish (pods)	2 cups		X			-1
Kohlrabi +	1 cup		X			-2
Leeks +	1 cup		X			-1
Lettuce, Bibb (5" head)	2 head		X			-2
Lettuce, Boston (5" head)	2 head		X			-2
Lettuce, Iceberg (6" head) +	1 head		X			-2
Lettuce, Mesclun +	1 head		X			-2
Lettuce, Romaine +	6 cups		X			-2
Mushrooms, Abalone	3 cups	1 cup	X			-1
Mushrooms, Domestic	3 cups	1 cup	X			-1
Mushrooms, Enoki	3 cups	1 cup	X			-1
Mushrooms, Portobello	3 cups	1 cup	X			-1

+ Organic Is Preferable   * Highly Glycemic   ⊕ Acid Neutralized   ■ Acceptable Fruits & Vegetables Only

Neutral:	1 Portion =		Yin	Neutral	Yang	Yin/Yang Score
	Raw	Cooked				
Mushrooms, Tree Oyster	3 cups	1 cup	X			-1
Onions, Green (scallions)	1 cup	1/2 cup	X			-1
Onions, Red	1 cup		X			-1
Onions, Spanish	1 cup		X			-1
Onions, Yellow	1 cup		X			-1
Peppers, Chili (chopped)	2/3 cup		X			-1
Potatoes, Red		1/3 cup	X			-1
Okra +		1 cup	X			-1
Radicchio	7 oz.		X			-2
Radishes +	2 cups		X			-1
Rapini	2 cups		X			-1
Red Algae	N/A		X			-1
Rutabaga +	3/4 cup	1/2 cup	X			-1
Sauerkraut		1 cup	X			-2
Seaweed		3 1/2 oz.	X			-2
Shallots	2 oz.		X			-1
Spinach +	4 cups		X			-2
Sprouts, Alfalfa	11 cups		X			-1
Squash, Acorn +		1/2 cup	X			-1
Squash, Butternut +		1/2 cup	X			-1
Squash, Yellow +		1 1/4 cups	X			-1
Swiss Chard +		1 cup	X			-2
Turnips (mashed) +		1 1/2 cups	X			-1
Turnip Greens +		1 1/2 cups	X			-2
Water Chestnuts	1/3 cup		X			-1
Watercress	22 1/2 cups		X			-2
Zucchini		1 1/2 cups	X			-1

Least Beneficial:	1 Portion =		Yin	Neutral	Yang	Yin/Yang Score
	Raw	Cooked				
Artichokes +	Small		X			-1
Jerusalem Artichokes +	Small		X			-1
Corn White		1/4 cup	X			-1
Corn Yellow		1/4 cup	X			-1
Fiddlehead Ferns	10 cups		X			-2
Hummus	1/4 cup		X			-1
Potatoes, White		1/3 cup	X			-1
Pumpkin (mashed)		3/4 cup	X			-1
Purslane +	6 1/2 cups	1 2/3 cups	X			-2
Radishes +	4 cups		X			-1
Sprouts, Mung	3 cups		X			-2
Sprouts, Radish	3 cups		X			-1
Taro	1/3 cup	1/5 cup	X			-1
Tomato +	2		X			-1

+ Organic Is Preferable   * Highly Glycemic   ⊕ Acid Neutralized   ■ Acceptable Fruits & Vegetables Only

FATS

NUTS AND SEEDS

Most Beneficial:	1 Portion =		Yin	Neutral	Yang	Yin/Yang Score
None						

Neutral:	1 Portion =		Yin	Neutral	Yang	Yin/Yang Score
	Raw	Cooked				
Almonds	1 tsp.		X			-2
Almond Butter	1/2 tsp.		X			-2
Brazil	1/2 nut		X			-2
Chestnuts	3/4 oz.		X			-2
Flax Seeds	3/4 tsp.		X			-1
Hemp Seeds	3/4 tsp.		X			-1
Hickory Nuts	1/2 tsp.		X			-2
Lychee Nuts (1C)	2 oz		X			-3
Macadamia	1 large		X			-2
Pecans	1/2 tsp.		X			-2
Radish Seeds	1 tsp.		X			-1
Walnuts	1/2 tsp.		X			-2
Watermelon Seeds	3/4 tsp.		X			-1

Least Beneficial:	1 Portion =		Yin	Neutral	Yang	Yin/Yang Score
	Raw	Cooked				
Cashews	2 nuts		X			-2
Cashew Butter	2/3 tsp.		X			-2
Filbert Nuts	1/2 tsp.		X			-2
Peanuts	6 nuts		X			-2
Peanut Butter	1/2 tsp.		X			-2
Pignolia (pine seeds)	1 tsp.		X			-2
Pistachios	2/3 tsp.		X			-2
Poppy Seeds	1 1/4 tsp.		X			-1
Pumpkin Seeds	3/4 tsp.		X			-1
Sesame Butter (Tahini)	1/3 tbsp.		X			-1
Sesame Seeds	1 tsp.		X			-1
Sunflower Butter	3/4 tsp.		X			-1
Sunflower Seeds	3/4 tsp.		X			-1

+ Organic Is Preferable   * Highly Glycemic   ⊕ Acid Neutralized   ■ Acceptable Fruits & Vegetables Only

FATS

OILS and OTHER FATS

Most Beneficial:	1 Portion =		Yin	Neutral	Yang	Yin/Yang Score
	Raw	Cooked				
Black Currant Oil	1/3 tsp.		X			-2
Olive Oil	1/3 tsp.		X			-2
Salmon Oil	1/3 tsp.		X			-2

Neutral:	1 Portion =		Yin	Neutral	Yang	Yin/Yang Score
	Raw	Cooked				
Borage Oil	1/3 tsp.		X			-2
Butter	1/3 tsp.		X			-1
Cod Liver Oil	1/3 tsp.		X			-2
Cream (half & half)	1 tbsp.		X			-1
Cream Cheese	1 tsp.		X			-1
Flax Seed Oil (linseed)	1/3 tsp.		X			-2
Ghee	1/3 tsp.		X			-1
Hemp Seed Oil	1/3 tsp.		X			-2
Sour Cream	1/2 tbsp.		X			-1
Sour Cream, Light	1 tbsp.		X			-1

Least Beneficial:	1 Portion =		Yin	Neutral	Yang	Yin/Yang Score
	Raw	Cooked				
Avocado	1 tbsp.		X			-2
Canola Oil	1/3 tsp.		X			-2
Coconut Oil	1/3 tsp.		X			-2
Corn Oil	1/3 tsp.		X			-2
Cottonseed Oil	1/3 tsp.		X			-2
Hydrogenated Oil	1/3 tsp.		X			-2
Lard	1/3 tsp.		X			-2
Olives (black)	3		X			-2
Olives (Greek)	3		X			-2
Olives (green)	3		X			-2
Olives (Spanish)	3		X			-2
Palm Oil	1/3 tsp.		X			-2
Peanut Oil	1/3 tsp.		X			-2
Safflower Oil	1/3 tsp.		X			-2
Sesame Seed Oil	1/3 tsp.		X			-2
Shortening, vegetable	1/3 tsp.		X			-2
Tahini	1/2 tsp.		X			-2
Sunflower Oil	1/3 tsp.		X			-2

+ Organic Is Preferable   * Highly Glycemic   ⊕ Acid Neutralized   ■ Acceptable Fruits & Vegetables Onl

MISCELLANEOUS

BEVERAGES

Most Beneficial:	1 Portion =		Yin	Neutral	Yang	Yin/Yang Score
	Raw	Cooked				
Green Tea	N/A			X		<
Green Tea (decaffeinated)	N/A			X		<
Purified Water	N/A			X		<

Neutral:	1 Portion =		Yin	Neutral	Yang	Yin/Yang Score
	Raw	Cooked				
Beer (light)	4 oz.			X		0
Beer (regular)	4 oz.			X		0
Cappuccino, Decaf	N/A				X	<
Cappuccino, Regular	N/A				X	<
Champagne	4 oz		X			-3
Coffee, Decaf	N/A				X	<
Coffee, Regular	N/A				X	<
Sparkling Water	N/A			X		<
Sports Drink (natural)	1/3 cup		X			-3
Tea, Black, Decaf	N/A				X	<
Tea, Black, Regular	N/A				X	<
Wine, Red	4 oz.		X			-3
Wine, White	4 oz.		X			-3

Least Beneficial:	1 Portion =		Yin	Neutral	Yang	Yin/Yang Score
	Raw	Cooked				
Club Soda	N/A				X	<
Latté	3/4 cup		X			-2
Liquors, Distilled	1 oz.			X		0
Soda, Diet	2 1/2 oz.		X			-3
Sodas (other)	2 1/2 oz.		X			-3
Seltzer Water	N/A			X		<
Sports Drink (artificial)	1/3 cup		X			-3

MISCELLANEOUS

CONDIMENTS

Most Beneficial: NONE	1 Portion =		Yin	Neutral	Yang	Yin/Yang Score

Neutral:	1 Portion =		Yin	Neutral	Yang	Yin/Yang Score
	Raw	Cooked				
Apple Butter	2 tsp.		X			-3
"Bragg's" Amino Acids	N/A				X	<
Jam * ■	2 tsp.		X			-3
Jelly * ■	2 tsp.		X			-3
Maple Syrup	2 tsp.		X			-3
Mayonnaise (dairy) (1F)	1 tsp.		X			-1
Mayonnaise (vegetarian) (1F)	1 tsp		X			-1
Mustard	N/A				X	<
Salad Dressing	N/A		X			-2
Soy Sauce	N/A					<
Tamarind	N/A					<

Least Beneficial:	1 Portion =		Yin	Neutral	Yang	Yin/Yang Score
	Raw	Cooked				
Barbecue Sauce	2 tbsp.		X			-3
Candy Bar *	1/4 bar		X			-3
Cocktail Sauce	2 tbsp.		X			-3
Dill Pickles	9		X			-1
Ketchup	2 tbsp.		X			-2
Kosher Pickles	9		X			-1
Plum Sauce	1 1/2 tbsp.		X			-3
Sweet Pickles	1 1/2		X			-1
Sour Pickles	9		X			-1
Relish	4 tsp.		X			-2
Teriyaki Sauce	1 tbsp.		X			-3
Worcestershire Sauce	N/A				X	<

MISCELLANEOUS

SPICES

Most Beneficial:	1 Portion =		Yin	Neutral	Yang	Yin/Yang Score
	Raw	Cooked				
Curry	N/A				X	<
Ginger	N/A				X	<
Horseradish	N/A				X	<
Parsley	N/A				X	<
Pepper Cayenne	N/A				X	<
Rosemary	N/A		X			<

Neutral:	1 Portion =		Yin	Neutral	Yang	Yin/Yang Score
	Raw	Cooked				
Agar	N/A		X			<
Anise	N/A		X			<
Arrowroot Starch	1 tsp.		X			-1
Basil	N/A		X			<
Bay Leaf	N/A		X			<
Bergamot	N/A		X			<
Black Strap Molasses *	1/2 tsp.		X			-3
Brewer's Yeast	N/A		X			<
Brown Rice Syrup *	3 tsp.		X			-3
Capers	N/A				X	<
Caraway Seeds	N/A		X			<
Cardamom	N/A				X	<
Carob	1 oz.		X			-3
Chervil	N/A				X	<
Chives	N/A		X			<
Chocolate *	1 oz.		X			-3

+ Organic Is Preferable   * Highly Glycemic   ⊕ Acid Neutralized   ■ Acceptable Fruits & Vegetables Only

Neutral:	1 Portion =		Yin	Neutral	Yang	Yin/Yang Score
	Raw	Cooked				
Cloves	N/A				X	<
Coriander	N/A				X	<
Cream of Tartar	N/A		X			<
Cumin	N/A				X	<
Dill	N/A		X			<
Dulse	N/A		X			<
Fennel	N/A		X			<
Garlic	N/A				X	<
Honey *	1/2 tbsp.		X			-3
Kelp	N/A		X			<
Marjoram	N/A		X			<
Mint	N/A				X	<
Miso	N/A			X		<
Mustard	N/A				X	<
Nutmeg	N/A				X	<
Paprika	N/A				X	<
Peppercorn Pepper	N/A				X	<
Red Pepper	N/A				X	<
Peppermint	N/A				X	<
Pimento	N/A				X	<
Rice Syrup *	3 tsp.		X			-3
Saffron	N/A			X		<
Sage	N/A				X	<
Salt	N/A		X			<
Savory	N/A				X	<
Spearmint	N/A		X			<
Stevia	N/A		X			<
Sucanat	2 tsp.		X			-3
Tarragon	N/A		X			<
Thyme	N/A			X		<
Turmeric (tuber)	N/A		X			<
Turmeric (rhizone)	N/A				X	<
Vanilla	N/A		X			<
Vinegar, Apple Cider	N/A				X	<
Vinegar, Balsamic	N/A				X	<
Vinegar, Red Wine	N/A				X	<
Vinegar, White	N/A				X	<
Wintergreen	N/A		X			<

+ Organic Is Preferable   * Highly Glycemic   ⊕ Acid Neutralized   ■ Acceptable Fruits & Vegetables Only

Least Beneficial:	1 Portion =		Yin	Neutral	Yang	Yin/Yang Score
	Raw	Cooked				
Allspice	N/A				X	<
Almond Extract	N/A		X			<
Barley Malt	3tsp.		X			-2
Cinnamon	N/A				X	<
Cornstarch	1 tsp.		X			-1
Corn Syrup *	2 tsp.		X			-3
Gelatin	N/A			X		<
Pancake Syrup *	2 tsp.		X			-3
Pepper, Ground Black	N/A				X	<
Pepper, White	N/A				X	<
Sugar, Brown *	2 tsp.		X			-3
Sugar, Confectionery *	1 tbsp.		X			-3
Sugar, White *	2 tsp.		X			-3
Tapioca	N/A		X			<

MISCELLANEOUS

TEAS and/or HERBS

Most Beneficial:	1 Portion =		Yin	Neutral	Yang	Yin/Yang Score
	Raw	Cooked				
Cayenne	N/A				X	<
Deglycyrrhizinated licorice	N/A			X		<
Echinacea	N/A		X			<
Ginger	N/A				X	<
Ginseng, American	N/A		X			<
Green Tea	N/A			X		<
Milk Thistle	N/A		X			<
Parsley	N/A				X	<
Peppermint	N/A		X			<
Raspberry Leaf	N/A			X		<
Rosehip	N/A			X		<
Sage	N/A				X	<

+ Organic Is Preferable   * Highly Glycemic   ⊕ Acid Neutralized   ■ Acceptable Fruits & Vegetables Only

Neutral:	1 Portion =		Yin	Neutral	Yang	Yin/Yang Score
	Raw	Cooked				
Alfalfa	N/A			X		<
Burdock	N/A		X			<
Cascara Sagrada	N/A		X			<
Catnip	N/A		X			<
Chamomile	N/A			X		<
Chickweed	N/A		X			<
Dandelion	N/A		X			<
Dong Quai	N/A				X	<
Elder	N/A				X	<
Gentian	N/A		X			<
Ginseng, Siberian	N/A				X	<
Goldenseal	N/A		X			<
Hawthorne	N/A				X	<
Horehound	N/A		X			<
Licorice Root	N/A			X		<
Mulberry	N/A		X			<
Sarsaparilla	N/A			X		<
Slippery Elm	N/A			X		<
Spearmint	N/A		X			<
St. John's Wort	N/A		X			<
Strawberry Leaf	N/A		X			<
Thyme	N/A			X		<
Valerian	N/A				X	<
Vervain	N/A		X			<
White Birch	N/A		X			<
White Oak Bark	N/A		X			<
Yarrow	N/A			X		<
Yellowdock	N/A		X			<

Least Beneficial:	1 Portion =		Yin	Neutral	Yang	Yin/Yang Score
	Raw	Cooked				
Aloe	N/A		X			<
Colt's Foot	N/A		X			<
Corn silk	N/A		X			<
Fenugreek	N/A				X	<
Hops	N/A			X		<
Linden	N/A		X			<
Mullein	N/A		X			<
Red Clover	N/A		X			<
Rhubarb	N/A			X		<
Senna	N/A		X			<
Shepherd's Purse	N/A			X		<
Skullcap	N/A		X			<

+ Organic Is Preferable   * Highly Glycemic   ⊕ Acid Neutralized   ■ Acceptable Fruits & Vegetables Only

Blood Type B Recipes

INSTRUCTIONS FOR USE:

The following pages provide five recipes specific for this particular blood type: breakfast, lunch, dinner, dessert and one snack. Each recipe takes into account the correct foods for this specific blood type, the proper ratio of proteins, carbohydrates and fats (Macrobalance™ Portions) and an acceptable Yin Yang energetic score. In compliance with the 4th piece of the New Millennium Diet puzzle, it is recommended that organic foods be used as much as possible. Each meal (breakfast, lunch and dinner) offers the user three, four, five or six Portion amounts.

The recipe consists of two parts. Part one, a shopping list that provides the correct amount of ingredients necessary according to the 4 different Portion sizes. The shopping list also shows the amount in which the various Portion sizes contribute towards the total Yin Yang score.

Part two is the Preparation section and provides simple to follow instructions in preparing the recipe.

It is very simple to use the recipes, it is done in three easy steps:
1. **Determine the correct amount of Portions needed (Chapter 7).**
2. **In the recipe, refer to the Grocery List, select the correct Portion column and obtain the ingredients in the amounts listed.**
3. **Prepare the recipe according to the Preparation instructions in Part two.**

It's that simple to enjoy a complete Macrobalanced™ meal. Bon appetit!

Breakfast: Tropical Orange Crepe
Blood Type B

Shopping List

Ingredients:	Portion Size			
	3	4	5	6
	Amount of Ingredient			
Proteins:				
Whole Egg(s)	1 egg	1 egg	2 eggs	2 eggs
Soy Flour	1/8 cup	1/6 cup	1/5 cup	1/4 cup
Soy Milk (unsweetened)	3/8 cup	1/2 cup	5/8 cup	3/4 cup
Soy Yogurt (plain)	3/8 cup	1/2 cup	1/2 cup	1/2 cup
Knox Gelatin (plain)	3/4 env.	3/4 env.	3/4 env.	1 env.
Carbohydrates:				
Mandarin Oranges	1/2 cup	1/2 cup	3/4 cup	3/4 cup
Arrowroot Powder **	1 1/2 tsp	2 tsp	2 1/2 tsp	3 tsp
Fats and Oils:				
Butter	1 tsp	1 1/2 tsp	1 2/3 tsp	2 tsp
Spices:				
Orange Extract	3/4 tsp	1 tsp	1 1/4 tsp	1 1/2 tsp
Yin (-)/Yang(+) (excess)	-1	-4	-3	-4

Preparation:

Mix eggs with soy flour and milk to form a crepe batter. Spray crepe pan with an olive oil non-stick spray. When the pan is heated add the batter to the pan. Once the bottom of the crepe is slightly brown, flip over and cook for approximately 1 minute. Place the crepe onto a serving plate. Mix the soy yogurt, arrowroot powder**, butter, and gelatin in a bowl. Lightly heat the mixture in a saucepan, then add the mandarin oranges and continue to cook until sauce thickens. Pour sauce into crep and fold over both sides. Serve warm.

** Arrowroot Powder should be well-mixed with 3 to 5 teaspoons of water before adding to ther ingredients.

Lunch: Ginger Curry Turkey Meatballs with Pineapple
Blood Type B

Shopping List

Ingredients:	Portion Size			
	3	4	5	6
	Amount of Ingredient			
Proteins:				
Turkey (ground)	4 1/2 oz	6 oz	7 1/2 oz	9 oz
Carbohydrates:				
Onions (diced)	1/3 cup	1/2 cup	2/3 cup	1 cup
Celery (diced	2/3 cup	1 cup	1 1/4 cup	1 1/2 cup
Kidney beans (cooked, chopped)	1/5 cup	1/4 cup	1/3 cup	1 cup
Arrowroot Powder *	1 1/2 tsp	2 tsp	2 1/2 tsp	3 tsp
Pineapple	3/8 cup	1/2 cup	5/8 cup	1 cup
Cherries or grapes	1/4 cup	1/3 cup	2/5 cup	1 cup
Fats and Oils:				
Olive Oil	1 tsp	1 1/3 tsp	1 2/3 tsp	2 tsp
Spices:				
Sea Salt	pinch	pinch	pinch	pinch
Pepper	pinch	pinch	pinch	pinch
Ginger (powdered)	1/8 tsp	1/2 tsp	3/4 tsp	1 tsp
Curry	1/4 tsp	1/2 tsp	2/3 tsp	1 tsp
Vegetable Broth	1/3 cup	1/2 cup	3/4 cup	1 cup
Orange Extract	1/8 tsp	1/4 tsp	1/3 tsp	3/8 tsp
Yin (-)/Yang(+) (excess)	-1	-1	-4	-4

Preparation:
Mix ground turkey with onions, celery, kidney beans, olive oil, pepper, curry and ginger. Using this mixture, form as many meatballs as available. Place in a baking pan. Bake in preheated 400° oven for 20 minutes or until cooked. In a saucepan slowly simmer cherries, pineapple and vegetarian broth, orange extract and arrowroot powder. Stir sauce constantly to prevent burning. After meatballs are cooked, place in fruit sauce. Serve immediately.

** Arrowroot Powder should be well-mixed with 3 to 5 teaspoons of water before adding to other ingredients.

Snack: Cucumber, Carrot and Mozzarella
Blood Type B

Shopping List

Ingredients:	Portion Size		
	1	2	3
	Amount of Ingredient		
Proteins:			
Mozzarella Cheese	1 oz	2 oz	3 oz
Carbohydrates:			
Cucumbers	1/2 cup	1 cup	1 1/2 cup
Carrots	1/2 cup	1 cup	1 1/2 cup
Fats and Oils:			
Almond butter	3/4 tsp	1 1/2 tsp	2 1/4 tsp
Spices:			
Sea Salt	pinch	pinch	pinch
Yin (-)/Yang(+) (excess)	-2	-1	0

Preparation:
Cut the mozzarella and vegetables into desired portions. Use almond butter as a spread on the cucumbers and carrots. Sprinkle with sea salt.

Dinner: Mandarin Orange Beef
Blood Type B

Shopping List

Ingredients:	Portion Size			
	3	4	5	6
	Amount of Ingredient			
Proteins:				
Beef (cubed)	3 oz	4 oz	5 oz	6 oz
Carbohydrates:				
Bell Peppers (Green)	5/6 cup	1 1/8 cup	1 1/2 cup	1 2/3 cup
Celery (chopped)	3 cups	4 cups	5 cups	6 cups
Arrowroot Powder *	1 1/2 tsp	2 tsp	2 1/2 tsp	2 1/2 tsp
Mandarin Oranges	1/4 cup	1/3 cup	1/2 cup	1/2 cup
Fats and Oils:				
Flax seeds	2 1/4 tsp	3 tsp	3 3/4 tsp	4 tsp
Butter	2/3 tsp	1 tsp	1 tsp	1 tsp
Spices:				
Red wine	3/4 tsp	1 tsp	1 1/4 tsp	1 1/2 tsp
Beef Stock	3/8 cup	1/2 cup	5/8 cup	3/4 cup
Soy Suace	3/4 tbsp	1 tbsp	1 1/4 tbsp	1 1/2 tbsp
Ginger	3/4 tsp	1 tsp	1 1/4 tsp	1 1/2 tsp
Yin (-)/Yang(+) (excess)	-2	-2	-3	-3

Preparation:

In a pan, sauté the beef in butter until browned and remove from pan. Add celery to pan and cook until tender, stirring frequently. In a separate saucepan cook the mandarin oranges, bell peppers, beef stock, red wine, soy sauce, ginger, flax seeds and arrowroot powder until thickened. Add beef-celery mixture to sauce and simmer for 7 to 9 minutes. Serve warm.

* Arrowroot Powder should be well-mixed with 3 to 5 teaspoons of water before adding to the other ingredients.

Dessert: Frozen Pineapple Cream
Blood Type A

Shopping List

Ingredients:	Portion Size		
	1	2	3
	Amount of Ingredient		
Proteins:			
Egg Whites	1 egg	2 eggs	3 eggs
Soy Yogurt	1/4 cup	1/2 cup	3/4 cup
Carbohydrates:			
Pineapple	1/4 cup	1/2 cup	3/4 cup
Arrowroot Powder*	1 1/3 tsp	2 tsp	2 1/4 tsp
Fats and Oils:			
Almonds (finely chopped)	2/3 tsp	1 1/3 tsp	2 tsp
Spices:			
Ginger	1/8 tsp	1/5 tsp	1/3 tsp
Orange Extract	1/4 tsp	1/3 tsp	1/3 tsp
Yin (-)/Yang(+) (excess)	-1	-3	-4

Preparation:

In a saucepan, place the pineapple, ginger, orange extract, yogurt and arrowroot powder*. Heat until warmed thoroughly. Set aside until cool. Place the egg whites in a mixing bowl and whip until firm. Add the egg whites and almonds to the cooled fruit mixture. Stir the mixture, place into freezer until frozen. Serve cold.

* Arrowroot Powder should be well-mixed with 3 to 5 teaspoons of cold water before adding to the other ingredients.

Chapter 11

Blood Type AB: Modern

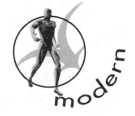

Health and Dietary Characteristics

- 25% Protein
  50% Carbohydrate
  25% Fat
- Combination of Both A and B Blood Types
- Immune System Tolerance
- Hypersensitive Digestive Tract
- Unknown Evolutionary Link

Personality Characteristics

- Mysterious
- Adaptive and Balanced
- Appealing Personalities

BLOOD TYPE AB—CHARACTERISTICS

PERSONALITY CHARACTERISTICS

Type AB individuals are said to have a "mysterious" personality, that is, difficult to describe precisely. We do know, however, that you are very adaptive and balanced individuals. You do not tend to be aggressive in the style of O types, nor do you overly intellectualize the issues of life as do A types. You tend to have attributes that make you appealing to most people. You are warm and welcoming with a tendency to forgive if things do not work out in the way that they were expected. Your type has the potential to be very charismatic and the ability to captivate your audience.

PHYSIOLOGY AND DIETARY CHARACTERISTICS

AB individuals possess the rarest blood type on the planet, making up approximately 2–5% of the population, a result of combining A and B bloodlines some 1,000 to 2,000 years ago. The mixture of B blood created a stronger individual than the Type A. You have a more durable immune system and greater adaptive ability relative to A individuals.

But you have to watch your step and follow your blood type diet as closely as possible. You have a much more limited range of foods than any of the other blood types. If you follow the recommendations, staying within the appropriate macronutrient ratio of 25% protein, 50% carbohydrate, and 25% fat, and eating foods that are beneficial for your blood type, you will be OK. In fact, you will generate significant fat loss and build up your immune system by watching your diet. The lower amount of protein that is recommended follows the Type A approach. If you consume large amounts of meat, you are likely to stimulate insulin production, leading to increased fat storage. A types fare better on a vegetarian diet, while B types handle meat well. You can eat meat, in moderation, but your best choices should favor game-based varieties.

You need to avoid foods on both the A and B food listings that are not beneficial. Tomatoes are an exception. Your AB constitution can tolerate tomatoes even though they are contraindicated for A and B types. Other foods to avoid are lima beans, kidney beans, corn, buckwheat, and sesame seeds. They all have negative effects in your body.

Weight Management

In addition, the lectins in the foods just mentioned cause binding to the insulin receptors, inducing fat storage. Wheat will do the same, even though it is tolerated by your blood type. Its high glycemic rating calls for moderation in consumption. Moreover, wheat can cause an acidizing effect on AB muscle tissue. Alkalinity is in your best interest.

Foods Encouraging Fat Gain:

Red meat, chicken, kidney beans, lima beans, seeds, corn, buckwheat, wheat.

Foods Encouraging Fat Loss:

Tofu, seafood, dairy, green vegetables, kelp, pineapple.

Exercise

Your best bet is to practice some form of stress reduction and pursue exercise similar to the A type. AB physiology promotes heightened anxiety, irritability, and poor focusing tendencies. To counteract this tendency, relaxation, yoga and meditation techniques are more beneficial for you than intense exercise, which adds stress to your body.

Outdoor activities such as hiking, swimming, or bicycling provide a natural relaxation effect, required for your system's optimum functioning, as well as important cardiovascular stimulation. Any type of exercise that promotes a meditative and relaxing effect should be performed at least three to four times a week. Excessive exercise or competitive activities weaken your immune and nervous systems, and will tend to generate fatigue and susceptibility to infections.

If the Type AB person is interested in intense competitive sports, I suggest taking small amounts of valerian or chamomile, herbs that will help put your body into a relaxed state after the activity. MSM (methylsulfonylmethane), a supplement that provides biologically active sulfur to the body, is useful to prevent muscle soreness caused by high-intensity training.

DIETARY SPECIFICS

PROTEINS

MEATS AND POULTRY

Game meats are the preferred meat protein for ABs. Reduce your consumption of other forms of meat. You have a lesser production of stomach acid, therefore red meats are poorly tolerated. Chicken is also not for you. It causes severe lectin reactions in Type AB individuals. Snails, an exotic delicacy, are acceptable and can be beneficial for AB blood types, especially those who are suffering with breast cancer.

Digestive enzymes or hydrochloric acid may be needed to facilitate the digestion of meat that is included in your diet. Not only will this help in the breakdown of protein, but also help prevent or reduce indigestion. Avoid smoked or cured meats. The nitrate additives in these foods are known carcinogens.

In regard to the Rh factor, AB negatives can eat small amounts of partridge and quail. AB positives should avoid them.

PROTEINS

SEAFOOD

Stay away from lobster, shellfish, clams, crabs, and shrimp. Many other seafoods are quite beneficial and should be eaten as a primary protein source. No smoked or pickled seafood. These foods are aggravating because of your reduced stomach acid production.

In regard to the Rh factor, domestic sea bass is acceptable for AB negative individuals. If you are AB positive, avoid it.

PROTEINS

DAIRY

AB blood types tolerate dairy, which is considered to be a neutral food group. Goat cheese is the preferred dairy food. Dairy should be eaten in sufficient quantities in order to obtain enough calcium and other minerals. Processed dairy, especially cheeses, should not be eaten frequently. Many commercially available cheeses contain chemical residues.

Eggs are an excellent source of protein for you and should be eaten on a regular basis. Eggs contain high amounts of essential nutrients, which are important for many physiological functions. If you are thinking eggs are a source of cholesterol, you are right. But keep in mind that most cholesterol, about 75%, is produced by the liver; the rest comes from the foods we eat. So, go ahead and eat eggs without worry.

Heart disease is caused by bad lectins and improper macronutrient ratios, making the person immunologically susceptible to infections such as chlamydia pneumoniae, not the cholesterol in food. If you are still concerned about the cholesterol in eggs, stick to the egg whites. Two small egg whites are equivalent to one protein Portion for ABs. Eggs do not contain the lectins found in chicken; another reason they should be included in the AB diet.

CARBOHYDRATES

BEANS AND LEGUMES

Lentils, especially green lentils, are acceptable for AB blood types, even though they are not recommended for B types. Avoid kidney and lima beans. Legumes and beans have a higher glycemic rating and should be consumed only in moderation. If you experience gas as a result of eating beans, try Beano. It is a product that is widely available and effective in reducing gas.

In regard to the Rh factor, AB negatives can eat fava and garbanzo beans. AB positives should avoid them.

CARBOHYDRATES

GRAINS AND CEREALS

Wheat is tolerated as long as it is not eaten frequently. Its high glycemic rating and lectin content can cause some disruptions when eaten too often or in too great a quantity. Wheat is a potential allergen for many people. If you're suffering with a wheat-based allergy, avoid any forms of wheat even if it is listed as a neutral food. If you are interested in losing fat, your best bet is to avoid most types of grains. They promote insulin release, which in turn promotes fat storage.

In regard to the Rh factor, kasha is acceptable for AB negative individuals. AB positives should avoid it.

CARBOHYDRATES

BREADS

Use Essene or Ezekiel breads. These contain sprouted wheat flour instead of whole wheat flour. Corn should be avoided. As noted above, reduce your consumption of grains (thus, breads) if you are interested in weight loss.

CARBOHYDRATES

PASTAS AND FLOURS

The same is true for pastas and flours made from grains. Pastas are highly glycemic foods and do not fit into the New Millennium–based concepts. Pastas made from semolina, spinach, rice, quinoa, and spelt are tolerated by AB types. They are preferable to artichoke or buckwheat pastas.

CARBOHYDRATES

VEGETABLES

Vegetables, especially organic produce, are an excellent source of vital nutrients and are important foods for your physiology. Many vegetables tolerated by A and B types are also acceptable for you. Tomatoes are an exception, they should be avoided by both Type A and Type B; however, they are tolerable for Type ABs.

In regard to the Rh factor, AB negatives tolerate yellow and green peppers. AB positives should avoid them.

CARBOHYDRATES

FRUITS

Avoid bananas. The lectin content is too high for you. Acidic fruits, such as oranges, should be avoided because they can irritate the sensitive AB digestive tract. Tropical fruits such as mangoes, guavas, and pineapples are excellent choices because of their high bromelain content, which is beneficial for digestion.

In regard to Rh factor, star fruit is acceptable for AB negatives. AB positives should avoid it.

CARBOHYDRATES

JUICES

High alkaline juices such as cranberry, grape, and black cherry are preferable over any other juices. One teaspoon of lemon juice mixed with an 8 oz. glass of water is an excellent morning drink. It helps purge the system of toxins and decreases mucus that has accumulated throughout the night when the system slows down. Orange juice should be avoided. Opt for apple, pineapple, or grapefruit juice when eating out for breakfast. Cabbage juice is an excellent detoxification juice, especially beneficial for fasting. One to two quarts or more a day of freshly juiced cabbage is a superb way to stimulate the release of toxins, especially in the liver, intestinal tract, and kidneys. In addition to detoxification, it also helps remove excess fluid weight and even reduces cellulite.

FATS

NUTS AND SEEDS

Refer to the food listings. There are a large number of nuts and seeds that should be avoided by AB types.

In regard to Rh factor, pumpkin seeds are acceptable for AB negative types but not for AB positives.

FATS

OILS

Olive oil is your preferred oil of choice. However, canola, flaxseed, and hemp seed oils are acceptable. The traditional safflower and sunflower oils should be avoided because of their lectin content. Cold water fish oils, such as imported cod or salmon, should be consumed on a regular basis in order to promote hormonal balance and cellular harmony.

MISCELLANEOUS

BEVERAGES

Coffee, both in a decaffeinated or caffeinated form, is a beneficial beverage for your blood type because it enhances stomach acid production. However, do not drink more than two cups a day of the caffeinated brew because it can weaken the adrenal glands, leading to chronic fatigue and perhaps contributing to fibrocystic breast disease.

Red wine and beer are acceptable alternatives to distilled liquors. Red wine has high levels of certain grape skin bioflavonoids, which have been shown to be highly beneficial for the immune and cardiovascular systems.

Sodas should be avoided as well as many of the black decaffeinated and caffeinated teas.

MISCELLANEOUS

CONDIMENTS

Most pickled condiments should be avoided. They are highly fermented and can induce digestive disturbances similar to vinegar substances. Avoid ketchup since it contains vinegar. Lemon juice mixed with other herbs is an excellent substitute for vinegar-based salad dressings. Vinegar is very acidic and can irritate AB's sensitive digestive tracts.

MISCELLANEOUS

SPICES

Kelp or other herbal salt substitutes are excellent replacements for salt. The iodine in kelp helps to stimulate the thyroid gland, which enhances fat loss and improves overall immune system and metabolic function. Cornstarch, corn syrups, and barley malt sweeteners should be avoided. They score high on the glycemic index. In addition, they harbor bad lectins, which can interfere with the immune system and normal physiological functioning.

MISCELLANEOUS

TEAS AND HERBS

Burdock, chamomile, and green tea can be potent liver detoxifying agents and immune stimulants.

In regard to the Rh factor, AB negatives can handle hops and red clover, but not AB positives.

MISCELLANEOUS

SUPPLEMENTS

Multivitamins

AB types should supplement their diets with vitamins, minerals, and phytonutrients in order to optimize their nutritional status, which helps them in the polluted environment and high stress of present-day living. The pollutants and stressors of modern life take a huge toll on nutrients. Regular supplementation with a blood type–specific multivitamin will significantly enhance the body's ability to fight disease and slow down the aging process.

Vitamin C

There is a high rate of cancer among AB blood types. Vitamin C is an important anticancer nutrient. Among other things, it can help neutralize various toxins that are found in our food, air and water. Smoked meats, for instance, have added nitrates for preservative effects. Vitamin C helps counteract the negative influence of these compounds, which have been associated with stomach cancers.

The best form of vitamin C is buffered (nonacidic) vitamin C. Usually, it is buffered with either calcium or sodium. The nonacidic form of vitamin C can be tolerated at higher levels. The customary ascorbic acid form of C may cause stomach upset. In cases of illness, vitamin C can be taken in divided doses throughout the day up to bowel tolerance. Bowel tolerance means that you take as much as necessary to cause temporary diarrhea, and then cut back slightly to a lesser dosage. Vitamin C is considered by many nutritionally oriented physicians to be most effective at this bowel tolerance level.

MSM (methylsulfonylmethane)

MSM (methylsulfonylmethane) is an excellent source of healing sulfur. The supplement reduces pain, inflammation and allergic reactions, in addition to promoting healthy skin, hair, and nails. Take between 2–5 grams on a daily basis.

Selenium

Selenium is a powerful antioxidant. It should be taken with caution because too much can be toxic. It is found to be very beneficial for individuals with prostate cancer. The recommended dosage is 200 mcg. daily.

Zinc

Zinc is a potent immune booster. Usually, 15 milligrams a day is sufficient for a protective effect. Higher doses can be toxic over time. If you plan on using more than the recommended amount, only do so under the supervision of a physician educated in nutritional medicine. Zinc, especially zinc methionine, is an excellent remedy for sore throats and ear infections. Usually, after four to five zinc tablets, a sore throat will be significantly improved. Typically, the zinc is mixed with a small amount of fruit sugar to make the tablet more palatable.

Herbs

Echinacea and Astragalus

Echinacea and astragalus are superb herbs for boosting immune system function. They are excellent in fighting colds and flu, as well as more serious immune deficiency illnesses such as cancer.

Hawthorn

Hawthorn berry is an outstanding herb, widely used in Europe for strengthening the cardiovascular system. AB types have a predisposition toward heart disease. Taken either in its tincture or tablet form, hawthorn usually can provide a cardioprotective effect.

If you have heart disease I suggest a supplement containing EDTA, a chelating agent shown in thousands of studies worldwide to remove calcium and plaque complexes that block arteries. One bottle of an EDTA chelating agent is approximately equivalent to one intravenous chelation therapy session. Typically, 24–30 bottles are required for optimum results, especially in cases of highly blocked arteries.

Chamomile and Valerian Root

These herbs are known for their ability to help induce sleep and relaxation. Valerian, in its homeopathic form, has a remarkable impact on insomnia and other sleep-related disorders. These remedies are natural tranquilizers that can often replace pharmaceutical drugs. However, always consult your physician before stopping or changing any medication.

Milk Thistle

This is a powerful liver-repairing herb. It improves blood flow to the liver and also helps repair liver damage. Milk thistle exerts a significant protective effect against many toxic chemicals found in our daily lives. It offers protection, for instance, from chemotherapeutic and other medications that are toxic to the liver. If you are receiving chemotherapy or radiation, taking this herb can significantly reduce the harm inflicted on the body by these chemicals. Milk thistle is also one of the few herbs that has been shown to have protective effects against poisonous mushrooms that are eaten. Dandelion is another excellent detoxifying herb that also has diuretic properties.

Quercetin

Quercetin is a bioflavonoid, that is, a natural compound found in plants, which has powerful antioxidant and anti-inflammatory effects. It should be used in conjunction with vitamin C. The recommended dosage is 250–500 milligrams. Quercetin is a useful agent for injuries to ligaments or tendons. The substance reduces inflammation in sprains and strains and helps to repair the collagen damage that occurs in these painful injuries. Quercetin is also used to treat histamine-related reactions such as asthma and allergies.

Bromelain

Bromelain is an enzyme found in pineapples. It helps improve digestion, while reducing gas and bloating. It has also been shown, when taken between meals, to be very effective at reducing inflammation. It is useful as an aid to the body in removing damaged tissue at the sites of injuries, which facilitates the healing process. As with quercertin, it is beneficial after injuries such as those involving ligaments or tendons.

Activin

Activin is a grape seed extract shown in clinical studies to kill cancer cells in the test tube. If you're suffering from any type of cancer condition, or a cardiovascular illness, I recommend 100–150 milligrams of Activin daily.

Blood Type AB Food Chart

25% Protein—50% Carbohydrate—25% Fat

Proper Food Ratio

The proper macronutrient ratio for blood Type AB is 25% protein, 50% carbohydrate and 25% fat. One portion of protein equals 5.75 grams, one portion of carbohydrates equals 11.5 grams and one portion of fat equals 2.5 grams. You will only use this information if you want to use a food not listed in the food groups. Otherwise, all food listings are designated in their appropriate portion requirements.

Classification of Foods

Three (3) food classifications are used in the New Millennium Diet Plan. They are most beneficial, neutral and least beneficial foods. These classifications are based on blood type compatibility, glycemic index, toxicity levels and other food characteristics.

These factors have been carefully analyzed and weighed against each other to determine their appropriate designation within the food classifications. For example, peanuts and peanut butter have been considered as a *favorable food* by other diet plans. In this diet plan, they have been rated as *least beneficial*, due to the fact that they contain over 183 chemical residues. Similar, reclassification of foods have been made on this basis.

It is important that you realize this distinction in your meal planning to achieve maximum results.

Most Beneficial Foods

These foods demonstrate optimum blood type compatibility and contain the lowest level of toxic chemical residues. They should be selected as your first choice in diet planning.

Neutral Foods

These foods are neutral in their blood type compatibility, but may contain slightly higher levels of toxic chemical residues. They should be selected as your second choice in diet planning.

Least Beneficial Foods

These foods demonstrate the least blood type compatibility and may contain the highest levels of toxic chemical residues. They should be considered as the last choice in diet planning and be consumed only on a very limited basis if at all.

Rh Factor—Type AB Positive and Type AB Negative

The Type AB positive and Type AB negative diets are very similar except for certain foods that are in bold type in the least beneficial section of the different food classifications. Type AB negatives can consider the bold type foods in the chart as neutral foods unless you have a known allergic reaction to the food. However, Type AB positives must look at those bold foods as least beneficial. This system applies to all blood types. This is the only pertinent difference between Type AB negatives and Type AB positives.

FOOD GROUPS USED IN THE CHART

PROTEINS
- MEAT • POULTRY • EXOTICS
- SEAFOOD
- DAIRY PRODUCTS

CARBOHYDRATES
- BEANS and LEGUMES
- GRAINS and CEREALS
- BREADS
- PASTAS and FLOURS
- VEGETABLES
- FRUITS
- JUICES

FATS
- NUTS and SEEDS
- OILS and other Fats

MISCELLANEOUS
- BEVERAGES
- CONDIMENTS
- SPICES • TEAS • HERBS

FOOD CHART LEGEND

+ Organic Is Preferable

* Highly Glycemic

⊕ Acid Neutralized

■ Acceptable Fruits & Vegetables Only

< This food possibly has a Yin or Yang energy, but for our diet planning is considered negligible

1P 1 Protein Portion

1C 1 Carbohydrate Portion

1F 1 Fat Portion

*1P/1C/1F This food contains 1 Portion of protein, 1 Portion of carbohydrate and 1 Portion of Fat in the serving size listed

* Note: The number before the letter will always signify the amount of Protein-Carbohydrates-Fat Portions in the serving size listed.

PROTEINS

MEAT • POULTRY • EXOTICS

Most Beneficial:	1 Portion =		Yin	Neutral	Yang	Yin/Yang Score
	Raw	Cooked				
Lamb		3/4 oz.			X	+2
Mutton		3/4 oz.			X	+2
Pheasant		1 1/4 oz.			X	+3
Rabbit		3/4 oz.			X	+2
Turkey		3/4 oz			X	+3
Turkey (breast, skinless)		3/4 oz.			X	+3
Turkey (breast, deli, ground)		1 1/4 oz.			X	+3
Turkey (hot dog)		3/4 link			X	+3

Neutral:	1 Portion =		Yin	Neutral	Yang	Yin/Yang Score
	Raw	Cooked				
Alligator		1 1/4 oz.			X	+2
Ostrich		1 1/4 oz.			X	+3
Soy Burger		1/3 patty			X	+1
Soy (hot dog)		3/4 link			X	+1
Soy Sausage		1 2/3 link			X	+1
Soy Sausage Patty		3/4 patty				+1
Tempeh (1P/1C)		1 1/4 oz.	X		X	+1/-1
Tofu (firm or extra firm)		2 1/2 oz.			X	+2
Tofu (soft or regular) (1P/1C)		2 1/2 oz.	X		X	+1/-1
Turkey Bacon		2 1/2 strips			X	+3

Least Beneficial:	1 Portion =		Yin	Neutral	Yang	Yin/Yang Score
	Raw	Cooked				
Bacon		2 1/2 strips			X	+1
Beef, Ground (10–15%)		1 1/4 oz.			X	+2
Beef (hot dog)		3/4 link			X	+2
Beef, Lean		3/4 oz.			X	+2
Buffalo		3/4 oz.			X	+2
Canadian Bacon		3/4 oz.			X	+1
Chicken (breast, deli, ground)		1 1/4 oz.			X	+3
Chicken (breast, skinless)		3/4 oz.			X	+3
Chicken, (dark, skinless)		3/4 oz.			X	+3
Chicken (hot dog)		3/4 link			X	+3
Cornish Hens		3/4 oz.			X	+3
Duck		1 1/4 oz.			X	+3
Goose		3/4 oz.			X	+3
Ham, Lean		3/4 oz.			X	+1
Ham, Deli		1 1/4 oz.			X	+1
Heart, Beef		3/4 oz.			X	+2
Kidney, Beef		3/4 oz.			X	+2
Kielbasa		1 2/3 oz.			X	+2
Liver, Beef		3/4 oz.			X	+2
Partridge		1 1/4 oz.			X	+3
Pepperoni		3/4 oz.			X	+2
Pork		3/4 oz.			X	+1
Pork Chop		3/4 oz.			X	+1
Pork (hot dog)		3/4 link			X	+1
Pork Sausage		1 2/3 links			X	+1
Quail		1 1/4 oz.			X	+3
Rattlesnake		1 1/4 oz.			X	+2
Salami		3/4 oz.			X	+2
Tripe (beef)		1 1/4 oz.			X	+2
Veal		3/4 oz.			X	+2
Venison (domestic)		3/4 oz.			X	+2
Venison (imported)		3/4 oz			X	+2

+ Organic Is Preferable   * Highly Glycemic   ⊕ Acid Neutralized   ■ Acceptable Fruits & Vegetables Only

PROTEIN

DAIRY PRODUCTS

(Protein-rich dairy sources unless otherwise noted)

Most Beneficial:	1 Portion =		Yin	Neutral	Yang	Yin/Yang Score
	Raw	Cooked				
Cheese, Goat	3/4 oz.				X	+2
Cottage Cheese	1 1/2 oz				X	+2
Eggs	1 small				X	+3
Egg white	2 small				X	+3
Farmer	3/4 oz.				X	+2
Feta	3/4 oz.				X	+2
Kefir (1P/1/2C/1F)	3/4 cup		X		X	+1/-1/-1
Milk, Goat (1P/1/2C/1F)	3/4 cup		X		X	+1/-1/-1
Mozzarella	3/4 oz.				X	+2
Ricotta	2 oz.				X	+2
Yogurt, Plain, lowfat (1P/1/2C)+	1/3 cup		X		X	+1/-1

Neutral:	1 Portion =		Yin	Neutral	Yang	Yin/Yang Score
	Raw	Cooked				
Casein	3/4 oz.				X	+2
Cheese, Almond	3/4 oz				X	+2
Cheese, Soy	3/4 oz.				X	+2
Colby	3/4 oz.				X	+2
Edam	3/4 oz.				X	+2
Emmenthal	3/4 oz.				X	+2
Gouda	3/4 oz.				X	+2
Gruyere	3/4 oz.				X	+2
Ice Cream, Soy (1C) *	1 cup		X			-3
Ice Cream, Rice (1C) *	1 cup		X			-3
Jarlsberg	3/4 oz.				X	+2
Milk, Almond (1C) *	1 cup		X			-2
Milk, Oat (1C) *	1 cup		X			-2
Milk, Rice (1C) *	1 cup		X			-2
Milk, Skim (1P/1/2C)	3/4 oz.		X		X	+1/-1
Milk, Soy (1C)	1 cup		X			+1
Monterey Jack	3/4 oz.				X	+2
Muenster	3/4 oz.				X	+2
Neufchatel	3/4 oz.				X	+2
String Cheese	3/4 oz.				X	+2
Swiss Cheese	3/4 oz.				X	+2
Whey	1/4 oz.				X	-+2
Yogurt, Frozen (1C) *	1/3 cup		X			-3
Yogurt w/fruit (1C) + ■	1/3 cup		X			-3
Yogurt, Goat (plain) (1P/1/2C/3F)	1/3 cup		X		X	+1/-1/-1
Yogurt, Soy (plain) (1P/1/2C)	1/3 cup		X		X	+1/-1

+ Organic Is Preferable   * Highly Glycemic   ⊕ Acid Neutralized   ■ Acceptable Fruits & Vegetables Only

Least Beneficial:	1 Portion =		Yin	Neutral	Yang	Yin/Yang Score
	Raw	Cooked				
American Cheese	3/4 oz.				X	+2
Blue Cheese	3/4 oz.				X	+2
Brie	3/4 oz.				X	+2
Buttermilk (1P/1/2C/3F)	3/4 cup		X		X	+1/-1/-1
Camembert	3/4 oz.				X	+2
Cheddar	3/4 oz.				X	+2
Egg (substitute)	1/5 cup				X	+2
Ice Cream (1C) *	1/3 cup		X			-3
Milk (evaporated)	1/3 cup		X			-1
Milk, Ice (1C) *	1/3 cup		X			-3
Milk Shake (1C) *	1/3 cup		X			-3
Milk, Whole (1P/1/2C/3F)	3/4 cup		X		X	+1/-1/-1
Parmesan	3/4 oz.				X	+2
Provolone	3/4 oz.				X	+2
Sherbet	1/3 cup		X			-3

PROTEINS

SEAFOOD

Most Beneficial:	1 Portion =		Yin	Neutral	Yang	Yin/Yang Score
	Raw	Cooked				
Albacore (tuna)		3/4 oz.			X	+1
Bream		1 1/4 oz.			X	+1
Cod (imported)		1 1/4 oz.			X	+1
Grouper		1 1/4 oz.			X	+1
Hake		1 1/4 oz.			X	+1
Mahi Mahi		1 1/4 oz.			X	+1
Marlin		1 1/4 oz.			X	+1
Menpachi		1 1/4 oz.			X	+1
Milkfish		1 1/4 oz.			X	+1
Monkfish		1 1/4 oz.			X	+1
Mullet (imported)		1 1/4 oz.			X	+1
Ocean Perch		1 1/4 oz.			X	+1
Palani		1 1/4 oz.			X	+1
Pickerel		1 1/4 oz.			X	+1
Pollock		1 1/4 oz.			X	+1
Porgy		1 1/4 oz.			X	+1
Red Snapper		1 1/4 oz.			X	+1
Sailfish		1 1/4 oz.			X	+1
Salmon (Pacific)		1 1/4 oz.			X	+1
Sardine		3/4 oz.			X	+1

+ Organic Is Preferable   * Highly Glycemic   ⊕ Acid Neutralized   ■ Acceptable Fruits & Vegetables Only

Most Beneficial: (continued)	1 Portion =		Yin	Neutral	Yang	Yin/Yang Score
	Raw	Cooked				
Shad		1 1/4 oz.			X	+1
Snail		1 1/4 oz.			X	+1
Tarpon		1 1/4 oz.			X	+1
Trout (imported)		3/4 oz.			X	+1
Trout, Sea		3/4 oz.			X	+1
Wahoo		1 1/4 oz.			X	+1
Whiting		1 1/4 oz.			X	+1

Neutral:	1 Portion =		Yin	Neutral	Yang	Yin/Yang Score
	Raw	Cooked				
Abalone		1 1/4 oz.			X	+1
Angle Shark		1 1/4 oz.			X	+1
Belt Fish		1 1/4 oz.			X	+1
Lobster, spiney		3/4oz.			X	+1
Mackerel		1 1/4 oz.			X	+1
Mud Fish		1 1/4 oz.			X	+1
Mussels		1 1/4 oz.			X	+1
Orange Roughy		1 1/4 oz.			X	+1
Scallops		1 1/4 oz.			X	+1
Sea Urchin (roe)		3/4 oz.			X	+1
Silver Perch		1 1/4 oz.			X	+1
Smelt		1 1/4 oz.			X	+1
Snapper		1 1/4 oz.			X	+1
Sole		1 1/4 oz.			X	+1
Squid (calamari)		2 oz.			X	+1
Tilefish		1 1/4 oz.			X	+1
Tuna (canned)		3/4 oz.			X	+1
Tuna (steak)		3/4 oz.			X	+1
White Fish		1 1/4 oz.			X	+1
White Perch		1 1/4 oz.			X	+1

Least Beneficial:	1 Portion =		Yin	Neutral	Yang	Yin/Yang Score
	Raw	Cooked				
Anchovy		3/4oz.			X	+1
Arctic Char		1 1/4 oz.			X	+1
Barracuda		1 1/4 oz.			X	+1
Beluga		1 1/4 oz.			X	+1
Black Cod		1 1/4 oz.			X	+1
Bluefish		1 1/4 oz.			X	+1
Bluegill Bass		3/4oz.			X	+1
Bonito		1 1/4 oz.			X	+1
Buffalo Fish		1 1/4 oz.			X	+1
Butterfish (imported)		1 1/4 oz.			X	+1

+ Organic Is Preferable   * Highly Glycemic   ⊕ Acid Neutralized   ■ Acceptable Fruits & Vegetables Only

Least Beneficial:	1 Portion =		Yin	Neutral	Yang	Yin/Yang Score
	Raw	Cooked				
Carp		1 1/4 oz.			X	+1
Catfish		1 1/4 oz.			X	+1
Caviar	1 1/4 oz.				X	+1
Clam		1 1/4 oz.			X	+1
Cod (domestic)		1 1/4 oz.			X	+1
Coho Salmon (Great Lakes)		1 1/4 oz.			X	+1
Conch		1 1/4 oz.			X	+1
Crab		1 1/4 oz.			X	+1
Crayfish		1 1/4 oz.			X	+1
Croaker		1 1/4 oz.			X	+1
Eel		1 1/4 oz.			X	+1
Flounder		1 1/4 oz.			X	+1
Frog		1 1/4 oz.			X	+1
Gray sole		1 1/4 oz.			X	+1
Haddock		1 1/4 oz.			X	+1
Halibut		1 1/4 oz.			X	+1
Herring (fresh)		1 1/4 oz.			X	+1
Herring (pickled)		1 1/4 oz.			X	+1
Lobster		3/4 oz.			X	+1
Lox (smoked salmon)		1 1/4 oz.			X	+1
Mullet (domestic)		1 1/4 oz.			X	+1
Octopus		1 1/4 oz.			X	+1
Oysters		1 1/4 oz.			X	+1
Pike		1 1/4 oz.			X	+1
Ribbonfish		1 1/4 oz.			X	+1
Sand Dabs		1 1/4 oz.			X	+1
Sea Bass (domestic)		3/4 oz.			X	+1
Sea Bass (imported)		3/4 oz			X	+1
Sea Herring		1 1/4 oz.			X	+1
Shark, Thresher		1 1/4 oz.			X	+1
Shark		1 1/4 oz.			X	+1
Sheephead		1 1/4 oz.			X	+1
Shrimp		1 1/4 oz.			X	+1
Spot		1 1/4 oz.			X	+1
Striped Bass		3/4 oz.			X	+1
Sturgeon		1 1/4 oz.			X	+1
Swordfish		1 1/4 oz.			X	+1
Talapia		1 1/4 oz.			X	+1
Trout (domestic)		3/4 oz.			X	+1
Turtle		1 1/4 oz.			X	+1
Walleye		1 1/4 oz.			X	+1
Weakfish		1 1/4 oz.			X	+1
White Bass		3/4 oz.			X	+1
Yellow Perch		1 1/4 oz.			X	+1
Yellowtail		3/4 oz.			X	+1

+ Organic Is Preferable   * Highly Glycemic   ⊕ Acid Neutralized   ■ Acceptable Fruits & Vegetables Only

CARBOHYDRATES

BEANS AND LEGUMES

Most Beneficial:	1 Portion =		Yin	Neutral	Yang	Yin/Yang Score
	Raw	Cooked				
Green Peas		1/2 cup	X			-1
Navy Beans		1/4 cup	X			-1
Red Beans		1/2 cup	X			-1
Red Soy Beans		1/2 cup	X			-1
Domestic Lentils	1/2 cup	1/3 cup	X			-1
Green Lentils	1/2 cup	1/3 cup	X			-1

Neutral:	1 Portion =		Yin	Neutral	Yang	Yin/Yang Score
	Raw	Cooked				
Bean Sprouts	12 1/2 cups		X			-1
Broad Beans		2/3 cup	X			-1
Cannellini Beans		1/2 cup	X			-1
Copper Beans		1/2 cup	X			-1
Green Beans		1 1/4 cup	X			-1
Green Peas		1/2 cup	X			-1
Jicama Beans		2/3 cup	X			-1
Northern Beans		1/2 xup	X			-1
Pinto Beans +		1/2 cup	X			-1
Red Lentils	1/2 cup	1/3 cup	X			-1
String Beans		1 1/4 cups	X			-1
White Beans		1/2 cup	X			-1
Pea Pods		1/2 cup	X			-1
Snow Peas		1/2 cup	X			-1
Tamarind Beans		1/2 cup	X			-1

Least Beneficial:	1 Portion =		Yin	Neutral	Yang	Yin/Yang Score
	Raw	Cooked				
Aduke Beans		1/5 cup	X			-1
Adzuki Beans		1/5 cup	X			-1
Black Beans		1/2 cup	X			-1
Black-eyed Peas		1/2 cup	X			-1
Fava Beans		1/2 cup	X			-1
Garbanzo Beans		1/3 cup	X			-1
Kidney Beans		1/2 cup	X			-1
Lima Beans		1/3 cup	X			-1
Mung Beans		1/2 cup	X			-1
Snap Beans		1/2 cup	X			-1

+ Organic Is Preferable   * Highly Glycemic   ⊕ Acid Neutralized   ■ Acceptable Fruits & Vegetables Only

CARBOHYDRATES

BREADS

Most Beneficial:	1 Portion =		Yin	Neutral	Yang	Yin/Yang Score
	Raw	Cooked				
Essene Bread	2 1/2 oz.			X		0
Ezekiel Bread	1 slice			X		0
Soya Flour Bread	1 1/4 slice			X		0
Sprouted Wheat Bread	2/3 slice			X		0

Neutral:	1 Portion =		Yin	Neutral	Yang	Yin/Yang Score
	Raw	Cooked				
Brown Rice Bread	2/3 slice			X		0
Brown Rice Cakes	1 1/4 cakes			X		0
Durum Wheat	2/3 slice			X		0
Fin Crisp	2 1/2 pieces			X		0
Gluten-Free Bread	2/3 slice			X		0
Flat Bread	2 1/2 pieces			X		0
High Protein Bread	2/3 slice			X		0
Matzos, Wheat	1/2 board			X		0
Melba Toast	2/3 slice			X		0
Millet Bread *	2/3 slice			X		0
Multi-Grain Bread	2/3 slice			X		0
Oat Bran Muffins	1/2 muffin			X		0
Pumpernickel.	3/4 slice			X		0
Rye Bread (100%) +	1 slice			X		0
Spelt Bread	2/3 slice			X		0
Wasa Bread	1 1/4 slice			X		0

Least Beneficial:	1 Portion =		Yin	Neutral	Yang	Yin/Yang Score
	Raw	Cooked				
Bagels, Wheat	1/3 bagel			X		0
Bread Sticks (hard)	1 1/4 stick			X		0
Bread Sticks (soft)	2/3 stick			X		0
Cake	1/2 piece		X			-2
Corn Muffins	1/3			X		0
Doughnut	1/2		X			-2
English Muffins	1/3 muffin			X		0
Graham Crackers	1 3/4 crackers			X		0
Kamut	1 1/4 slice			X		0
Pancakes (wheat) 4"	2/3			X		0
Pita Bread	1/3 pocket			X		0
Rice Cakes, white	1 1/4			X		0
Rice Crackers	7 crackers			X		0
Rye Crisps	4 pieces			X		0

+ Organic Is Preferable   * Highly Glycemic   ⊕ Acid Neutralized   ■ Acceptable Fruits & Vegetables Only

Least Beneficial:	1 Portion =		Yin	Neutral	Yang	Yin/Yang Score
	Raw	Cooked				
Saltine Crackers	4			X		0
Vita, Rye	4 pieces			X		0
Waffle, Wheat	2/3			X		0
Wheat Bran Muffins	1/3			X		0
Whole Wheat Bread	2/3 slice			X		0

CARBOHYDRATES

FRUITS

Most Beneficial:	1 Portion =		Yin	Neutral	Yang	Yin/Yang Score
	Raw	Cooked				
Cherries +	10		X			-3
Figs (fresh) *	1 1/4 piece		X			-3
Gooseberries	1 1/4 cup		X			-3
Grapefruit	2/3		X			-3
Grapes, Black +	2/3 cup		X			-3
Grapes, Concord +	2/3 cup		X			-3
Grapes, Green +	2/3 cup		X			-3
Grapes, Red +	2/3 cup		X			-3
Kiwi	1 1/4		X			-3
Lemons	1 1/4		X			-3
Loganberries	1 cup		X			-3
Pineapple (cubed)	2/3 cup		X			-3
Plums, Dark +	1 1/4		X			-3
Plums, Green +	1 1/4		X			-3
Plums, Red +	1 1/4		X			-3

Neutral:	1 Portion=		Yin	Neutral	Yang	Yin/Yang Score
	Raw	Cooked				
Apples +	2/3		X			-3
Apricots +	3 3/4		X			-3
Blackberries +	1 cup		X			-3
Blueberries +	2/3 cup		X			-3
Boysenberries	2/3 cup		X			-3
Cranberries +	1 cup		X			-3
Currants, Black	1 cup		X			-3
Currants, Red	1 cup		X			-3
Currants, White	1 cup		X			-3
Dates +	2 1/2		X			-3
Elderberries	2/3 cup		X			-3
Feiojas (medium) +	2 1/2		X			-3
Figs (dried) *	1 1/4 piece		X			-3

+ Organic Is Preferable   * Highly Glycemic   ⊕ Acid Neutralized   ■ Acceptable Fruits & Vegetables Only

Neutral:	1 Portion=		Yin	Neutral	Yang	Yin/Yang Score
	Raw	Cooked				
Kumquat	3 3/4		X			-3
Limes	1 1/4		X			-3
Melon, Bitter	1/2		X			-3
Melons, Canang	3/4 cup		X			-3
Melon, Cantaloupe +	1/2		X			-3
Melons, Casaba +	3/4 cup		X			-3
Melons, Christmas	3/4 cup		X			-3
Melons, Crenshaw +	3/4 cup		X			-3
Melon, Honeydew +	1/2		X			-3
Melons, Musk	3/4 cup		X			-3
Melons, Spanish	3/4 cup		X			-3
Watermelons	1 cup		X			-3
Nectarines (medium)+	2/3		X			-3
Papaya	1 1/4 cup		X			-3
Peaches, (medium) +	1 1/4		X			-3
Peaches (canned) +	2/3 cup		X			-3
Pears (medium) +	2/3		X			-3
Pears (canned) +	2/3 cup		X			-3
Plantains	1 2/3 oz.		X			-3
Prunes +	2 1/2		X			-3
Raisins (organic only) + *	1 1/4 tbsp.		X			-3
Raspberries	1 1/4 cup		X			-3
Strawberries +	1 1/4 cup		X			-3
Tangerines	1 2/3		X			-3

Least Beneficial:	1 Portion =		Yin	Neutral	Yang	Yin/Yang Score
	Raw	Cooked				
Bananas	1/2		X			-3
Cactus	1/2 cup		X			-1
Coconut	6 2/3 oz.		X			-3
Guava	2/3 cup		X			-3
Mangoes	2/3 cup		X			-3
Oranges	3/4		X			-3
Persimmons (medium)+	1 1/4		X			-3
Pomegranates (medium) +	1/2		X			-3
Prickly Pears	1/2		X			-3
Raisins (commercial) *	1 1/4 tbsp.		X			-3
Rhubarb (diced)	3 cups		X			-3
Star Fruit (medium)	1 1/2		X			-3

+ Organic Is Preferable   * Highly Glycemic   ⊕ Acid Neutralized   ■ Acceptable Fruits & Vegetables Only

CARBOHYDRATES

GRAINS & CEREALS

Most Beneficial:	1 Portion =		Yin	Neutral	Yang	Yin/Yang Score
	Raw	Cooked				
Oat Bran	1/2 oz.			X		0
Oatmeal (slow cooking)	2/3 oz.	1/2 cup		X		0
Rice Bran	1/2 cup			X		0
Spelt (flakes)	2/3 oz.			X		0

Neutral:	1 Portion =		Yin	Neutral	Yang	Yin/Yang Score
	Raw	Cooked				
Amaranth	2/3 oz.			X		0
Barley	2/3 tbsp.			X		0
Cream of Brown Rice *		1/2 cup		X		0
Cream of Wheat	2/3 oz.	1/2 cup		X		0
Familia	2/3 oz.	1/2 cup		X		0
Farina	2/3 oz.	1/2 cup		X		0
Granola	2/3 oz.			X		0
Grape nuts	2/3 oz.			X		0
Grits	2/3 oz	1/2 cup		X		0
Millet *	2/3 oz.			X		0
Rice, Brown, Puffed *	1/2 oz.			X		0
Seven Grains *	3/4 oz.			X		0
Shredded Wheat *	2/3 oz.			X		0
Wheat Bran	2/3 oz.			X		0
Wheat Germ	1 1/4 oz.			X		0

Least Beneficial:	1 Portion =		Yin	Neutral	Yang	Yin/Yang Score
	Raw	Cooked				
Buckwheat	2/3 oz.			X		0
Cornflakes *	1/2 oz.			X		0
Cornmeal *	2/3 oz.			X		0
Cream of White Rice *	2/3 oz.	1/2 cup		X		0
Kamut (flakes)	2/3 oz.			X		0
Kasha	2/3 oz.			X		0
Rice, White Puffed *	1/2 oz.			X		0

+ Organic Is Preferable   * Highly Glycemic   ⊕ Acid Neutralized   ■ Acceptable Fruits & Vegetables Only

CARBOHYDRATES

JUICES

Most Beneficial:	1 Portion =		Yin	Neutral	Yang	Yin/Yang Score
	Raw	Cooked				
Black Cherry + *	1/2 cup		X			-3
Cabbage	1/4 cup		X			-2
Carrot *	1/2 cup		X			-1
Celery +	1 cup		X			-1
Cranberry *	1/3 cup		X			-3
Water w/ Lemon	N/A			X		<

Neutral:	1 Portion =		Yin	Neutral	Yang	Yin/Yang Score
	Raw	Cooked				
Apple + *	1/2 cup		X			-3
Apple Cider + *	1/2 cup		X			-3
Apricot	1/3 cup		X			-3
Boysenberry -	1/3 cup		X			-3
Cucumber	1 cup		X			-1
Grape *	1/3 cup		X			-3
Grapefruit + *	1/2 cup		X			-3
Orange ⊕	1/2 cup		X			-3
Papaya *	1/3 cup		X			-3
Pineapple *	1/3 cup		X			-3
Prune + *	1/4 cup		X			-3
Vegetable Juice* ■	1 1/4 cup		X			-2

Least Beneficial:	1 Portion =		Yin	Neutral	Yang	Yin/Yang Score
	Raw	Cooked				
Orange, (regular) *	1/2 cup		X			-3
Guava *	1/2 cup		X			-3
Pomegranate	1/2 cup		X			-3
Tomato	1 1/4 cups		X			-1
V-8 Juice	1 cup		X			-2

+ Organic Is Preferable   * Highly Glycemic   ⊕ Acid Neutralized   ■ Acceptable Fruits & Vegetables Only

CARBOHYDRATES

PASTAS AND FLOURS

Most Beneficial:	1 Portion =		Yin	Neutral	Yang	Yin/Yang Score
	Raw	Cooked				
Kamut Flour	2/3 oz.			X		0
Oat Flour	2/3oz.			X		0
Rice, Brown *		1/4 cup		X		0
Rice Flour, Brown *		2/3 oz.		X		0
Rye Flour	1 oz.			X		0
Rice, Wild *		1/4 cup		X		0
Soy Flour	2/3 oz.			X		0
Sprouted Wheat Flour	2 oz.			X		0

Neutral:	1 Portion =		Yin	Neutral	Yang	Yin/Yang Score
	Raw	Cooked				
Couscous	2/3 oz.			X		0
Barley Flour	3/4 oz.			X		0
Bulgur Wheat Flour	2/3 oz.			X		0
Durum Wheat Flour	2/3 oz.			X		0
Gluten Flour	1 1/4 oz.			X		0
Quinoa Flour	2/3 oz.			X		0
Rice, Basmati *		1/4 cup		X		0
Semolina Pasta		1/3 cup		X		0
Spinach Pasta		1/3 cup		X		0
Spelt Flour	3/4 oz.			X		0
Spelt Noodles		1/3 cup		X		0
Whole Wheat Flour *	1 1/4 oz.			X		0

Least Beneficial:	1 Portion =		Yin	Neutral	Yang	Yin/Yang Score
	Raw	Cooked				
Artichoke Pasta (Jerusalem)		1/3 cup		X		0
Buckwheat Flour	2/3 oz.			X		0
Graham Flour *	2/3 oz.			X		-2
Kasha	2/3 oz			X		0
White Flour *	1 oz.			X		0
Rice, White *		1/4 cup		X		0
Soba Noodles		1/3 cup		X		0
White Rice Flour *	2/3 oz.			X		0

+ Organic Is Preferable   * Highly Glycemic   ⊕ Acid Neutralized   ■ Acceptable Fruits & Vegetables Only

CARBOHYDRATES

VEGETABLES

Most Beneficial:	1 Portion =		Yin	Neutral	Yang	Yin/Yang Score
	Raw	Cooked				
Barley Greens	N/A	N/A	X			-1
Beet Greens	7cups		X			-2
Beets		2/3 cups	X			-1
Blue Green Algae	N/A	N/A	X			-2
Broccoli +	2 1/2 cups		X			-1
Cauliflower		2 1/2 cups	X			-1
Celery +	2 1/2 cups		X			-2
Chicory Greens	1 1/4 cups		X			-2
Collard Greens +	1 1/4 cups		X			-2
Cucumber (whole) +	1 1/4		X			-1
Cucumber (sliced)	1 1/4 cups		X			-1
Dandelion Greens +	2 cups		X			-2
Dill Weed +	18 3/4 cups		X			-1
Garlic	12 1/2 cloves		X			-1
Kale +	1 1/4 cup		X			-2
Kelp	5 oz.		X			-2
Mustard Greens	4 cups	3 cups	X			-2
Parsley +	6 1/4 cups		X			-2
Parsnips *	1/2 cup		X			-1
Potatoes, Sweet	1/2 cup		X			-1
Pumpkins (mashed)		1 cup	X			-1
Red Algae	N/A	N/A	X			-1
Red Chard		1 1/4 cup	X			-2
Peppers, Serrano+	3/4 cup		X			-1
Sprouts, Alfalfa	13 3/4 cups		X			-1
Yams (medium)		2/3	X			-1

Neutral:	1 Portion =		Yin	Neutral	Yang	Yin/Yang Score
	Raw	Cooked				
Arugula	14 cups		X			-1
Asparagus		15 spears	X			-1
Bamboo Shoots	4 3/4 cups	1 1/4 cup	X			-2
Bok Choy +		3 3/4 cups	X			-1
Carrots *	4 1/2 oz.	2/3 cup	X			-1
Chicory Roots	1 1/4 cup		X			-2
Choy Sum +	2 1/2 cups		X			-1
Cilantro (coriander)		3 cups	X			-1
Daikon Radish	3 cups		X			-1
Endive	9 cups		X			-2
Escarole +	6 1/3 cups		X			-2
Hominy (grits)		1/2 cup	X			-1

+ Organic Is Preferable   * Highly Glycemic   ⊕ Acid Neutralized   ■ Acceptable Fruits & Vegetables Only

Neutral:	1 Portion =		Yin	Neutral	Yang	Yin/Yang Score
	Raw	Cooked				
Horseradish (pods)	2 1/2 cups		X			-1
Kohlrabi +	1 1/4 cup		X			-2
Leeks +	1 1/4 cup		X			-1
Lettuce Bibb (5" head)	2 1/2 head		X			-2
Lettuce, Boston (5" head)	2 1/2 head		X			-2
Lettuce, Iceberg (6" head) +	1 1/4 head		X			-2
Lettuce, Mesclun +	1 1/4 head		X			-2
Lettuce, Romaine +	9 cups		X			-2
Mushrooms, Domestic	3 3/4 cups	1 cup	X			-1
Mushrooms, Enoki	3 3/4 cups	1 cup	X			-1
Mushrooms, Portobello	3 3/4 cups	1 cup	X			-1
Mushrooms, Oyster	3 3/4 cups	1 cup	X			-1
Mushrooms, Tree	3 3/4 cups	1 cup	X			-1
Okra +		1 1/3 cups	X			-1
Onions, Red	1 1/4 cups		X			-1
Onions, Spanish	1 1/4 cups		X			-1
Onions, Yellow	1 1/4 cups		X			-1
Onions, Green (scallions)	1 1/4 cups	1/2 cup	X			-1
Peppers, Chili	3/4 cup		X			-1
Peppers, Poblano +	3 3/4 oz.		X			-1
Potatoes, Red +	1/2 cup		X			-1
Purslane +	8 cups	1 2/3 cups	X			-2
Radicchio.	8 3/4 oz		X			-1
Rapini	2 1/2 cups		X			-1
Rutabaga +	3/4 cup	1/2 cup	X			-1
Sauerkraut	1 1/4 cups		X			-2
Seaweed		4 1/2 oz.	X			-2
Shallots	2 1/2 oz.		X			-1
Spinach +	5 cups		X			-2
Spirulina	2 oz.		X			-2
Sprouts, Brussels	1 1/2 cups		X			-1
Squash, Acorn +		2/3 cup	X			-1
Squash, Butternut +		2/3 cup	X			-1
Squash, Yellow +		1 1/2 cups	X			-1
Swiss Chard +		1 1/4 cup	X			-2
Tomatillo	1 1/4 cups		X			-1
Tomato +	2 1/2		X			-1
Turnip Greens +		2 cups	X			-2
Turnips (mashed) +		1 1/4 cup	X			-1
Water Chestnuts	1/2 cup		X			-1
Watercress	28 cups		X			-1
Zucchini		2 cups	X			-1

+ Organic Is Preferable   * Highly Glycemic   ⊕ Acid Neutralized   ■ Acceptable Fruits & Vegetables Only

Least Beneficial:	1 Portion =		Yin	Neutral	Yang	Yin/Yang Score
	Raw	Cooked				
Artichokes, Domestic+	Medium		X			-1
Artichokes, Jerusalem +	Medium		X			-1
Chinese Cabbage	3 3/4 cups	1 2/3 cups	X			-2
Cabbage, Red	3 3/4 cups	1 2/3 cups	X			-2
Cabbage, White	3 3/4 cups	1 2/3 cups	X			-2
Corn, White		1/3 cup	X			-1
Corn, Yellow		1/3 cup	X			-1
Eggplant +	2 cups		X			-1
Fiddlehead Ferns	12 1/2 cups		X			-2
Hummus	1/3 cup		X			-1
Mushrooms, Abalone	3 3/4 cups	1 cup	X			-1
Mushrooms, Shitake	3 3/4 cups	1 cup	X			-1
Peppers, Green	2 3/4 cups		X			-1
Peppers, Jalapeno	3 3/4 oz.		X			-1
Peppers, Red	2 3/4 cups		X			-1
Peppers, Yellow	2 3/4 cups		X			-1
Potatoes, White	1/2 cup		X			-1
Radishes +	5 cups		X			-2
Sprouts, Mung	3 3/4 cups		X			-1
Sprouts, Radish	3 3/4 cups		X			-1
Taro	1/2 cup	1/4 cup	X			-1

FATS

NUTS AND SEEDS

Most Beneficial:	1 Portion =		Yin	Neutral	Yang	Yin/Yang Score
	Raw	Cooked				
Chestnuts	2/3 oz.		X			-2
Hemp Seeds	2/3 tsp.		X			-1
Walnuts	1/3 tsp.		X			-2

Neutral:	1 Portion =		Yin	Neutral	Yang	Yin/Yang Score
	Raw	Cooked				
Almond Butter	1/3 tsp.		X			-2
Almond Nuts	3/4 tsp.		X			-2
Brazil Nuts	1/3 nut		X			-2
Cashews	1 1/2 nuts		X			-2
Flax Seeds	2/3 tsp.		X			-1
Hickory Nuts	1/3 tsp.		X			-2
Lychee Nuts (1C)	2 1/2 oz		X			-3
Macadamia Nuts	1 small		X			-2

+ Organic Is Preferable   * Highly Glycemic   ⊕ Acid Neutralized   ■ Acceptable Fruits & Vegetables Only

Neutral:	1 Portion =		Yin	Neutral	Yang	Yin/Yang Score
	Raw	Cooked				
Pignolia (pine nuts)	3/4 tsp.		X			-1
Pistachios	1/2 tsp.		X			-2
Radish Seeds	3/4 tsp.		X			-1
Watermelon Seeds	2/3 tsp.		X			-1

Least Beneficial:	1 Portion =		Yin	Neutral	Yang	Yin/Yang Score
	Raw	Cooked				
Cashew Butter	2/3 tsp.		X			-2
Filbert Nuts	1/3 tsp.		X			-2
Peanuts	5 nuts		X			-2
Peanut Butter	1/3 tsp.		X			-2
Poppy Seeds	1 tsp.		X			-1
Pumpkin Seeds	2/3 tsp.		X			-1
Sesame Seeds	3/4 tsp.		X			-1
Sesame Butter (tahini)	1/4 tbsp.		X			-1
Sunflower Butter	2/3 tsp.		X			-1
Sunflower Seeds	2/3 tsp.		X			-1

FATS

OILS AND OTHER FATS

Most Beneficial:	1 Portion =		Yin	Neutral	Yang	Yin/Yang Score
	Raw	Cooked				
Hemp Seed Oil	1/4 tsp.		X			-2
Olive Oil	1/4 tsp.		X			-2
Salmon Oil	1/4 tsp.		X			-2

Neutral:	1 Portion =		Yin	Neutral	Yang	Yin/Yang Score
	Raw	Cooked				
Black Currant Oil	1/4 tsp.		X			-2
Borage Oil	1/4 tsp.		X			-2
Canola Oil	1/4 tsp.		X			-2
Cod Liver Oil	1/4 tsp.		X			-2
Flax Seed Oil	1/4 tsp.		X			-2
Olives (green)	2 1/2		X			-2
Olives (Greek)	2 1/2		X			-2
Olives (Spanish)	2 1/2		X			-2

+ Organic Is Preferable   * Highly Glycemic   ⊕ Acid Neutralized   ■ Acceptable Fruits & Vegetables Only

Least Beneficial:	1 Portion =		Yin	Neutral	Yang	Yin/Yang Score
	Raw	Cooked				
Avocado	3/4 tbsp		X			-2
Butter	1/4 tsp.		X			-1
Coconut Oil	1/4 tsp.		X			-2
Corn Oil	1/4 tsp.		X			-2
Cottonseed Oil	1/4 tsp.		X			-2
Cream (half & half)	3/4 tbsp.		X			-1
Cream Cheese	3/4 tsp.		X			-1
Ghee	1/4 tsp.		X			-1
Hydrogenated Oil	1/4 tsp.		X			-2
Lard	1/4 tsp.		X			-2
Olives (black)	2 1/2		X			-2
Palm Oil	1/4 tsp.		X			-2
Peanut Oil	1/4 tsp.		X			-2
Safflower Oil	1/4 tsp.		X			-2
Sesame Seed Oil	1/4 tsp.		X			-2
Shortening, Vegetable	1/4 tsp.		X			-2
Sour Cream	1/3 tbsp.		X			-1
Sour Cream, Light	3/4 tbsp.		X			-1
Sunflower Oil	1/4 tsp.		X			-2
Tahini	1/3 tsp		X			-2

MISCELLANEOUS

BEVERAGES

Most Beneficial:	1 Portion =		Yin	Neutral	Yang	Yin/Yang Score
	Raw	Cooked				
Coffee, Decaf	N/A				X	<
Green Tea	N/A			X		<
Green Tea (decaffeinated)	N/A			X		<
Wine, Red	5 oz.		X			-3
Purified Water	N/A			X		<

Neutral:	1 Portion =		Yin	Neutral	Yang	Yin/Yang Score
	Raw	Cooked				
Beer (light)	5 oz.			X		0
Beer (regular)	5 oz.			X		0
Coffee, Regular	N/A				X	<
Cappuccino, Decaf	N/A				X	<
Champagne	5 oz.		X			-3
Seltzer Water	N/A			X		<
Sports Drink (natural)	1/2 cup		X			-3
Sparkling Water	N/A					<
Wine, White	5 oz.		X			-3

+ Organic Is Preferable   * Highly Glycemic   ⊕ Acid Neutralized   ■ Acceptable Fruits & Vegetables Only

Least Beneficial:	1 Portion =		Yin	Neutral	Yang	Yin/Yang Score
	Raw	Cooked				
Cappuccino (regular)	N/A				X	<
Club Soda	N/A				X	<
Latte'	1 cup		X			-2
Liquors, Distilled	1 1/4 oz.			X		0
Soda, Diet	3 oz.		X			-3
Sodas (other)	3 oz.		X			-3
Sports Drink (artificial)	1/2 cup		X			-3
Tea, Black, Decaffeinated	N/A				X	<
Tea, Black (regular)	N/A				X	<

MISCELLANEOUS

CONDIMENTS

Most Beneficial:	1 Portion =		Yin	Neutral	Yang	Yin/Yang Score
	Raw	Cooked				
"Bragg's" Amino Acids	N/A				X	<

Neutral:	1 Portion =		Yin	Neutral	Yang	Yin/Yang Score
	Raw	Cooked				
Apple Butter	2 1/2 tsp.		X			-3
Fruit Jams ■ *	2 1/2 tsp.		X			-3
Fruit Jellies ■ *	2 1/2 tsp.		X			-3
Mayonnaise (dairy) (1F)	3/4 tsp.		X			-1
Mayonnaise (vegetarian) (1F)	3/4 tsp		X			-1
Mustard	N/A				X	<
Salad Dressing	N/A		X			<
Soy Sauce	N/A					<
Tamarind	N/A					<

Least Beneficial:	1 Portion =		Yin	Neutral	Yang	Yin/Yang Score
	Raw	Cooked				
Candy Bar *	1/3 Bar		X			-3
Barbecue Sauce *	2 1/2 tbsp.		X			-3
Cocktail Sauce *	2 1/2 tbsp.		X			-3
Dill Pickles	11 1/2		X			-1
Ketchup *	2 1/2 tbsp.		X			-1
Kosher Pickles	11 1/2		X			-1
Maple Syrup *	2 1/2 tsp.		X			-3
Plum Sauce *	1 1/2 tbsp.		X			-3
Relish *	5 tsp.		X			-2
Sour Pickles	11 1/2		X			-1
Sweet Pickles *	2		X			-1
Teriyaki Sauce	1 1/4 tbsp.		X			-3
Worcestershire Sauce	N/A		X			<

+ Organic Is Preferable   * Highly Glycemic   ⊕ Acid Neutralized   ■ Acceptable Fruits & Vegetables Only

MISCELLANEOUS

SPICES

Most Beneficial:	1 Portion =		Yin	Neutral	Yang	Yin/Yang Score
	Raw	Cooked				
Curry	N/A				X	<
Garlic	N/A				X	<
Ginger	N/A				X	<
Horseradish	N/A				X	<
Miso	N/A			X		<
Parsley	N/A				X	<
Sage	N/A				X	<

Neutral:	1 Portion =		Yin	Neutral	Yang	Yin/Yang Score
	Raw	Cooked				
Agar	N/A		X			<
Arrowroot Starch	1 1/4 tsp.		X			-1
Basil	N/A		X			<
Bay Leaf	N/A		X			<
Bergamot	N/A		X			<
Black Strap Molasses	2/3 tsp.		X			-3
Brewer's Yeast	N/A		X			<
Brown Rice Syrup	3 3/4 tsp.		X			-3
Caraway Seeds	N/A		X			<
Cardamom	N/A				X	<
Carob	1 1/4 oz.		X			-3
Chervil	N/A				X	<
Chives	N/A		X			<
Chocolate *	1 1/4 oz.		X			-3
Cinnamon	N/A				X	<
Cloves	N/A				X	<
Coriander	N/A				X	<
Cream of Tartar	N/A		X			<
Cumin	N/A				X	<
Dill	N/A		X			<
Dulse	N/A		X			<
Fennel	N/A		X			<
Kelp	N/A		X			<
Marjoram	N/A				X	<
Mint	N/A		X			<
Mustard	N/A				X	<
Nutmeg	N/A				X	<
Paprika	N/A				X	<
Pepper, Cayenne	N/A				X	<

+ Organic Is Preferable   * Highly Glycemic   ⊕ Acid Neutralized   ■ Acceptable Fruits & Vegetables Only

Neutral: (continued)	1 Portion =		Yin	Neutral	Yang	Yin/Yang Score
	Raw	**Cooked**				
Peppermint	N/A		X			<
Pimento	N/A				X	<
Rice Syrup *	3 3/4 tsp.		X			-3
Rosemary	N/A		X			<
Saffron	N/A			X		<
Salt	N/A		X			<
Savory	N/A				X	<
Spearmint	N/A		X			<
Stevia	N/A		X			<
Sucanat	2 1/2 tsp.		X			-3
Tarragon	N/A		X			<
Thyme	N/A			X		<
Turmeric (Tuber)	N/A		X			<
Turmeric (rhizone)	N/A				X	<
Vanilla	N/A		X			<
Wintergreen	N/A		X			<

Least Beneficial:	1 Portion =		Yin	Neutral	Yang	Yin/Yang Score
	Raw	**Cooked**				
Allspice	N/A				X	<
Almond Extract	N/A		X			<
Barley Malt *	3 3/4 tsp.		X			-2
Anise	N/A		X			<
Capers	N/A				X	<
Cornstarch *	1 1/4 tsp.		X			-1
Corn Syrup *	2 1/2 tsp.		X			-3
Gelatin	N/A			X		<
Honey *	2/3 tbsp.		X			-3
Pancake Syrup *	2 1/2 tsp.		X			-3
Pepper, Ground Black	N/A				X	<
Pepper, Red	N/A				X	<
Pepper, White	N/A				X	<
Peppercorn	N/A				X	<
Sugar, Brown *	2 1/2 tsp.		X			-3
Sugar, Confectionery *	1 1/4 tbsp.		X			-3
Sugar, White *	2 1/2 tsp.		X			-3
Tapioca	N/A		X			<
Vinegar, Apple Cider	N/A				X	<
Vinegar, Balsamic	N/A				X	<
Vinegar, Red Wine	N/A				X	<
Vinegar, White	N/A				X	<

+ Organic Is Preferable   * Highly Glycemic   ⊕ Acid Neutralized   ■ Acceptable Fruits & Vegetables Only

MISCELLANEOUS

TEAS and/or HERBS

Most Beneficial:	1 Portion =		Yin	Neutral	Yang	Yin/Yang Score
	Raw	Cooked				
Alfalfa	N/A			X		<
Burdock	N/A		X			<
Chamomile	N/A			X		<
Deglycyrrhizinated Licorice	N/A			X		<
Echinacea	N/A		X			<
Ginger	N/A				X	<
Ginseng, American	N/A		X			<
Green Tea	N/A			X		<
Hawthorne	N/A				X	<
Rosehip	N/A			X		<
St. John's Wort	N/A		X			<
Strawberry Leaf	N/A		X			<

Neutral:	1 Portion =		Yin	Neutral	Yang	Yin/Yang Score
	Raw	Cooked				
Cayenne	N/A				X	<
Chickweed	N/A		X			<
Dandelion	N/A		X			<
Dong Quai	N/A				X	<
Elder	N/A				X	<
Goldenseal	N/A		X			<
Horehound	N/A		X			<
Licorice Root	N/A			X		<
Milk Thistle	N/A		X			<
Mulberry	N/A		X			<
Parsley	N/A				X	<
Peppermint	N/A		X			<
Raspberry Leaf	N/A			X		<
Sage	N/A				X	<
Sarsaparilla	N/A			X		<
Slippery Elm	N/A			X		<
Spearmint	N/A		X			<
Thyme	N/A			X		<
Valerian	N/A				X	<
Vervain	N/A		X			<
White Birch	N/A		X			<
White Oak Bark	N/A		X			<
Yarrow	N/A			X		<
Yellowdock	N/A		X			<

+ Organic Is Preferable   * Highly Glycemic   ⊕ Acid Neutralized   ■ Acceptable Fruits & Vegetables Only

Least Beneficial:	1 Portion =		Yin	Neutral	Yang	Yin/Yang Score
	Raw	Cooked				
Aloe Vera	N/A		X			<
Catnip	N/A		X			<
Cascara sagrada	N/A		X			<
Colt's Foot	N/A		X			<
Corn silk	N/A		X			<
Fenugreek	N/A				X	<
Gentian	N/A		X			<
Ginseng, Siberian	N/A				X	<
Hops	N/A			X		<
Linden	N/A		X			<
Mullein	N/A		X			<
Red Clover	N/A		X			<
Rhubarb	N/A			X		<
Senna	N/A		X			<
Shepherd's Purse	N/A			X		<
Skullcap	N/A		X			<

+ Organic Is Preferable　　* Highly Glycemic　　⊕ Acid Neutralized　　■ Acceptable Fruits & Vegetables Only

Blood Type AB Recipes

INSTRUCTIONS FOR USE:

The following pages provide five recipes specific for this particular blood type: breakfast, lunch, dinner, dessert and one snack. Each recipe takes into account the correct foods for this specific blood type, the proper ratio of proteins, carbohydrates and fats (Macrobalance™ Portions) and an acceptable Yin Yang energetic score. In compliance with the 4th piece of the New Millennium Diet puzzle, it is recommended that organic foods be used as much as possible. Each meal (breakfast, lunch and dinner) offers the user three, four, five or six Portion amounts.

The recipe consists of two parts. Part one, a shopping list that provides the correct amount of ingredients necessary according to the 4 different Portion sizes. The shopping list also shows the amount in which the various Portion sizes contribute towards the total Yin Yang score.

Part two is the Preparation section and provides simple to follow instructions in preparing the recipe.

It is very simple to use the recipes, it is done in three easy steps:
1. **Determine the correct amount of Portions needed (Chapter 7).**
2. **In the recipe, refer to the Grocery List, select the correct Portion column and obtain the ingredients in the amounts listed.**
3. **Prepare the recipe according to the Preparation instructions in Part two.**

It's that simple to enjoy a complete Macrobalanced™ meal. Bon appetit!

Breakfast: Italian Scramble
Blood Type AB

Shopping List

Ingredients:	Portion Size			
	3	4	5	6
	Amount of Ingredient			
Proteins:				
Whole Egg(s)	2 eggs	3 eggs	4 eggs	5 eggs
Mozzarella Cheese	1 oz	1 oz	1 1/4 oz	1 1/3 oz
Carbohydrates:				
Broccoli (chopped	3/4 cup	1 1/5 cup	1 1/2 cup	1 2/3 cup
Zucchini (chopped)	1 1/3 cup	1 2/3 cup	2 1/4 cup	2 2/3 cup
Onions (chopped)	3/5 cup	4/5 cup	1 cup	1 1/5 cup
Apples (sliced)	1/2 cup	3/4 cup	1 cup	1 1/4 cup
Fats and Oils:				
Olive Oil	1 tsp	1 1/3 tsp	1 2/3 tsp	2 tsp
Butter	2/3 tsp	1 tsp	1 1/8 tsp	1 1/3 tsp
Spices:				
Sea Salt	pinch	pinch	pinch	pinch
Oregano (dried)	pinch	pinch	pinch	pinch
Turmeric	pinch	pinch	pinch	pinch
Basil (dried)	pinch	pinch	pinch	pinch
Marjoram	pinch	pinch	pinch	pinch
Yin (-)/Yang(+) (excess)	-2	-3	-4	-3

Preparation:

In a saute pan, cook the vegetables in the olive oil until soft. Once cooked, add the five spices, eggs, butter and grated mozzarella to the vegetable mixture. Scramble until eggs have solidified. Cook the apple slices in a separate pan lightly sprayed with olive oil. Serve immediately while warm.

Lunch: Thai Red Curry Fish
Blood Type AB

Shopping List

Ingredients:	Portion Size			
	3	4	5	6
	Amount of Ingredient			
Proteins:				
Fish	2 3/4 oz	3 2/3 oz	4 1/2 oz	5 1/2 oz
Yogurt (low fat)	3 3/4 oz	5 oz	6 1/4 oz	7 1/2 oz
Carbohydrates:				
Snow Peas	1 cup	1 1/2 cup	1 2/3 cup	1 2/3 cup
Onions (chopped	1 cup	1 1/3 cup	1 2/3 cup	1 2/3 cup
Peppers (green, chopped)	5/8 cup	1 cup	1 cup	1 1/4 cup
Arrowroot Powder*	2 tsp	2 1/4 tsp	3 1/4 tsp	3 3/4 tsp
Fats and Oils:				
Olive Oil	1/4 tsp	1/3 tsp	1/2 tsp	1/2 5sp
Butter	2 tsp	2 2/3 tsp	3 1/3 tsp	4 tsp
Spices:				
Garlic	1 1/2 clove	2 clove	2 1/2 clove	3 clove
Vinegar	1 1/2 tsp	2 tsp	2 1/2 tsp	3 tsp
Turmeric	3/8 tsp	3/4 tsp	1 tsp	1 1/4 tsp
Red Curry Powder	1/2 tsp	1/2 tsp	5/8 tsp	3/4 tsp
Yin (-)/Yang(+) (excess)	-1	-1	-4	-4

Preparation:

In a saucepan add the oil and butter and cook all the vegetables until tender. Add spices, fish, yogurt and approximately 1 cup water and continue to cook until fish is poached and tender. Add arrowroot powder* and continue to cook 5 to 7 minutes longer. Serve hot.

** Arrowroot Powder should be well-mixed with 3 to 5 teaspoons of water before adding to other ingredients.

Snack: Tomato Mozzarella
Blood Type AB

Shopping List

	Portion Size		
	1	2	3
Ingredients:	**Amount of Ingredient**		
Proteins:			
Mozzarella Cheese	3/4 oz	1 1/2 oz	2 1/4 oz
Carbohydrates:			
Tomato	1 1/3 tom.	2 2/3 tom.	4 tom.
Fats and Oils:			
Flax Seeds	2/3 tsp	1 1/3 tsp	2 tsp
Spices:			
Sea Salt	pinch	pinch	pinch
Yin (-)/Yang(+) (excess)	-1	-1	1

Preparation:
Slice tomatoes and mozzarella. Sprinkle flax seeds on top. Lightly season with sea salt.

Dinner: Mandarin Orange Beef
Blood Type AB

Shopping List

Ingredients:	Portion Size			
	3	4	5	6
	Amount of Ingredient			
Proteins:				
Beef (cubed)	3 oz	4 oz	5 oz	6 oz
Carbohydrates:				
Bell Peppers (Green)	5/6 cup	1 1/8 cup	1 1/2 cup	1 2/3 cup
Celery (chopped)	3 cups	4 cups	5 cups	6 cups
Arrowroot Powder *	1 1/2 tsp	2 tsp	2 1/2 tsp	2 1/2 tsp
Mandarin Oranges	1/4 cup	1/3 cup	1/2 cup	1/2 cup
Fats and Oils:				
Flax seeds	2 1/4 tsp	3 tsp	3 3/4 tsp	4 tsp
Butter	2/3 tsp	1 tsp	1 tsp	1 tsp
Spices:				
Red wine	3/4 tsp	1 tsp	1 1/4 tsp	1 1/2 tsp
Beef Stock	3/8 cup	1/2 cup	5/8 cup	3/4 cup
Soy Suace	3/4 tbsp	1 tbsp	1 1/4 tsbsp	1 1/2 tbsp
Ginger	3/4 tsp	1 tsp	1 1/4 tsp	1 1/2 tsp
Yin (-)/Yang(+) (excess)	-2	-2	-3	-3

Preparation:

In a pan, sauté the beef in butter until browned and remove from pan. Add celery to pan and cook until tender, stirring frequently. In a separate saucepan cook the mandarin oranges, bell peppers, beef stock, red wine, soy sauce, ginger, flax seeds and arrowroot powder until thickened. Add beef-celery mixture to sauce and simmer for 7 to 9 minutes. Serve warm.

* Arrowroot Powder should be well-mixed with 3 to 5 teaspoons of water before adding to the other ingredients.

Dessert: Frozen Cherry Cream
Blood Type AB

Shopping List

Ingredients:	Portion Size		
	1	2	3
	Amount of Ingredient		
Proteins:			
Egg Whites	1/4 egg	1/2 eggs	3/4 eggs
Unflavored Gelatin	1/4 env.	1/2 env.	3/4 env.
Soy Yogurt*	1/4 cup	1/2 cup	3/4 cup
Carbohydrates:			
Cherries	1/2 cup	1 cup	1 1/2 cup
Arrowroot Powder*	1 1/3 tsp	2 tsp	2 1/4 tsp
Fats and Oils:			
Almonds (finely chopped)	3/4 tsp	1 1/2 tsp	2 1/4 tsp
Spices:			
Ginger	1/6 tsp	1/5 tsp	1/3 tsp
Orange Extract	1/4 tsp	1/3 tsp	1/3 tsp
Yin (-)/Yang(+) (excess)	-1	-3	-4

Preparation:

In a saucepan, place the cherries, gelatin, arrowroot powder*, ginger, orange extract and yogurt. Heat until warmed thoroughly. Set aside until cool. Place the egg whites in a mixing bowl and whip until firm. Add the egg mixture and almonds to the cooled fruit mixture. Stir the mixture, place into freezer until frozen. Serve cold.

* Arrowroot Powder should be well-mixed with 3 to 5 teaspoons of cold water before adding to the other ingredients.

CHAPTER 12

Candida: The Hidden Epidemic

C andidiasis is a condition that involves the widespread overgrowth of yeast in the intestines, bloodstream, vaginal tract, and other bodily tissues. To date, the medical establishment has refused to acknowledge the existence of this widespread disease; however, literally millions of people throughout the United States and the world are suffering with this condition on a daily basis. It's estimated that one-third of the entire population of the United States has a mild-to-moderate degree of systemic candida, and most medical doctors fail to accurately diagnose and treat the symptoms that are associated with this condition.

The New Millennium Diet offers a systematic approach to improving one's health and well-being by removing dangerous food lectins, balancing the macronutrient percentages, creating a harmony between Yin and Yang, and reducing the chemicals and toxins found in our daily food choices. For 80% of the population, this approach will rapidly eliminate fatigue, improve digestion, enhance muscle tone, increase fat loss, reverse the physical signs of aging, and improve mental clarity; however, somewhere between 10–20% of the population, additional advice must be considered because of a tiny parasitic organism known as *Candida albicans*.

Candida has been called the missing diagnosis because it truly presents a wide variety of symptoms that can be associated with numerous different medical conditions, such as dry skin and itching, toenail or fingernail fungus, bad breath, colitis, PMS, water retention, acne, thyroid disturbances, chemical sensitivities, allergies, hair loss, low sex drive, rapid premature aging, and numerous other conditions that medical doctors attempt to classify in order to treat the condition. Many times their efforts are fruitless and even damaging to the patient because of their general lack of knowledge regarding this condition.

Most medical doctors believe that only patients with severe immunological weakness, such as those that are undergoing cancer chemotherapy or suffering with AIDS, can be susceptible to overgrowth of this particular yeast species. However, every person on the planet has candida overgrowth to one degree or another, depending upon the strength of their immune system. The onslaught of numerous immune-destroying chemicals in our environment, excessive prescription of antibiotics, birth control pills, Western medications, as well as emotional and psychological stressors, is placing a huge burden on many people's immune systems, allowing the candida bug to grow.

The New Millennium Diet, as I have stated, can significantly reduce many symptoms that could be associated with ill health or even candidiasis; however, greater clarification when the symptoms do not fully resolve is required for complete clearance of this problem. I believe it is important for me to mention this condition because very few people even realize that their health is being compromised by this tiny fungus.

Candida is one of many organisms that is constantly fighting to be the dominant organism inhabiting the human body. Most of this fight occurs between the good beneficial bacteria and the budding yeast organisms. Initially, this infestation occurs in the intestinal tract and then will move from the intestinal tract to the liver via the portal circulation and then on to other internal organs. You may ask how candida can actually move from the intestinal tract into the bloodstream. Leaky gut syndrome is the answer.

Intestinal Permability/Leaky Gut Syndrome

Leaky gut syndrome is a condition in which small tears or holes are made in the intestinal tract by a disturbed intestinal environment. This disturbance in the intestinal floor comes about because of the overgrowth of candida and other foreign or parasitic agents. These organisms eat at the intestinal lining and create toxins that damage the delicate structures which make up the lining of the intestinal tract. After years of constant wear and tear on this delicate system, tiny holes begin to appear. These holes allow undigested food particles, foreign, bacterial or yeast organisms, chemical toxins and other colon by-products into the bloodstream. Once in the bloodstream, these dangerous factors can migrate or circulate to the liver, which is supposed to remove them. However, if the liver comes under too much stress, the rain barrel effect predominates. The rain barrel effect occurs when the barrel is full of rain; excess water then pours over the sides of the barrel. In a similar sense, the liver allows the same type of scenario to occur. If the liver becomes too congested with these yeasts, fungal, or bacterial toxins or if too many undigested food particles circulate to this organ and clog its various detoxification pathways, then those toxins that come after this clogging will then be allowed to pass through the portal circulation into the general bloodstream. This can lead to symptoms of fatigue, diffuse allergic reactions, atopic dermatitis, brain fog, and a general body poisoning, which are commonly seen as the symptoms of the yeast syndrome.

Many times if candida is able to pass through the intestinal wall, it can then become a permanent resident of other internal organs. It also can very effectively attach to the intestinal wall and can parasitize the digestive tract lining for years. I believe that this organism will affect or does affect every person on the planet over the course of their lifetime to one degree or another. Nail fungus, which literally effects millions of people in the later years of life develop, is one of the symptoms of this condition. So, if you have nail fungus, realize that the problem is not just localized to the nail bed but is a systemic condition, and nail fungus is just one of its many symptoms.

Yeast Toxins

Yeast is all over, found in almost every part of our life. Yeast is found on the exposed surfaces of furniture in our homes. It's found in our cars, in the dirt, in the air that we breathe and in the water we drink. You can't avoid it. You just need to control it — and you can!

It is estimated that there are approximately 250 different species of candida, many of which can parasitize the body and lead to the condition known as candidiasis. Mycotoxins are the toxins produced by the yeast, which can be very harmful. Many patients suffering with chronic fatigue, immune dysfunction syndrome or environmental illness syndrome (chemical toxicity syndrome) can become very sensitized to mold or yeast in their home or work environments. In Chapter 5, I discussed the importance of having healthy living and working environments. These principles have been widely applied in Europe, and particularly in Germany, where they are known as "bau-biologie," German for building biology. These concepts are now being introduced in the United States. Refer to Chapter 5 for more information on this important issue.

Researchers have identified some 80–90 different yeast toxins which can contribute to a general poisoning of the body. Among other things, these toxins can seriously weaken the immune system. As mentioned earlier, they impact the liver's ability to remove toxic and foreign substances. If the immune system and the liver become overwhelmed, the spillover of circulating toxins and antigens causes a derangement in the body's innate intelligence. Exaggerated immune responses take place, a hypersensitivity that leads to food and environmental allergies and chemical sensitivities. People who had no such problems before begin to report sensitivity to pollens, chemicals, odors, perfumes, and to a wide variety of foods, including foods that are even allowed on the New Millennium Diet.

Fatigue, one of the major complaints associated with this condition, is caused by candida toxins. This toxic waste can also be produced from what is called "the die-off" reaction. This occurs when large numbers of candida are killed by the body or through medicinal agents used in treatment. The fatigue results from disturbances created by the toxins at the cellular level. Among other things, they interfere with normal energy generation. They skew the sodium and potassium pump, the mechanism that controls fluid balance within the cells. The result is poor bio-electrical conductivity in the system. Disturbances spread from cells to tissues, to organs, and finally involves the entire body, causing malaise and fatigue. In the treatment of candidiasis, I have found that acupuncture offers significant help to reestablish disturbed electrical communication between the cells in the body. I use this method, along with diet and natural antifungal medicines, to strengthen the body's ability to overcome candidiasis.

In addition to the toxins, yeast cell activity also produces acetaldehyde. This substance is converted by the liver into ethanol, which is an alcohol. This is probably why patients report feeling drunk, while having poor memory and what they refer to as brain fog, an inability to think clearly. I hear many complaints of anxiety, depression, irritability, disorientation, dizziness, and panic attacks, all of which may be connected to the body's inability to deal with acetaldehyde. This substance also interferes with proper cell enzymatic and nutrient function, leading to extreme fatigue, poor stamina, and low sex drive. Acetaldehyde rapidly consumes antioxidants, compounds produced in the body that act like policemen, protecting the system against damage from stress and chemical reactions. You do not want any reduction in your body's antioxidant level. When antioxidant power is lost, aging and disease acceleration takes place.

If you suffer with candidiasis, please follow the anti-candida recommendations in this section for at least the first six weeks, or longer if necessary, before starting on the full New Millennium program. How much longer depends on the severity of your condition. This initial six-week phase is designed to cleanse your body, that is, reduce the level of yeast infestation sufficiently enough so that you can then move into our regular New Millennium Diet.

Immune System Breakdown

In our bodies, candida organisms work around the clock. No breaks. No holidays. Once there is a weakening of the body's normal defenses, the yeasts proliferate and bombard the immune system continually, leading to a gradual but systematic degradation of our health. If this goes on for an extended period, the immune system becomes dysfunctional and ineffective, setting the stage for more serious conditions. Candida does the original dirty work, so to speak. You experience symptoms. Then more problems and breakdowns follow: to the intestinal absorptive processes, to hormonal function, to the nervous system. All can become affected in a cascade of dysfunction, which can be extremely challenging to treat.

The immune system can break down from emotional issues and trauma such as a divorce or death of a loved one. When this occurs, the opportunistic candida finds the defenses weakened, and many times the infection spreads or worsens in the body. Typically, three to six months later, people begin to notice loss of memory, extreme gas and bloating, generalized fatigue, chemical sensitivities, and constant headaches. Often, people do not relate these developments with the specific emotional or mental upset that occurred months before, which perhaps now at this later date are no longer being experienced. As I tell patients, however, a real recovery has not taken place. The cells remember. They have recorded the trauma, the upset, the disturbance. This imprint on the cellular level, or even perhaps on an energetic level, needs to be erased. Many times simply riding out the initial emotional or mental trauma is only half the battle. Patients often say they have been to therapy and successfully resolved their grief or other emotions, yet they continue to experience physical imbalance and symptoms. After treating thousands of patients over the years I have learned that the body remembers every experience, be it positive or negative, and if it is negative, the imprint must be eliminated from the cellular machinery in order to restore optimum functioning.

Antibiotics

We know that a course of antibiotics can destroy the good bacteria in the intestinal tract and create a ripe environment for the proliferation of yeast. Candida patients often say they have never taken antibiotics or drugs. Yet they fail to recognize that most of our meat, chicken, and fish contain chemicals, hormones, steroids, or antibiotics. These are substances that do not belong in our food supply. But drugs and antibiotics are widely used in commercial livestock methods, and fish are becoming increasingly tainted with agrochemicals because of toxic runoff into our streams, lakes, and oceans. So, even if you haven't seen a doctor in the last 30 years and have never received an antibiotic, your body may still be accumulating antibiotics, as well as other disruptive chemicals, leading to the proliferation of candida.

As you can see, there are many, many symptoms associated with candidiasis. I've just mentioned a few. Not every person develops all of the symptoms associated with candidiasis. Most chronic patients develop somewhere between 10–50% of the symptoms I am listing below. Let's go ahead and break them up into subcomponents so that they can be more fully understood.

Table 12-1 Symptoms of Candidiasis

Digestive Symptoms:

Abdominal Distension	Heartburn
Abdominal Pains or Cramps	Hemorrhoids
Anal Itching	Hunger
Bloating	Indigestion
Constipation	Mouth Ulcers
Diarrhea	Mucus in the Stools
Digestive Symptoms	Parasites
Food Allergies	Piles
Gas	Poor Nutrient Absorption
Green or Malodorous Stools	Tongue Coated Yellow
Halitosis (Bad Breath)	

Brain Symptoms:

Anger	Headaches
Anxiety	Insomnia
Brain Fog	Irritability
Decreased Attention Span	Mood Swings
Dizziness	Poor Concentration
Drowsiness	Poor Coordination
Frustration	Reduced Memory

Hormonal Symptoms:

PMS	Menstrual Irregularities
Impotence	Peri-Menopausal Symptoms
Infertility	Vaginal Yeast
Low Sex Drive	Vaginitis

Additional Symptoms:

Anxiety Attacks	Nasal Congestion
Blurred Vision	Nervousness
Brain Fog	Night Sweats
Burning Eyes	Nightmares
Cold Hands and Feet	Palpitations
Earaches	Postnasal Drip
Eczema	Prostatitis
Excess Mucus	Psoriasis
Fatigue	Recurrent Colds
Frequency or Burning of Urination	Syncope, or Fainting
Hay Fever	Tightness in the Chest
Hives	Tremors
Itching or Scaling Skin Lesions	Unrefreshed Sleep
Lethargy	Water Retention
Muscle and Joint Pains	Weakness

Weak Digestion and Poor Assimilation of Nutrients

Candida interferes with the normal digestion of food and assimilation of nutrients. As a result, most patients rarely get adequate nourishment to fuel good body function. After some time, the many systems working with such precision in the body start to fail. Energy production falls. Fatigue develops. Low blood sugar and hypoglycemia occur. The liver cannot store sufficient levels of glycogen, leading to insufficient supplies of glucose for the muscles and brain.

You may wake up in the morning and feel as heavy as lead, the result of excessive toxic buildup in the muscle tissue or a lack of glycogen to the muscles. Either way, there's a fuel shortage in your body and your muscles can't operate in a normal fashion.

The interference with proper nutrient assimilation has a particularly strong impact on the satiety centers of the brain. Normally, when you have eaten enough food, your body passes the satiety message on to your brain. The brain, in its wisdom, then signals the stomach and intestinal tract, which gives you the sensation of fullness. Candida patients, however, are constantly hungry. The body actually calls for more food because it is not receiving the necessary nutrients to function. Candida infestation can lead to many gastrointestinal disturbances, such as nausea, heartburn, gas, bloating, pain, and inflammation. These are signs and symptoms that the candida organism is on the loose in your intestinal tract and is interfering with the spleen, pancreas, liver, stomach, and intestinal linings.

Consuming large amounts of fiber, either in the form of psyllium husks or bentonite clay, helps to purge and cleanse the colon of this organism and its by-products so that good bacteria can then be reintroduced. It is estimated that 50% of the population is digesting less than half of the food they eat. I believe the main reason for this poor digestive performance is linked to intestinal candidiasis. If you are unable to derive adequate nourishment and energy from your food, your body will suffer in many ways. Candidiasis, as widespread as it is, is a major, yet unrecognized, underlying cause of much of the chronic illness that afflicts society today.

Role of Spleen and Pancreas

In Chinese medicine, disturbances in the spleen-pancreas organ system are taken quite seriously. The spleen is important in the *transportation and transformation* of food and is vital for a properly functioning digestive tract. The smooth running of the spleen is undermined by excessive consumption of sweets, too much worry, toxins from the environmental, and genetic weaknesses. If the spleen isn't performing as it should you can experience bloating, diarrhea alternating with constipation, weight loss, heartburn, indigestion, bad breath, and mucus in the stools. Spleen weakness also happens to be one of the major factors in candida infections. Part of my approach to eliminate candida includes acupuncture. I use it to strengthen the spleen and pancreas.

Avoiding raw or cold foods is another way to help the spleen. Such foods can actually "shock" the spleen. Many people are being advised to consume large amounts of raw vegetables and fruit. This practice should be minimized if you suffer from digestive disturbances. Even if the foods contain high levels of enzymes, the coldness of the food depletes the energy of the spleen. How can you tell if your spleen is weak? Look in the mirror and stick out your tongue. If it appears pale in the center with a slight yellowish coating on top, that's an indicator that your spleen is weak. The food-related symptoms you are experiencing are likely the spleen's message to you that it doesn't have the strength to perform its job well. After you start the anti-candida program outlined later in this chapter, monitor the color of your tongue. If the yellow coating becomes lighter, that means you are making progress. You can use your tongue as a gauge of your improving health.

Most candida patients are aware that humidity plays a role in aggravating their condition. The reason is that humidity influences the functioning of the spleen. Increased dampness causes increased dampness in the organ itself, and weakens its energy. Climatic factors also affect other organs. For example, the kidney is affected by cold, the heart by heat, the lungs by dryness and the liver by wind.

Just as there is an association between climate and the various organs, there is also a relationship with taste and organ function. Spleen energy is influenced by the element of sweetness. This is one reason why patients with candida often crave sweet foods. Such craving is a warning sign that the spleen is seriously damaged and in need of repair. As generally harmful as regular sugar is to the body, aspartame, a common ingredient in many substitute sweeteners, is about 200 times sweeter than sugar and can have a much more detrimental effect on the spleen. Stay away from sweeteners with aspartame. The calories don't matter as much as the intensity of the taste. The sweeter the taste, the more damage is inflicted on the spleen.

Neurological and Emotional Complaints

Neurological and emotional symptoms are common. They include mood swings, irritability, anger, brain fog, confusion, and dizziness. Neuromuscular disturbances include muscle spasms, radiculopathies, and neuropathies. Problems mimicking multiple sclerosis can develop, such as poor muscular coordination or numbness in the extremities. Physicians rarely link these symptoms to candida. One of my patients who was diagnosed previously with multiple sclerosis had complete reversal of all symptoms after I placed her on the anti-candida diet. Even the white patches appearing on her brain, as seen on her Magnetic Resonance Imaging (MRI) test and considered typical signs of MS, resolved after three months on the program.

The acetaldehyde that is produced as a waste product of yeast organisms is converted to alcohol in the liver. And alcohol, as we know, is deadly. Among other things, it can damage nerve tissue. Alcohol is thus said to be neurotoxic. Candida-induced neurotoxicity can affect nerve function throughout the entire nervous system of the body. Such damage can create emotional disturbances. I see that often when patients break down in front of me and cry as they describe their condition. This is not a mental disorder — "it's all in your head" — as many physicians suggest. It is real, one of many manifestations of a systemic infestation.

Patients who feel drunk and are having brain fog are being literally poisoned by alcohol. In the liquor industry, yeast is actually used to make alcohol. And, if given the opportunity, it will create a harmful alcohol tide within our body. Imagine being intoxicated 24 hours a day. Many candida patients have to reread a paragraph four or five times before they're able to understand or retain the information. The alcohol and other toxins affecting the nerves leads to real mental impairment and emotional instability. In severe cases, candidiasis can trigger paranoia, schizophrenia, or other types of neurotic or psychotic behavior. I'm not saying these conditions are solely caused by candidiasis, but it can certainly accelerate such tendencies or aggravate an existing condition. Tragically, the processed and refined food served to most institutionalized patients in the United States encourages the growth of candida. The chemical imbalances that occur in the body as a result of this overgrowth further deteriorates the relatively poor status of these patients.

Impact on Sex Organs

As many women can unfortunately attest to, candida causes many gynecological problems. They include vaginal yeast infections, menstrual irregularities, infertility, endometriosis, and chronic urinary tract infections. Men are not spared. They can experience impotence and/or prostatitis.

If you are using over-the-counter antifungal creams to treat female problems associated with candida, be very careful. Attempting to continually suppress episodes can weaken the immune system and actually lead to a further spread of the organism in the body. The creams will begin to have less and less effect. If you're experiencing this dilemma, it means that the immune system is weakening. Your body is unable to provide the complementary support needed for any antibiotic or antifungal agent to work.

Candidiasis and Children

Children are very susceptible to candida. Many infants are exposed to yeast during birth because the organism is almost always present to some degree in the vaginal canal. The yeast is thus transferred to infant during the birthing process. Pregnant women should supplement their diets with good bacteria such as acidophilus that can help reduce the presence of candida in the intestines, vaginal tract, and bloodstream. Diaper rash, tonsillitis, ear infections, constipation, diarrhea, a white coating in the mouth, and poor development could be related to childhood candidiasis.

Emotional issues, such as hyperactivity, aggressiveness, irrational behavior, learning disabilities, and poor attention span may also have a yeast connection. One infant, diagnosed with cystic fibrosis as well as severe childhood eczema and asthma, had a significant improvement of all symptoms after the parents instituted an anti-candida program. Herbs and nutrients for immune system support were incorporated, but the biggest role in the boy's recovery was played by diet. Hyperactivity and attention deficit disorders have also responded to diet. A typical diet high in sugar and processed carbohydrates encourages yeast growth, and is one of the main factors behind many behavioral disorders. Reducing the consumption of sugar usually improves attention and decreases restlessness.

Antifungal and Antibiotic resistance

Full recovery requires more than just a super antibiotic or antifungal agent. It requires an intact, functioning immune system. The right medication may kill up to 99% of the marauding microbes, but such agents always leave resistant organisms remaining that will multiply if the immune system does not eradicate them. This is one reason why I do *not* recommend that patients use Diflucan, Sporanox, Nystatin, Monistat, or any other antifungal medications. In the long run, they lead to fungal resistance. They may work initially; however, in time they will fail to work, and you are then left with a tougher, more entrenched fungal infection than when you started. It is better to treat candidiasis with diet, and natural medications that build up your own immune system's ability to fight the disease.

Summary

The spread of candida in the body is caused by four major factors:

1. A weakened or impaired immune system originating from the use of drugs such as birth control pills, antibiotics, or steroids, as well as toxins in our food and environment.

2. A genetic susceptibility or weakness in certain organs that can interfere with the body's natural resistance.

3. Emotional or mental trauma, such as death, divorce, heartbreaks, or job stress, all of which can interfere with the natural function of organs and the flow of energy. This can lead to disease in general, including candida.

4. The typical Western diet of processed and refined foods, in addition to all the toxins, antibiotics and hormones that is found in food, failing to adequately nourish the body. It contains, however, the precise raw materials required by yeast organisms to thrive.

The Challenge of Diagnosis

Over 80% of the physicians in the United States fail to acknowledge, let alone diagnose, patients with candida infections. Many patients actually diagnose themselves and seek out holistic physicians who can confirm or refute the diagnosis through a number of blood, stool, and other tests. From a clinical perspective, the overall picture of complaints and symptoms is probably the most solid way to determine candidiasis.

When I was in medical school, my professors always emphasized the importance of making a diagnosis based on the history of the patient and then using laboratory tests for confirmation. The tables have been turned in our present-day medical system. Many diagnoses are based solely on laboratory results and history used only for confirmation. I'm sorry to say that this is not the way that medicine should be practiced. Many blood tests, including the standard CBC and chemistry profiles, only provide limited information. If abnormalities are picked up, they usually relate only to severe disturbance. Subtle changes, indicative of early illness or irregularities in a person's energy flow, are often missed.

Many of my patients have had extensive laboratory and diagnostic analyses performed that have come back showing all is well and normal. The patients, however, are describing a whole host of symptoms that are totally destroying any semblance of a normal life.

Many doctors, confronted by differing evidence, often choose to believe the lab results. They will suggest that the patient has a psychosomatic disorder, or that there is a stress problem, and then refer you to a psychiatrist for further evaluation. Many candida sufferers know this scenario all too well. Many have been told, "it's all in your head."

Physicians also discount the effectiveness of the various candida blood tests that are available today. They believe these tests do not provide an accurate assessment of candida infection. This has some basis in truth. There are a number of diagnostic tests available to us, but none really provide a fully accurate answer. We all harbor varying amounts of yeast in our body, and determining whether or not there are enough of these organisms equivalent to an infection can be difficult. Normal levels of candida in the blood have been determined in the general population; however, some people may be more sensitive to lesser than normal levels than others, thereby making any findings difficult to interpret.

Some lab tests may be of benefit. They include the following:

- **Urine D-arabinitol Tests**. This analysis monitors a carbohydrate metabolite produced by the candida organism, and is a general toxic substance in the body. You may have difficulty finding a lab that actually performs the test, but it is worthwhile to ask your physician.

- **Blood Tests.** Blood tests check for elevated antibody activity, specifically IgG, IgM, and IgA antibodies. The IgM level is regarded as the most significant marker of acute or active candida infection. IgG is associated with past or chronic infection. An elevated IgG antibody result indicates you may have had a past infection but are not currently affected. IgA relates to mucosal involvement. If the IgA antibody is elevated, then you may have a current infestation of the mucous membrane linings within your body, such as the intestines, vagina, or the throat or mouth.

- **Stool Examinations**. You must, however, specifically request this. Many stool tests do not include candida reporting. Gram staining of yeast along with direct microscopic examination of the stool is one of the best diagnostic approaches for assessing candidiasis. If a stool examination is performed, it is important to do a digestive analysis of the stool as well. Many laboratories, such as the Great Smokies Laboratories in Asheville, North Carolina (phone: (828) 285-2223), provide both forms of testing. Stool collection should take place at home at a time when symptoms are heightened, and preferably before treatment is instituted.

- **Microscopic Blood Analysis.** Analysis of the blood using a high-powered microscope. Often a candida overgrowth in the blood can be seen, and its intensity measured, directly through visual means. Repeated microscopic examination of the blood can track the progress of the treatment.

- **Chinese Medicine.** Traditional practitioners of Chinese medicine are able to perform pulse diagnosis as well as other effective diagnostic techniques.

- **Skin Sampling**. A small amount of skin is scraped from affected areas. These samples can be submitted for laboratory culturing and evaluation.

- **Blood Alcohol Content**. This is an infrequently used test that can provide valuable information. If the blood alcohol level is greater than 0, this may be a sign of a candida overgrowth. Remember the connection between yeast and the production in the body of acetaldehyde, a candida by-product that is converted into alcohol. You need to avoid any alcoholic beverages or medications containing alcohol prior to this test.

- The candida questionnaire (see below). Scoring high on this test can be a strong indication that you are infected. In such case, you should see a competent health professional for treatment.

The Candida Questionnaire

The candida questionnaire is a useful way to identify the presence of a yeast overgrowth. I've included it here in the chapter for anyone who may suspect they have candidiasis. It can also serve as an indicator of susceptibility for developing an infection. The questionnaire covers aspects of medical history that can provide important candida clues. The questionnaire is not intended for childhood cases. A special questionnaire for youngsters can be obtained through the New Millennium Medicine Institute at (800) 969-9914.

Candida Questionnaire Instructions:

SECTION A: HISTORY

For every "Yes" response, circle the numeric score that is associated with the question. Total all points for that section.

SECTION B: PREDOMINANT SYMPTOMS

If the response is "none," score 0 for the question.
If the response is "mild," score 4 for the question.
If the response is "moderate," score 7.
If the response is "severe," score 10.
Total all points for this section.

SECTION C: ADDITIONAL SYMPTOMS

If the response is "none," score 0 for the question.
If the response is "mild," score 2 for the question.
If the response is "moderate," score 3.
If the response is "severe," score 4.
Total all points for this section.

The Candida Questionnaire

Section A: History	Score
Have you used broad-spectrum antibiotics in the past?	8
Have you ever taken antibiotics for acne for a month or longer, such as Tetracycline?	40
Have you ever taken any type of broad-spectrum antibiotic for a two-month or longer period of time or have you taken any short courses of antibiotics one month or less, four or more times in a one-year period?	40
Have you ever suffered with prostatitis, vaginitis or any other types of reproductive organ disturbances?	30
Have you ever been pregnant?	
a) Three or more times?	7
b) Two times or less?	4
Have you ever used prednisone or other types of corticosteroids, such as Decadron?	
a) One week or longer?	12
b) One week or less?	5
Do you use birth control pills or have you used birth control pills in the past?	
a) One year or longer?	12
b) One year or less?	7
Do you react to perfumes, chemicals, household fumes, insecticides?	
a) To a mild degree?	4
b) To a moderate or severe degree?	18
Do your symptoms react with damp or humid weather or do you find that you have some sort of sensitivity to molds or moldy places?	18
Do you have an increased craving for sugar or breads or any type of refined carbohydrate?	20
Do you crave alcoholic beverages or any type of refined beverages?	10
Are you affected by tobacco smoke or any other type of chemical odors?	10

Do you suffer from ringworm, jock itch, athlete's foot or do you have any type of chronic infection of your toenails, fingernails or skin?	
a) Mild to moderate?	12
b) Severe to chronic?	18
Total Score for Section A:	

Section B: Predominant Symptoms **INSTRUCTIONS:**	**Score**
For each symptom that you are affected with, enter the appropriate numbered score in the column at the right. If the symptom is MILD, score ....4 If the symptom is MODERATE, score.....7 If the symptom is SEVERE, score.........10	
Lethargy or Fatigue	
Sensation of Being Drained	
Memory Disturbances	
Confusion	
Disturbed Decision Making	
Neurological Complaints such as Numbness, Tingling or Paresthesias	
Sleep Disturbance	
Muscle Aches or Pains	
Paralysis or Muscular Weakness	
Digestive Disturbances or Pains	
Joint Disturbances, including Pain or Swelling	
Constipation	
Diarrhea	
Gas, Bloating or Indigestion	
Vaginal Disturbances, including Itching, Discharges or Burning	
Inflammation of the Prostate, also known as Prostatitis	
Impotence	
Infertility or Endometriosis	
Lowered Sex Drive	
Menstrual Disturbances	
Premenstrual Complaints	
Body Coldness, espcially the Extremities	
Emotional Liability, including Crying Jags or Anger	
Hypoglycemia or Poor Food Tolerance	
Total Score for Section B:	

Section C: Additional Symptoms	**Score**
If a symptom occurs enter the appropriate score in the column at the right. If the symptom is MILD, score ....2 If the symptom is MODERATE, score ....3 If the symptom is SEVERE, score..........4	
Tremors or Bodily Shaking	
Drowsiness	
Coordination Difficulties	
Concentration Disturbances	
Mood Swings	
Headaches	
Equilibrium Disturbances	
Easy Bruising	
Ear Congestion	
Body Rashes or Hives	
Eczema, Psoriasis or Atopic Dermatitis	
Food Allergies or Intolerances	
Disturbed Stool Formation including Mucus or Blood in the Stool	
Rectal Itching	
Frequent Thirst or Dry Mouth or Throat	
Oral Ulcers	
Halitosis (Bad Breath)	
Body, Foot or Hair Odors	
Postnasal Drip or Nasal Congestion	
Nose Itching	
Frequent or Recurrent Sore Throat	
Hoarseness of the Voice or Laryngitis	
Frequent or Recurrent Bronchitis or Persistent Cough	
Asthma or Wheezing	
Chest Pains or Tightness	
Frequency of Urination or Incontinence or Urgency	
Burning on Urination	
Tearing or Burning of the Eyes	
Floaters or Poor Vision	
Conjunctival Infections or Recurrent Infections of the Ears or Eyes	
Ear or Head Pains	
Total Score for Section A:	
Total Score for Section B:	
Total Score for Section C:	

Grand Total of Three Sections, A, B, C:

The Grand Total score provides an indication of the level of candida involvement in your body. **Scores between 0–60 for women, and 0–40 for men, are indicative of no candida involvement.**

Scores totaling from 61 to 120 for women, and 41 to 90 for men, indicate mild candida infection. If your score falls in this range, you should follow the anti-candida diet program of this chapter for a minimum of 6 weeks before moving to the standard New Millennium Diet.

Results between 121 and 185 for women and 91 to 145 for men suggest a moderate to intermediate candida infection. The anti-candida diet combined with the "natural candida fighters"(special supplements described later in the chapter) should be followed for a minimum of 3 months before transitioning to the standard New Millennium diet.

A result higher than 185 for women and more than 145 for men indicates a severe candida infection. The anti-candida diet, "natural candida fighters," and guidance from a qualified holistic practitioner are necessary for long-term eradication of the infection. Treatment for severe infections usually lasts 6 months to 2 years.

Treatment

There are many treatments used to battle this unrelenting disease. A wide variety of natural and chemical approaches are available. I do not recommend conventional anti-fungal drugs such as Diflucan or Sporanox, unless you are suffering also with AIDS or other serious immune-compromising conditions. The use of such drugs often leads to the proliferation of more virulent and resistant strains of candida. A natural approach can be very effective and provide lasting benefits in up to 95% of cases.

The first and most important step is the anti-candida protocol of the New Millennium Diet. This program should be followed from six weeks to one year, depending on the severity of the condition, as indicated by your questionnaire scores above.

If you undergo treatment by a knowledgeable holistic practitioner, the length of treatment depends on how long you have suffered with candida. You can make a rough estimate by multiplying the number of years you have had candida by 1 to 2 months. If, for instance, you have had the disease for 10 years, it may require upwards of 10–20 months for a full recovery. In general, you can expect to begin feeling better within 2 to 6 weeks after beginning the program. A complete cure requires more time. So be patient, and be diligent in following the program. Candida often invades the organs and deep tissues of the body. A determined and prolonged fight may be necessary to completely detoxify and heal the system.

The Anti-Candida Program of the New Millennium Diet

This powerful anti-candida program is superimposed on your specific blood type New Millennium Diet. What is required is that you temporarily place the foods listed below in the least beneficial food category, and try to avoid them. Do this regardless of whether they are considered neutral or even most beneficial in your specific blood type plan. Keep them in this to-be-avoided category until such time as your candida problem is under control.

Table 12-2 Candida Diet Protocol—Food Avoidance List

- All breads, including yeast-free, wheat and rye breads, rice crackers and cakes and any other grain-based food because of the high glycemic nature of grains.
- All dairy products, including milk, cheeses, cottage cheese, yogurts, buttermilks except for goat's milk. Only if goat's milk is acceptable for your individual blood type.
- All mushrooms. Mushrooms are a fungus and can introduce more fungal elements into your bloodstream. Prevents healing.
- All fermented foods, such as miso, soy sauce, tamari, vinegar, tempeh, any foods that contain these products. Condiments such as mustard, pickles, mayonnaise, ketchup, olives, barbecue sauce, chile sauce, salad dressings, tomato sauces.
- All alcoholic beverages, especially the fermented ones, such as beer, wine and champagne.
- Any and all processed foods, most of which are already eliminated from the New Millennium Diet.
- All malted products.
- All salad dressings, including natural salad dressings. These products contain vinegar and other fermented ingredients.
- All teas except for the most beneficial ones as specified in your specific food listing.
- All coffee products, including decaffeinated coffee. These products put additional stress on the liver. A good alternative is a herbal-based coffee substitute.
- All products that are made with refined sugars, molasses, honey, corn syrup, maple syrup or any type of artificial sweetener such as Nutrasweet. These products feed yeast, parasites and bacteria.
- All ice creams, cookies, pastries, cakes or any other types of dessert.
- Any foods containing additives or preservatives.
- Most carbonated beverages except for naturally carbonated products.
- All smoked meat products.
- Peanuts and pistachios. These nuts contain aflatoxin, a highly toxic mold by-product that interferes with the immune system.
- All tap water unless filtered with a carbon or reverse osmosis system.
- All white or refined flour products, including pastas.

- All pork-containing products including sausages, ham, pork chops. Pork is not good for any blood type. It contains an antigen that can ruin your immune system and destroy your internal organs.

This special anti-candida program is designed to eradicate the yeast in your body. It eliminates all yeast-containing foods from your diet. You will want to avoid many breads and cereals, crackers, bagels, beer, and wine, as well as fermented foods like soy sauce and vinegar. You will also find highly processed, refined foods on the list. Avoid them, too.

As restrictive as this program seems, it is critical that you follow it for full recovery. I recommend you go even one step further, and eat only organically grown meat, vegetables and fruit, in order to minimize the chemicals and additives in your diet. If you are unable to obtain organic quality vegetables and fruits, then be sure to use an organic food rinse to remove the surface pesticides and sprays. The less exposure you have to chemicals in the food supply, the better your health will be.

Natural Candida Fighters

Along with the special diet, there are a number of supplements that I routinely recommend to patients with candida. They either kill yeast directly or strengthen your body's ability to rid itself of yeast. The supplement program is the second major element in your battle against candida.

Beneficial Bacteria

Yeast colonies often flourish after the destruction of the normal beneficial bacteria population in the body. Drugs, as we have seen, can cause this. The rise of yeast in this vacuum is also associated with an overgrowth of many other harmful bacterial and parasitic species. The names of the other opportunistic organisms that can rush in and create problem include a veritable who's-who of the "microbial Mafia" — *Staphylococcus aureus, beta-hemolytic streptococcus, Diplococcus pneumoniae, Klebsielleae, Proteus vulgaris, Pseudomonas aeruginosa,* salmonella, *E. coli, Bacillus subtilis, Mycobacterium avium, Aspergillus niger, H. pylori, Giardia lamblia, Entamoeba histolytica, Cryptosporidium,* and *Blastocystis hominis.* A replacement of the good bacterial strains — such as *Lactobacillus acidophilus* — is a critical measure. You want to reestablish their dominant role again in the body. As they reestablish themselves, they go to war against the bad guys. When selecting probiotics, many companies make available two forms, one derived from a dairy source or the other from a nondairy source. I recommend the nondairy source. Also, be sure to purchase products containing fructo-oligosaccharides (FOS), indigestible sugars that feed the good bacteria but are not absorbed into the bloodstream. You don't have to be concerned about excess sugar. FOS does not add any calories to your diet.

Caprylic Acid

Sodium caprylate, also known as caprylic acid, is an effective candida killer. It is widely available in health food stores, usually in capsule form. I suggest 4 capsules of 300 milligram strength each, taken with meals 3 times a day during the first 1 to 3 months of treatment. Subsequently, and after the infection has been significantly reduced, the dosage can be lowered to 2 capsules 3 times a day. Continue in this fashion for another 2 to 4 months to prevent recurrence. Caprylic acid is taken with meals so as to minimize the possibility of an upset or burning stomach, which might occur on an empty stomach. The presence of food in the system helps prevent such a reaction. The product is otherwise safe, nontoxic, and is very effective in killing candida in all parts of the body, especially the intestinal tract.

Biotin

Biotin is a member of the B complex vitamin family. It helps to stop the development of yeast tentacles, also known as tendrils, which the organisms use to bind to the gut wall. Once they affix to the wall, they commence the breakdown of the intestinal tissue. This eventually leads to the "leaky gut syndrome." By interrupting this process, you are interfering with the life cycle of candida. Usually a daily dose of 5 milligrams (5,000 micrograms) of biotin will do the job. Biotin can be taken once a day with meals and has no known negative side effects. It does have a side benefit: hair growth. Some candida patients mention an accompanying problem of hair loss, so you may experience some positive hair developments as a result of taking the vitamin.

Pau d'Arco

Pau d'Arco is a South American herb containing two natural compounds — lapachol and xyloidine — that directly kill candida. The herb, prepared from bark, is most effective in the form of a tea. It is used not only for candida but also against snake bites, and in general as a powerful agent to enhance the immune system and eliminate parasites from the intestinal tract. Pau d'Arco has a relatively low toxicity level. It could cause loose stools, but this would be beneficial for someone with constipation, which sometimes occurs during the initial stages of candida detoxification. I will be talking about detoxification in a moment. In most cases, one to three cups of tea per day is beneficial, depending upon the severity of your infection. Pau d'Arco is also available in health food stores.

Citrus Seed Extracts

Citrus Seed Extracts are combinations of grapefruit, lemon and tangerine seed extracts. They have a very powerful killing effect on candida. Typically, 2–10 drops taken 3 times a day is recommended. It may cause some upset, but is most effective on an empty stomach. The drops should be added to 4–8 ounces of water and taken 15–30 minutes prior to eating or at bedtime. If your stomach is too sensitive, take the drops with food.

Kolorex

Kolorex is a remedy created out of two unique candida-busting herbal compounds. The first is polygodial, a substance found in the leaves of *Pseudowintera colorata*, a native New Zealand plant traditionally used by the Maoris for many digestive disorders. Research at New Zealand's Canterbury University, beginning in 1982, isolated the medicinally active polygodial, which inhibits candida yeast cells by damaging their cellular membranes, thus causing a lethal "leaking" of internal fluids.

Kolorex also contains aniseed, a spice used in South America. The active ingredients in aniseed is anethole, shown to have antifungal activity. When polygodial and aniseed are combined, there is a huge increase in antifungal potency. The combination, in fact, is 32 times more potent against candida than polygodial alone.

Kolorex is powerful natural medicine, more effective in my opinion than the drug amphotericin B, commonly used to treat systemic yeast infections. Amphotericin B is extremely toxic, however, and is generally indicated only for extreme cases.

Colloidal Silver

This natural antibiotic and antifungal remedy is made up of tiny, microscopic particles of silver in solution. The particles are electrically charged and suspended in the solution, and when taken orally, circulate through the blood, organs, and lymphatic system to destroy invading organisms. Colloidal silver kills candida, bacteria and viruses on contact. Some studies suggest that more than 650 different organisms may be susceptible to its killing effect. There are no known resistant strains to colloidal silver. This is a powerful natural remedy and belongs in every anti-candida program. In the past, before refrigeration, people used to put silver dollars into their milk to keep it fresh at room temperature and prevent spoilage from bacterial activity.

Colloidal silver is regarded as a safe substance by the FDA. No known side effects have been observed, according to a University of Toronto study. The product is safe for children and animals. It has hundreds of uses, including disinfecting drinking water and swimming pools. Or it can be applied to the body on skin, eye or mucosal surfaces. Colloidal silver products are available in health food stores, but tend to be expensive. One to two ounces can cost twenty to thirty dollars. Colloidal silver generators are now available for home use so that gallons of silver solution can be produced for pennies a day.

Pancreatic Enzymes

Many patients report having indigestion and/or undigested food particles in their stool. This is a sign of insufficient pancreatic enzyme secretion or low stomach acid production. Digestive enzyme supplements can be useful in the beginning of the program. Two to three pancreatic enzymes taken 10–15 minutes before eating aids the digestive process. Hydrochloric acid should be used in moderation, and preferably under a physician's guidance, because it can cause a rebound loss of stomach acid production if used for too long of a period of time.

Aspergillus-derived enzymes have less suppressive effect on pancreas enzyme production. This is why I use and recommend them over animal-derived pancreatic enzymes. Especially avoid pancreatic enzymes that are derived from pork.

Leaky Gut Syndrome

Repair of a leaky gut is vital in order to reduce the flow of toxic by-products and undigested food particles into the bloodstream. These substances cause allergic and other hyperimmune responses. To accomplish this critical healing, I recommend two types of products.

The first product should contain two essential intestinal repairing ingredients, the amino acid L-glutamine and hypoallergenic rice protein. The L-glutamine is used by the intestinal lining as fuel for cellular repair. the hypo allergenic rice protein helps to reduce allergenic activity contributing to further destruction of the intestinal lining.

The second special healing product is manufactured under the name "Seacure," a predigested fish protein in capsule form that has been shown to rapidly repair and heal tissue damage in the digestive tract. Such damage occurs with ulcerative colitis, Crohn's disease, and the leaky gut syndrome. The cells lining the intestinal tract rapidly take up this high-quality protein source for healing the microtears and holes.

Activated Charcoal

Activated charcoal is a safe, time-tested remedy that draws toxic material to itself, forms a permanent bond with the substance, and then escorts it out of the body. Charcoal is the black part of partially burned wood. Activated charcoal refers to wood that has been specially processed in a pit under oxygen deprivation, which gives it several times the "binding power" of normal charcoal. The agent is widely used in fish tank filters as well as in purification systems to extract toxins from water. Taken as a supplement, it does a similar job in your intestinal tract. The charcoal binds up the toxins for elimination in the stool.

Alka-Seltzer Gold

This popular over-the-counter remedy acts as a buffering agent. It helps keep the body's pH, which should be in the 7.1–7.4 range, from becoming too acidic and is a useful product during the detoxification process.

Recovery and Maintenance

Now that I've laid out the information you need to understand the diagnosis, treatment, dietary modifications and supplement program, there remains another important issue to consider. It is called "die-off," or, in medical terms, the Herxheimer reaction. Simply put, when your body is full of yeast and its toxins, and you start eliminating the infection, you are likely to experience symptoms of detoxification. Countless yeast cells are dying. They, and their toxins, are essentially being rounded up and delivered through the channels of elimination and excreted. You may experience headache, nausea, flulike symptoms, muscle aches, joint pains, extreme fatigue, diarrhea, severe constipation, and abdominal discomfort. Some patients also report increased brain fog, poor memory, palpitations, and dry mouth. For a while, you may in fact feel worse than you felt before. The old adages, "You become worse before you become better," or "No pain, no gain," are often quite applicable.

But don't despair. There are very practical steps you can take to minimize discomfort. You can facilitate the "die-off" and reduce the symptoms of detoxification through colonics, enemas, lymphatic massage, activated charcoal, or the use of Alka-Seltzer Gold. All of these measures help speed the release of these poisons from the body and minimize potential detoxification symptoms.

When you begin the program, get in the habit of drinking a full glass of spring water with ten drops of lemon juice added to it. Do this daily, first thing in the morning. Start supplementing with a probiotic, that is, a quality product with beneficial bacteria, as well as biotin and Pau d'Arco. Usually, it's a good idea to drink 1 to 3 cups of Pau d'Arco tea per day, depending upon the severity of your infection. If the die-off symptoms become too severe, you can reduce the consumption of the tea as well as the other herbs and supplements I recommend in order to lower the intensity of the die-off reaction, slow it down, and make the process more tolerable. The remedies in this program are very potent.

Start taking 4-6 capsules of activated charcoal 4 times a day during the first week. In the following week, begin reducing the amount. Take 4–6 capsules 3 times a day. The third week, twice a day. During the fourth week, take 2–3 capsules 2 or 3 times a day. Always take activated charcoal an hour from food. If taken with food, it will bind up vitamins and minerals, and any medications you may be taking. Be sure to use it on an empty stomach.

The Alka Seltzer Gold should be taken once or twice a day during the first several weeks of detoxification. This product helps maintain a normal pH level in the body. If the body becomes too acidic, flulike symptoms and malaise can result. Alka Seltzer Gold sometimes even eliminates any detoxification reactions at all.

Wait for week or two after starting the program before adding the caprylic acid, citrus seed extracts and Kolorex.

During this detoxification period, the body needs to evacuate the accumulated dead yeast and toxins that will be deposited in the colon. You don't want them hanging out in the colon where they can be reabsorbed into the body. You definitely want them out. Sometimes, however, the detoxification process can cause constipation. What is happening is that the toxins create excessive heat in the large intestine. The heat burns up the fluids necessary for waste material to flow through the intestine and out the body. If the wastes lose their moisture content, dry stools and constipation can occur. If you experience this problem, take 2–4 aloe vera capsules or 1–4 capsules of magnesium peroxide at bedtime. Either agents acts as an effective stool softener and facilitates elimination. Home enemas or colonics administered by a qualified colon therapist are also beneficial for eliminating large quantities of toxins. A small amount of acidophilus or other beneficial bacteria added to an enema can help to inoculate the colon directly with good microbial flora.

Recovering from candida has its high and low points. Sometimes you begin to feel almost completely normal and then within a few hours or days later, the symptoms return. You will find, however, that when symptoms return they last for shorter and shorter periods. Don't let relapses discourage you. They are frequently part of the healing process, part of clearing out far-flung pockets of yeast and toxins from your system. As you progress and become healthier, you will find that the good days increase and bad days decrease. Just be patient. Candida can be a nasty problem when you have it and while you are getting it out.

Frequently Asked Questions About Candida

Patients who embark on the anti-candida program often have many questions. I'm sure you will have questions as well. Following are the most frequent questions I am asked:

Q. Do I have to give up sweets?
A. Many people have grown accustomed to using food — sweets, in particular — as a tool to help them through stressful times and when these foods are eliminated, it is as if a major coping mechanism has been removed. It is important to keep in mind the period of abstinence from such favorite foods is only temporary, but still a necessary part of the program designed to help the body and immune system through the stress of recovery. We all typically crave sugar and sweets, and overcoming the craving can be a challenge. Sugar is found in almost every meal in the standard American diet and when it's eliminated, you feel something is missing, that you've lost an old friend. Sugar feeds the yeast that you are trying to eliminate, so giving in to your craving is counterproductive. Try to stay as sugar-free as possible. Stick as close to the program as possible for at least the first six weeks and then begin to slowly introduce foods that are acceptable for your individual blood type. In

doing so, watch for possible reactions to the newly introduced foods. A reaction could be as subtle as increased gas and bloating, or as severe as a migraine headache.

Q. How does the New Millennium Diet relate to the anti-candida diet?

A. The anti-candida diet is superimposed on the specific blood type food plan. There are additional foods that need to be avoided, as outlined in this chapter, for at least six weeks. Usually when these foods are reintroduced into your diet after this period of time, you should be able to tolerate them. However, if you find that any one particular food is not tolerated, continue to avoid it for at least another six weeks and then try introducing it again. You may find that certain foods are readily reintroduced into your diet, while others may take more time before your body can tolerate the specific qualities or nature of an individual food.

Q. How long do I have to follow this program?

A. There's no way to know how much time each individual requires to overcome candida and recover from the illness. The answer depends on the severity of the condition. Usually, patients who have had candida symptoms for less than 6 months are able to recover within 3 or less months. Patients with candida for more than 6 months usually require 3 to 9 months. Longer than 5 years may require 1 to 3 years of healing time. For more long-term, deep-seated cases, I recommend seeking the help of a holistically trained physician who can add individualized treatment with homeopathy, acupuncture, and advanced nutritional prescriptions.

Q. I see other people eating poorly. Why don't they react to the foods that I'm reacting to?

A. Many factors influence a person's response to negative foods. Some people are genetically stronger. Some may be able to cope with emotions or life stressors better. Others may have a better living or working environment. Whatever the particulars, we all have different levels of tolerance, and thus some people can apparently get away with eating poorly without any signs of negative effects. I say *apparently* because it's very difficult to determine symptoms that friends or family members may be experiencing as a result of their eating habits. You can't tell whether or not they may have diarrhea alternating with constipation because of their food or whether their cola habit is causing them seriously disturbed sleep. All people eventually respond in a negative fashion to poor eating habits. As soon as their body runs out of its allotted tolerance and buffering ability, they, too, will show symptoms one way or another. Focus on your own health and what you do for yourself and for your recovery. When others see your improvement they may — or may not — get the message. If they do, they'll come to you and ask what you did.

Q. Why do I have to eliminate all grains from my diet? I have nothing to eat!

A. Most grains are highly glycemic foods. As you now know from reading this book, glycemic foods are rapidly converted into sugar in the bloodstream. Like pouring gasoline on a fire, the sugar feeds the candida, promoting candida overgrowth. Removing grains for a short period of time from your diet can give your body that extra breathing room in order to more rapidly recover from this condition.

Q. Can I use many of the meal replacement shakes or food bars presently available as a snack, or as an entire meal replacement. when following the anti-candida diet?

A. Many shakes and bars contain high concentrations of sugars, which can aggravate candida and further weaken your immune system. It is important to select products containing low glyceimic sugars, ingredients free of common allergants including eggs, wheat and dairy, and ideally fortified with antioxidants and herbs which are appropriate for your specific blood type.

Q. I thought I was supposed to feel better, not worse. What's going on?

A. As I have just discussed, the diet and the supplement program generate a detoxification reaction. See the section above for details. Symptoms frequently are experienced within the first two to five days. Do not stop the program because you are feeling worse. Just know your body is reacting as it should. It is cleaning house, and you are actually healing and becoming healthier in the process. Don't return to your old diet. If you do, then you will simply be allowing the disease process to rage on. Try not to be too physically active during this period. Your body will appreciate any extra rest and sleep you can give it as it goes through the stress of detoxification. Drink plenty of pure water and stay as strictly on the diet as possible. Use activated charcoal and Alka-Seltzer Gold as described above to reduce the symptoms associated with this cleansing. In some unusual cases, the cleanse can continue to occur for weeks after beginning the program. If you undergo acupuncture treatment, or when new antifungal preparations are added to your supplement program, you may experience renewed symptoms as deeper and deeper levels of toxicity and infection are being eliminated.

Q. What should I do if I go on vacation, or if I travel to another location, where it's difficult to follow the diet?

A. Do the best you can. Bring as many of the supplements as possible on your trip and try to stay as close to the prescribed program as possible. When you go off the diet, you'll experience severe reactions again to the foods you shouldn't be eating. Going off the diet may not be worth the discomfort. The goal is to have fun on your vacation, but following the diet as closely as possible is usually the best way to prevent setbacks and maximize your fun.

Q. Why can't I take the antifungal Western drugs available for candida?

A. Many of these drugs contain chemicals that can cause side effects and symptoms that may, in the long run, be harmful to your body. If you look in the *Physician's Desk Reference*, antifungal drugs such as Diflucan and Sporanox create potentially significant liver-related toxicity that can place an additional burden on an already weakened liver. In addition, these drugs can lead to fungal resistance, putting you into a worse position after you discontinue them. After more than ten years of working with natural products,

I find that most patients can overcome candida, unless they are suffering with AIDS or some other severe immunologically suppressive condition, without using these synthetic chemical-based medications. If you are interested in true recovery, I recommend starting with the natural approach. Follow the diet. Take the supplements. Do this before using the synthetic medications, unless your physician advises otherwise.

Q. What is the relationship between Epstein-Barr virus, cytomegalovirus, herpes type 6, and candida?

A. Patients with candida suffer from generalized immune suppression. Many times, viral, bacterial or other parasitic conditions are concurrently present because the body's defenses have been weakened and are unable to control pathogens. A good anti-candida program not only fortifies your ability to counteract candida but simultaneously improves your immune system and allows it to start effectively combating other harmful microorganisms as well.

Q. What is chronic fatigue syndrome and how does it relate to candidiasis?

A. Once again, patients with candida-related problems and the weakness it generates often suffer from other symptoms and disorders. Among them is a form of chronic fatigue. It is not, however, "the dreaded" chronic fatigue immune dysfunction syndrome (CFIDS), which is a separate condition. Many disease processes cause fatigue as a symptom. Candida is one. Epstein-Barr virus, HIV, cancer, hypothyroidism, lupus, and CFIDS are some of the others.

If I have not covered an issue or a question regarding the program, please feel free to call, write or e-mail me. The clinic phone number is (310) 828-3096, and a staff member can take your question. To write, we are located at 1821 Wilshire Boulevard, Suite 100, Santa Monica, California 90403.

If you have Internet access, our website address is http://www.newmedinstitute.com E-mail at info@newmedinstitute.com

For information on where to obtain products recommended by Dr. DeOrio, contact ProSana at (877) PROSANA (877-776-7262)

Method of Calculating Fat and Lean Body Mass—Female

Your body fat is that portion of your total body which is made up of fat tissue. Your total body tissue less the body fat is your lean body mass. For example, if a female's body fat is 20%, then her lean body mass is 80%. Expressed in weight, a 160-pound female would have 32 pounds of body fat and 128 pounds of lean body mass. One method to estimate your body fat is to use a cloth tape measure, a bathroom scale and conversion tables. The measurements should be made on the your bare skin and not around clothing. Take care that the tape fits snugly, but does not compress your skin. It is recommended that you take at least three measurements and compute the average to the nearest 1/2 inch.

GUIDELINES FOR CALCULATING FEMALE BODY FAT AND LEAN BODY MASS PERCENTAGES

1. Measure your height without shoes.

2. Measure your hips at their widest point.

3. Measure your waist at the belly button.

4. Take each of the above measurements at least 3 times and record the average on the worksheet provided below.

5. Find your height in Table A-1 (Constant A) and record the constant value on the worksheet.

6. Find your hip size in Table A-2 (Constant B) and record the constant value on the worksheet.

7. Find your waist size in table A-3 (Constant C) and record the constant value on the worksheet.

8. Add Constants B and C, then subtract Constant A. This figure rounded to the nearest whole number equals your percentage of body fat.

9. Deduct your percentage of body fat from 100%. The difference is your lean body mass percentage.

FEMALE BODY FAT AND LEAN BODY MASS

WORKSHEET

MEASUREMENTS	HEIGHT	HIP	WAIST
	(in inches)	(in inches)	(in inches)
First			
Second			
Third			
Average			
CONSTANT	A	B	C
Value From Table			
PERCENTAGE OF BODY FAT	B+C-A = %	PERCENTAGE OF LEAN MASS %	

EXAMPLE:

FEMALE BODY FAT AND LEAN BODY MASS WORKSHEET

MEASUREMENTS	HEIGHT	HIP	WAIST
	(in inches)	(in inches)	(in inches)
First	66 1/2	36 1/2	26 1/2
Second	66 1/2	36 1/2	26 1/2
Third	66 3/4	36 3/4	26 3/4
Average	66 1/2	36 1/2	26 1/2
CONSTANT	A	B	C
Value From Table	40.4	42.2	18.7
PERCENTAGE OF BODY FAT	B+C-A = 20.5 = 21%	PERCENTAGE OF LEAN MASS %	79%

TABLE A-1

Female Body Fat Determination Chart

Height Conversion: Constant (A)

Inches	Constant (A)	Inches	Constant (A)
55	33.5	67	40.8
55.5	33.7	67.5	41.0
56	34.1	68	41.4
56.5	34.3	68.5	41.6
57	34.7	69	42.1
57.5	34.9	69.5	42.2
58	35.3	70	42.7
58.5	35.5	70.5	42.8
59	36.0	71	43.3
59.5	36.1	71.5	43.4
60	36.6	72	43.9
60.5	36.7	72.5	44.0
61	37.2	73	44.5
61.5	37.3	73.5	44.6
62	37.8	74	45.1
62.5	38.0	74.5	45.3
63	38.4	75	45.7
63.5	38.7	75.5	45.9
64	39.0	76	46.3
64.5	39.2	76.5	46.5
65	39.6	77	47.0
65.5	39.8	77.5	47.2
66	40.2	78	47.7
66.5	40.4	78.6	47.9
67	40.8	79	48.1

TABLE A-2

Female Body Fat Determination Chart

Hip Conversion: Constant (B)

Inches	Constant (B)	Inches	Constant (B)
30	33.5	45.5	54.8
30.5	33.8	46	55.8
31	34.9	46.5	56.2
31.5	35.2	47	57.2
32	36.3	47.5	57.8
32.5	36.6	48	58.6
33	37.7	48.5	59.0
33.5	38.0	49	60.0
34	39.1	49.5	60.4
34.5	39.4	50	61.4
35	40.5	50.5	61.8
35.5	40.8	51	62.8
36	41.9	51.5	63.2
36.5	42.2	52	64.2
37	42.3	52.5	64.6
37.5	43.6	53	65.6
38	44.7	53.5	66.0
38.5	45.3	54	67.0
39	46.1	54.5	67.3
39.5	46.4	55	68.4
40	47.4	55.5	68.8
40.5	47.8	56	69.8
41	48.8	56.5	70.1
41.5	49.2	57	71.2
42	50.2	57.5	71.5
42.5	50.6	58	72.6
43	51.6	58.5	72.9
43.5	52.0	59	74.0
44	53.0	59.5	74.3
44.5	53.4	60.0	75.4
45	54.5	60.5	75.8

TABLE A-3

Female Body Fat Determination Chart

Abdomen Conversion: Constant (C)

Inches	Constant (C)	Inches	Constant (C)
20	14.2	35.5	25.1
20.5	14.4	36	25.6
21	14.9	36.5	25.8
21.5	15.1	37	26.3
22	15.6	37.5	26.5
22.5	15.8	38	27.0
23	16.3	38.5	27.2
23.5	16.5	39	27.7
24	17.1	39.5	27.9
24.5	17.2	40	28.4
25	17.8	40.5	28.6
25.5	18.0	41	29.1
26	18.5	41.5	29.3
26.5	18.7	42	29.9
27	19.2	42.5	30.0
27.5	19.4	43	30.6
28	19.9	43.5	30.8
28.5	20.3	44	31.3
29	20.6	44.5	31.5
29.5	20.8	45	32
30	21.3	45.5	32.2
30.5	21.5	46	32.7
31	22.0	46.5	32.9
31.5	22.2	47	33.4
32	22.8	47.5	33.6
32.5	22.9	48	34.1
33	23.5	48.5	34.3
33.5	23.6	49	34.8
34	24.2	49.5	35.0
34.5	24.4	50	36.5
35	24.9	50.5	36.7

Method of Calculating Fat and Lean Body Mass—Male

Your body fat is that portion of your total body which is made up of fat tissue. Your total body tissue less the body fat is your lean body mass. For example, if a male's body fat is 20%, then his lean body mass is 80%. Expressed in weight, a 200-pound male would have 40 pounds of body fat and 160 pounds of lean body mass. One method to estimate your body fat is to use a cloth tape measure, a bathroom scale and conversion tables. The measurements should be made on the your bare skin and not around clothing. Take care that the tape fits snugly, but does not compress your skin. It is recommended that you take at least three measurements and compute the average to the nearest 1/2 inch.

GUIDELINES FOR CALCULATING MALE BODY FAT AND LEAN BODY MASS PERCENTAGES

1. Measure your waist at the belly button.

2. Measure the wrist of your dominant hand at the space between the wrist bone and where the wrist bends.

3. Take each of the above measurements at least 3 times and record the average on the worksheet provided below.

4. Measure your weight on an accurate bathroom scale (only once) and record on the worksheet.

5. Subtract your wrist measurement from your waist measurement and record this number on the worksheet.

6. Using Table B , find your weight (left-hand side of table) and find your "waist minus wrist" number (top of table). Where the two columns intersect is your percentage of body fat.

7. Deduct your percentage of body fat from 100%. The difference is your lean mass percentage.

MALE BODY FAT AND LEAN BODY MASS WORKSHEET

MEASUREMENTS	Waist (In inches)	Wrist (in inches)	Weight (in lbs)
First			
Second			
Third			
Average			
Waist minus Wrist			
PERCENTAGE OF BODY FAT FROM TABLE B	%	PERCENTAGE OF LEAN MASS%	

EXAMPLE:

MALE BODY FAT AND LEAN BODY MASS WORKSHEET

MEASUREMENTS	Waist (In inches)	Wrist (in inches)	Weight (in lbs)
First	34 1/2	6 3/4	185
Second	34 5/8	7	-
Third	34 1/2	6 3/4	-
Average	34 1/2	7	185
Waist minus Wrist	27 1/2		
PERCENTAGE OF BODY FAT FROM TABLE B	15%	PERCENTAGE OF LEAN MASS%	85%

TABLE B (1 OF 4)

Body Fat Determination Chart

WAIST-WRIST (IN INCHES)

WEIGHT (in lbs)	22	22.5	23	23.5	24	24.5	25	25.5	26	26.5	27	27.5	28	28.5	29
120	4	6	8	10	12	14	16	18	20	21	23	25	27	29	31
125	4	6	7	9	11	13	15	17	19	20	22	24	26	28	30
130	3	5	7	9	11	12	14	16	18	20	21	23	25	27	28
135	3	5	7	8	10	12	13	15	17	19	20	22	24	26	27
140	3	5	6	8	10	11	13	15	16	18	19	21	23	24	26
145		4	6	7	9	11	12	14	15	17	19	20	22	23	25
150		4	6	7	9	10	12	13	15	16	18	19	21	23	24
155		4	5	6	8	10	11	13	14	16	17	19	20	22	23
160		4	5	6	8	9	11	12	14	15	17	18	19	21	22
165		3	5	6	8	9	10	12	13	15	16	17	19	20	22
170		3	4	6	7	9	10	11	13	14	15	17	18	19	21
175			4	6	7	8	10	11	12	12	15	16	17	19	20
180			4	5	7	8	9	10	12	13	14	16	17	18	19
185			4	5	6	8	9	10	11	13	14	15	16	18	19
190			4	5	6	7	8	10	11	12	13	15	16	17	18
195			3	5	6	7	8	9	11	12	13	14	15	16	18
200			3	4	6	7	8	9	10	11	12	14	15	16	17
205				4	5	6	8	9	10	11	12	13	14	15	17
210				4	5	6	7	8	9	11	12	13	14	15	16
215				4	5	6	7	8	9	10	11	12	13	16	16
220				4	5	6	7	8	9	10	11	12	13	14	15
225				3	4	6	7	8	9	10	11	12	13	14	15
230				3	4	5	6	7	8	9	10	11	12	13	14
235				3	4	5	6	7	8	9	10	11	12	13	14
240					4	5	6	7	8	9	10	11	12	13	14
245					4	5	6	7	8	9	9	10	11	12	13
250					4	5	6	6	7	8	9	10	11	12	13
255					3	4	5	6	7	8	9	10	11	12	13
260					3	4	5	6	7	8	9	10	10	11	12
265						4	5	6	7	8	8	9	10	11	12
270						4	5	6	7	7	8	9	10	11	12
275						4	5	5	6	7	8	9	10	11	11
280						4	4	5	6	7	8	9	9	10	11
285						4	4	5	6	7	8	8	9	10	11
290						3	4	5	6	7	7	8	9	10	11
295						3	4	5	6	6	7	8	9	10	10
300						3	4	5	5	6	7	8	9	9	10

TABLE B (2 OF 4)

Male Body Fat Determination Chart

WAIST-WRIST (IN INCHES)

WEIGHT (in lbs)	29.5	30	30.5	31	31.5	32	32.5	33	33.5	34	34.5	35	35.5	36	36.5
120	33	35	37	39	41	43	45	47	49	50	52	54			
125	32	33	35	37	39										
130	30	32	34	36	37	39	41	43	44	46	48	50	52	53	55
135	29	31	32	34	36	38	39	41	43	44	46	48	50	51	53
140	28	29	31	33	34	36	38	39	41	43	44	46	48	49	651
145	27	28	30	31	33	35	36	38	39	41	43	44	46	47	49
150	26	27	29	30	32	33	35	36	38	40	41	43	44	46	47
155	25	26	28	29	31	32	34	35	37	38	40	41	43	44	46
160	24	25	27	28	30	31	33	34	35	37	38	40	41	43	44
165	23	24	26	27	29	30	31	33	34	36	37	38	40	41	43
170	22	24	25	26	28	29	30	32	33	34	36	37	39	40	41
175	21	23	24	25	27	28	29	31	32	33	35	36	37	39	40
180	21	22	23	25	26	27	28	30	31	32	34	35	36	37	39
185	20	21	23	24	25	26	28	29	30	31	33	34	35	36	38
190	19	21	22	23	24	26	27	28	29	30	32	33	34	35	37
195	19	20	21	22	24	25	26	27	28	30	31	32	33	34	35
200	18	19	21	22	23	24	25	26	28	29	30	31	32	33	35
205	18	19	20	21	22	23	25	26	27	28	29	30	31	32	34
210	17	18	19	21	22	23	24	25	26	27	28	29	30	32	33
215	17	18	19	20	21	22	23	24	25	26	28	29	30	31	32
220	16	17	18	19	20	22	23	24	25	26	27	28	29	30	31
225	16	17	18	19	20	21	22	23	24	25	26	27	28	29	30
230	15	16	17	18	19	20	21	22	23	24	25	26	27	28	30
235	15	16	17	18	19	20	21	22	23	24	25	26	27	28	29
240	15	16	17	17	18	19	20	21	22	23	24	25	26	27	28
245	14	15	16	17	18	19	20	21	22	23	24	25	26	27	27
250	14	15	16	17	18	18	19	20	21	22	23	24	25	26	27
255	14	14	15	16	17	18	19	20	21	22	23	24	24	25	26
260	13	14	15	16	17	18	19	19	20	21	22	23	24	25	26
265	13	14	15	15	16	17	18	19	20	21	22	22	23	24	25
270	13	13	14	15	16	17	18	19	19	20	21	22	23	24	25
275	12	13	14	15	16	16	17	18	19	20	21	22	22	23	24
280	12	13	14	14	15	16	17	18	19	19	20	21	22	23	24
285	12	12	13	14	15	16	17	17	18	19	20	21	21	22	23
290	11	12	13	14	15	15	16	17	18	19	19	20	21	22	23
295	11	12	13	14	14	15	16	17	17	18	19	20	21	21	23
300	11	12	12	13	14	15	16	16	17	18	19	19	20	21	22

TABLE B (3 OF 4)

Body Fat Determination Chart

WAIST-WRIST (IN INCHES)

WEIGHT (in lbs)	37	37.5	38	38.5	39	39.5	40	40.5	41	41.5	42	42.5	43	43.5	44
120															
125															
130															
135	55														
140	53	54													
145	51	52	54	55											
150	49	50	52	53	55										
155	47	49	50	52	53	55									
160	46	47	48	50	51	53	54								
165	44	45	47	48	50	51	52	54	55						
170	43	44	45	47	48	49	51	52	54	55					
175	41	43	44	45	47	48	49	51	52	53	55				
180	40	41	43	44	45	47	48	49	50	52	53	54			
185	39	40	41	43	44	45	46	48	49	50	51	53	54	55	
190	38	39	40	41	43	44	45	46	48	49	50	51	52	54	55
195	37	38	39	40	41	43	44	45	46	47	49	50	51	52	53
200	36	37	38	39	40	41	43	44	45	46	47	48	50	51	52
205	35	36	37	38	39	40	41	43	44	45	46	47	48	49	51
210	34	35	36	37	38	39	40	42	43	44	45	46	47	48	49
215	33	34	35	36	37	38	39	40	42	43	44	45	46	47	48
220	32	33	34	35	36	37	38	39	41	42	43	44	45	46	47
225	31	32	33	34	35	36	37	38	40	41	42	43	44	45	46
230	31	32	33	34	35	36	37	38	39	40	41	42	44	44	45
235	30	31	32	33	34	35	36	37	38	39	40	41	42	43	44
240	29	30	31	32	33	34	35	36	37	38	39	40	41	42	43
245	28	29	30	31	32	33	34	35	36	37	38	39	40	41	42
250	28	29	30	31	31	32	33	34	35	36	37	38	39	40	41
255	27	28	29	30	31	32	33	34	34	35	36	37	38	39	40
260	27	27	28	29	30	31	32	33	34	35	35	36	37	38	39
265	26	27	28	29	29	30	31	32	33	34	35	36	36	37	38
270	25	26	27	28	29	30	31	31	32	33	34	35	36	37	37
275	25	26	27	27	28	29	30	31	32	32	33	34	35	36	37
280	34	25	26	27	28	29	29	30	31	32	33	33	34	35	36
285	34	25	26	26	27	28	29	30	30	31	32	33	34	34	35
290	23	24	25	26	27	27	28	29	30	31	31	32	33	34	35
295	23	24	25	25	26	27	28	28	29	30	31	32	32	33	34
300	22	23	24	25	26	26	27	28	29	29	30	31	32	33	33

TABLE B (4 OF 4)

Male Body Fat Determination Chart

WAIST- WRIST (IN INCHES)

WEIGHT (in lbs)	44.5	45	45.5	45.5	46	46.5	47	47.5	48	48.5	49	49.5	50		
120															
125															
130															
135															
140															
145															
150															
155															
160															
165															
170															
175															
180															
185															
190															
195	55														
200	53	54	55												
205	52	53	54	55											
210	50	51	53	54	55										
215	49	50	51	52	53	54	55								
220	48	49	50	51	52	53	54	55							
225	47	48	49	50	51	52	53	54	55						
230	46	47	48	49	50	51	52	53	54	55					
235	45	46	47	48	49	50	51	51	52	53	54	55			
240	44	45	46	46	47	48	49	50	51	52	53	54			
245	43	44	44	45	46	47	48	49	50	51	52	53			
250	42	43	44	44	45	46	47	48	49	50	51	52			
255	41	42	43	44	44	45	46	47	48	49	50	51			
260	40	41	42	43	43	44	45	46	47	48	49	50			
265	39	40	41	42	43	43	44	45	46	47	48	49			
270	38	39	40	41	42	43	43	44	45	46	47	48			
275	38	38	39	40	41	42	43	43	44	45	46	47			
280	37	38	38	39	40	41	42	43	43	44	45	46			
285	36	37	38	39	39	40	41	42	43	43	44	45			
290	35	36	37	38	39	39	40	41	42	43	43	44			
295	35	36	36	37	38	39	39	40	41	42	43	43			
300	34	35	36	36	37	38	39	39	40	41	42	43			

Commonly Asked Questions

S tarting any new program is filled with gaps in ones full understanding of the material. Usually many of the same questions are asked repeatedly. In order to understand this nutritional plan more thoroughly and to appreciate the subtleties, complexities, and simplicities of this approach I have dedicated this section to answering your questions to help you understand how this diet can improve the quality of your life for a lifetime.

1. **Is it important to make all the necessary changes immediately when beginning the New Millennium Diet?**

   The New Millennium Diet essentially consists of three main systems: One system incorporates the use of specific macronutrient ratios based on blood type. The second system incorporates blood type lectin compatible foods, and the third system consists of yin and yang's relation to the energetics of food. The most important thing to do is to attempt to follow the basic dietary listings for your individual blood type. Once you understand how blood type relates to food, I would then begin to incorporate the percentages for your specific blood type. If you're A or AB, then you need to follow a 25% protein, 50% carbohydrate, 25% fat ratio. If you're O or B, you need to follow a 30% protein, 40% carbohydrate, 30% fat ratio. Ideally, incorporating all of the three different systems into a synergistic whole is going to be the ideal and long term goal of all people interested in the New Millennium dietary approach. However, starting slow, learning the basics of the program, and mastering each section one at a time is a much better approach to prevent you from giving up entirely on the overall concept. Yin and yang concepts basically are there to help you better understand how foods actually contain an energetic quality, and those qualities need to be balanced at every meal as do the macronutrient ratios and the individual foods compatible with your blood type.

2. **If I'm blood type B and my wife is blood type AB, how do we cook for both blood types? I don't want to cook two separate meals.**

   This is an important question. Since blood type B's and AB's must avoid chicken, obviously chicken is not a favorable food group; consequently, most meals will not have chicken as their main protein source. It's a good idea to emphasize those foods that are beneficial for both blood types when preparing a meal. If your spouse or partner or even children have different blood types than yourself, it's a good idea to become familiar, especially if you're the food preparer in the family, and be aware of the foods that all the other blood types can enjoy. In addition, many people are fearful that they're not going to be able to eat the foods that they traditionally eat; however, there are over 200 different foods listed for each blood type, most people do not eat more than 30-40 different foods during their daily life.

3. **What does least beneficial mean?**

   Least beneficial means the food essentially is a poison. That means that when you eat this food, it's going to cause ill health in your body on many different levels; therefore, you should definitely try to consume more neutral and beneficial foods.

4. **Should all of the foods that I consume be on the most beneficial list?**

The most beneficial foods act as medicines in your body. Those specific foods should be eaten if you are suffering with any type of disease-like condition in an attempt to heal your body; however, make sure that they are appropriately balanced in terms of the macronutrient ratios and that you are consuming a sufficient number of portions at every meal.

5. **I noticed most of your herbal and supplement recommendations have brand names. Where can I find many of these different products?**

ProSana offers a wide variety of different and often times specialty products designed to augment some of the products that are commonly found at your local health food store. I have tested most of these products for purity and efficacy both in a research setting as well as in clinical practice. It's advised that you use the specific brand names recommended because they have been shown to have the most efficacy. A catalog can be obtained from ProSana by contacting (877) 776-7262 or see their Web site at **www.prosana.com**.

6. **This concept of yin and yang seems a bit confusing. How can I incorporate all of these concepts into one synergistic approach?**

The concepts of yin and yang are being presented to help you appreciate the fact that foods have an energetic quality. It's is not enough just to look at foods as proteins, carbohydrates, and fats. We also have to realize that there are heating and cooling elements that are also part of the inherent nature of food and these heating and cooling qualities can have an impact on the yin and yang states within the body.

7. **I'm blood type O and have recently had coronary artery bypass surgery. My doctor has recommended that I avoid all fat containing products, especially red meat. What can I do?**

Blood type O's fare poorly on a high carbohydrate diet because their bodies respond negatively to higher glycemic foods. O blood types in general have high stomach acids and a strong ability to breakdown and digest meat based products, including the fat contained within the meat. If an O blood type individual consumes excessive amounts of grains and dairy products, he would be setting himself up for the development of heart disease; whereas, if an A blood type individual was to consume excessive amounts of red meat or meats in general, they would be setting themselves up to develop heart disease. So, one cannot make a general statement that all people who have heart disease should avoid red meat because none of us have been created the same. We are all individuals, and our diets should reflect that individuality.

8. **I'm blood type AB, and you recommend that I perform isometric and other more relaxation types of exercise techniques; however, I love to mountain bike and find that this tends to be a very physically exhausting experience. What should I do?**

Blood type A's in general do better with more relaxing types of movements, such as tai chi, yoga, and chi kung; however, if you enjoy mountain biking or running, these types of activities can be incorporated into your daily lifestyle as long as after performing an exhaustive ride, that you follow it up with some form of relaxation technique in order to calm your nervous system and re-balance your body. In addition, you can use certain calming herbs, such as Kava Kava or valerian, to keep your body in a relaxed state which accelerates the recuperative processes.

9. **I find it difficult to find snacks that are both blood type compatible and macronutrient balanced. Do you have any recommendations?**

ProSana has developed a whole line of blood type compatible and macro balanced shakes and bars, and even multi-vitamins for ease of use in following this diet. The bars contain two macrobalanced portions, while being totally blood type compatible as well as yin-yang synergized. This also applies to the ProSana shakes.

10. **What happens if there are certain least beneficial foods in a recipe that are in low quantities but they are still present in the overall ingredient listing?**

    Depending upon the severity of your condition or your overall physical health, following the New Millennium dietary approach 100% is not practical. I would recommend that if you're able to follow the diet 80% or 90% of what's written, then you can receive an A+ on our rating scale. Therefore, if there's a least beneficial food that's listed as a specific ingredient in a recipe, as long as you don't have any serious food allergies to that particular ingredient, it would probably be okay. However, if you are suffering with some type of physical condition or disease for which there are no known therapies to heal it, I would definitely attempt to follow this dietary approach 95% or more of the time and therefore avoid that recipe.

11. **What if I have sweet cravings after I begin to follow the New Millennium Diet?**

    Often times, the sweet cravings will persist for two to six weeks after beginning the diet in certain individuals, especially if they had abused sugar in the past. Typically, the body adjusts to the requirements of this particular plan as the body accommodates many of the cravings will diminish for either sugar or chocolate or whatever your fancy may be. The body usually craves foods that it tends to be allergic to. It's a quirky kind of response, but I have seen it in thousands of patients over the years. As your body eliminates the antibodies, which are reacting to those types of foods, the body's desire for the food usually diminishes. In addition, there are certain types of aromatherapies that can be utilized to impact the limbic systems in the brain and can many times temporarily relieve excessive cravings for sugar or food. These types of products can be found at your local health food store underneath the listings of aromatherapy. If you're still craving food or you're finding that the cravings persist even after six weeks on the diet and using the aromatherapy techniques, I would recommend that you increase your fat portions by one. In other words, if you're consuming one portion of carbohydrate and one portion of protein, then you should consume two portions of fat. Many time, by consuming the extra fat, the carbohydrate is diluted, reducing further spikes in your insulin response. This helps to moderate the release of insulin, preventing swings in your blood sugar levels, which often times can lead to sugar cravings.

12. **Many people talk about the New Millennium Diet as being a high protein diet especially for O's and B's.**

    The New Millennium Diet is pretty much of a moderate protein diet. High protein diets usually are in the range of 40+ percentage points of protein with 30% or less of carbohydrate and fat. In addition, because of the balancing of protein amounts with carbohydrates and fats in the New Millennium dietary approach, the protein has a positive effect on the body actually supporting muscle mass development and hormonal balance.

13. **Will I lose fat or weight while following the New Millennium Diet?**

    Preferably, you will lose fat and not weight. Weight is made up of many different constituents, including bone, muscle, fat, water, and even waste products of metabolism. Excess fat, however, is the substance that has the most negative effect on the human body and is what predominantly leads to disease within our systems. The New Millennium Diet promotes fat loss and not weight loss. It enhances muscle mass development while decreasing overall fat percentages.

14. **Should I also incorporate food combining with the New Millennium Diet?**

    Our ancestors rarely, if ever, combined foods. When they ate, they had fruits, vegetables, and meats all at the same time typically. However, in less than five percent of the people that follow the new millennium diet food combining may have to be instituted temporarily until their digestive track can heal sufficiently enough to tolerate a more normal approach to eating .

APPENDIX D

References

Addi, GJ. Blood groups in acute rheumatism. *Scottish Med J,* 1959:4:547.

Aird, I. et al. Blood group in relation to peptic ulceration and carcinoma of the breast, colon, bronchus and return. *Brit Med J,* 1954:315-342.

American Association of Blood Banks. *Technical Manual, 10th ed.,* 1990.

An insight is gained on how ulcers develop. *The New York Times,* Dec. 17, 1993.

American Diabetes Association, 1997.

Anderson, R. et al. Elevated intake of supplemental chromium improves glucose and insulin variables in individuals with type 2 diabetes. *Diabetes,* 1997;46:1786-1791.

Ali, L. et al. Characterization of the hypoglycemic effects of *Trigonella foenum graccum* seed. *Planta Med,* 1995:61:358-360.

Ali, L. et al. Studies on hypoglycemic effects of fruit pulp, seed, and whole plant of *Momordia charantia* on normal and diabetic model rats. *Planta Med,* 1993: 59:408-411.

Atkins, R. and Herwood, RW. *Dr. Atkins' Diet Revolution.* New York: Bantam, 1972.

Berkow, R. *The Merck Manual.* Rathway, NJ: Merck & Co., Inc., 1992.

Blood groups and susceptibility to disease: A review. *Brit J Prev Soc Med II,* 1957:107-125.

Blood groups and intestine: An editorial. *Lancet,* 7475 Dec. 3, 1966.

Bordia, A. et al. Effect of ginger (*Zingiber officinale Rose.*) and fenugreek (*Trigonella foemum graecum L.*) on blood lipids, blood sugar and plarelet aggregation in patients with coronary artery disease. *Prost Leuko EFA,* 1997:56:379-384.

Brooks, SA. Predictive value of lectin binding on breast cancer recurrence and survival. *Lancet,* May 9, 1987:1054-1056.

Brown, D. *Encyclopedia of Herbs and Their Uses.* Dorling Kindersley: New York, 1995.

Brues, AM. Tests of blood group selection. *Amer J Forensic Med,* 1929:287-289.

Buchanan, JA and Higley, ET. The relationship of blood groups to disease. *Brit J Exper Pathol.* 1921:2:247-253.

Buckwalter, et al. Ethnologic aspects of the ABO blood groups: Disease Association. *JAMA,* 1957:327.

Buckwalter, et al. ABO blood groups and disease. *JAMA* 1956:1210-1214.

Cameron, C. et al. Acquisition of a B-like antigen by red blood cells. *Brit Med Journal,* July 11, 1959:29-34.

Dahiya, R. et al. ABH blood group antigen expression, synthesis and degradation in human colonic adenocarcinoma cell lines. *Cancer Res,* 1989:49:16:4550-4556.

D'Adamo, J. *The D'Adamo Diet.* Montreal: McGraw-Hill Ryerson, 1989.

D'Adamo, P. Gut ecosystems III: The ABO and other polymorphic systems. *Townsend Letter for Doctors,* August 1990.

D'Adamo, P. Possible alteration of ABO blood group observed in non-Hodgkin's lymphoma. *J Naturopath Med,* 1990:1:39-43.

Fenlon, S. et al. *Helix pomatia* and *Ulex europeus* lectin binding in human breast cancer. *J Pathology,* 1987:152:169-176.

Fiocchi, A., Borelola, E., Riva, E., et al. (1986). "A double-blind clinical trial for the evaluation of the therapeutic effectiveness of a calf thymus derivative (Thymomodulin) in children with recurrent respiratory infections." *Thymus;* 8: 831-839.

Food and Drug Administration Pesticide Monitoring Crop Reports for Fruits and Vegetables, 1985-1988, Washington D.C.

Fraser Roberts, JA. Some associations between blood types and disease. *Brit Med Bull,* 1959:15:129-133.

Freed, DLF. Dietary lectins and disease. *Food Allergy and Intolerance,* 1987:375-400.

Genova, R., and Guerra, A. (1986). "Thymomodulin in management of food allergy in children." *Int J Tissue Reac;* 8: 239-242.

Gunderson, E. FDA *Total Diet Study,* Apr 1982-Apr 1986: Dietary Intakes of Pesticides, Selected Elements and Other Chemicals. Arlington, Va: Association of Official Analytical Chemists.

Havlik, R. et al. Blood groups and coronary heart disease. A letter. *Lancet,* August 2, 1969:269-270.

Helm, R. and Froese, A. Binding of receptors for IgE by various lectins. *Int Arch Allergy Appl Immunology,* 1981:65:81-84.

Hentges, DJ. *Human Intestinal Microflora in Health and Disease.* New York: Academic Press 1983.

Industrial Chemical/Pesticide Monitoring Reports for Seafood, 1982-88. U.S. Food and Drug Administration, Wash. D.C.

Imported Meat and Poultry Samples Analyzed for Radiocesium by the Food Safety and Inspection Service Following the Chernobyl Accident. U.S. Department of Agriculture, May 1986-December 1988, Wash. D.C.

Koskins, LC, et al. Degradation of blood group antigens in human colon ecosystems. *J Clin Invest,* 1976:57:63-73.

Kushi, M and Jack, A. *The Cancer Prevention Diet.* New York: St. Martin's, 1983.

Karunanayake, EH, et al. Effects of *Momordica charantia* fruit juice on streptozotocin-induced diabetes in rats. *J Ethnopharmacol,* 1990:30: 199-204.

Langkilde, NC. et al. Binding of wheat and peanut lectins to human transitional cell carcinoma. *Cancer,* 1989:64:4:849-853.

Leatherdale, BA. et al. Improvement in glucose tolerance due to *Momordia charantia* (Karela). *BR Med J,* 1981:15:107-117.

Linder, M. *Nutritional Biochemistry and Metabolism with Clinical Applications* 2nd ed., Appleton & Lange: Norwalk, CT, 1991.

Madar, Z. et al. Glucose-lowering effect of fenugreek in non-insulin dependent diabetics. *Eur J Clin Nutr,* 1988:42:51-54.

Marcus, DM, The ABO and Lewis blood group system. *New Eng J Med,* 1969:280:994-1005.

Marles, FJ. Farnsworth, NR. Antidiabetics plants and their active constituents; an update. *Protocol J Nat Med,* Winter 1996:85-111.

Marth, C. and Daxenbichiler, G. Peanut agglutinin inhibits proliferation of cultured breast cancer cells. *Oncology,* 1988:45:47-50.

McConnell, RB. et al. Blood groups in diabetes mellitis. *Brit Med J,* 1956:1:772-776.

Mitchell, C. and Jacobson, M. *Tainted Booze: The Consumer's Guide to Urethane in Alcoholic Beverages.* Center for Science in the Public Interest, Wash. D.C., 1989:172-177.

Morecki, S. et al. Removal of breast cancer cells by soybean agglutinin in experimental model for purging human marrow. *Canc Res,* 1988:48: 18:4573-4577.

Motzer, RJ. et al. Blood group related antigens in human germ cell tumors. *Cancer Res,* 1988:48:18:5342-5347.

Mourant, AE. *Blood Relations: Blood Groups and Anthropology.* Oxford, England: Oxford University Press, 1983.

Murray, M., and Pizzorno, J. (1993). "Chronic Mononucleosis." *Textbook of Natural Medicine.* VI: Mono Ch-7. Seattle, WA: Bastyr Publications.

Muschel, L. Blood groups, disease and selection. *Bateriological Rev,* 1966:30:2:427-441.

Nachbar, MS. et al. Lectins in the U.S. diet: A survey of lectins in commonly consumed foods and a review of the literature. *Amer J Clin Nut,* 1980:33:233-245.

Nachbar, MS. et al. Lectins in the U.S. diet: Isolation and characterization of a lectin from the tomato (lycopersicon esculentum). *J Biol Chem,* 1980:255:2056-2061.

Nomi, T. and Besher, A. *You Are Your Blood Type.* New York: Pocket, 1983.

Ohbayashi, A., Akioka, T., and Tasaki, J. (1972). "A study of effects of liver hydrolysate on hepatic circulation." *J Therapy,* 54: 1582-1585.

Paolisso, G. et al. Pharmacologic doses of vitamin E improve insulin action in healthy subjects and non-insulin-dependent diabetic patients. *Am J Clin Nutr,* 1993:57:650-656.

Paolisso, G. et al. Daily magnesium supplements improve glucose handling in elderly subjects. *Am J Clin Nutr,* 1992:55:1161-1167.

Price, Weston A. *Nutrition and Physical Degeneration.* Connecticut: Kents Publishing, 1998.

Pritikin, N. and McGrady. P. *The Pritikin Program for Diet and Exercise.* New York: Grosset & Dunlap, 1979.

Race, RR. and Sanger, R. *Blood Groups in Man.* Oxford, England: Blackwell Scientific, 1975.

Ratner, et al. ABO group uropathogens and urinary tract infection. *Amer L Med Sci,* 1986:292:84-92.

Roath, S. et al. Transient acquired blood group B antigen associated with diverticular bowel disease. *Acta Haematologica,* 1987:77:88-90.

Ruttenburg, M. Safe Sushi: (letter). *New Eng J Med,* 1989:900.

Schell, O. *Modern Meat: Antibiotics, Hormones and the Pharmaceutical Farm.* New York: Random House, 1988.

Schinfeld, JS. PMS and candidiasis: Study explores possible link. *The Female Patient,* July 1987.

Shanmugasundaram, ERB, et al. Enzyme changes and glucose utilization in diabetic rabbits: The effect of Gymnema sylvestre. RBR. *J Ethnopharmacol,* 1983:7:205-234.

Shanmugasundaram, ERB, et al. Possible regeneration of the islets of langerhans in streptozotocin-diabetic rats given sylvestere leaf extract. *J Ethnopharmacol,* 1990:30:295-305.

Sharma, RD, et al. Effect of fenugreek seeds and leaves on blood glucose and serum insulin reponses in human subjects. *Nutr Res,* 1986:6: 1353-1364.

Sharon, N. and Halina, L. The biochemistry of plant lectins (phyto-hemaglutinins A) *Ann Rev Biochem,* 1973:42:541-574.

Shechter, Y. Bound lectins that mimic insulin produce persistent insulin-like effects. *Endocrinology*, 1983:113:1921-1026.

Shorter, RB and Kirsner, JB. Gastrointestinal Immunity for the Clinician. Florida: Grune & Stratton Inc., 1985.

Soulsby, EHL. Antigen-antibody reactions in helminth infections. *Adv Immunol*, 1962:2:265-308.

Srivastava, Y. et al. Antidiabetic and adaptogenic properties of *Momordica charantia* extract: An experimental and clinical evaluation. *Pharmacol Res Comm*, 1988:20:285-289.

Srivastava, Y. et al. Effect of *Momordica charantia* Linn. Pomous aqueous extract on cataractogenesis in murine alloxan diabetes. *Pharmacol Res Comm*, 1988:20:201-209.

The Lectins: Properties, Functions and Applications in Biology and Medicine. New York: Harcourt Brace Jovanovich/Academic Press, 1986.

Steinman, David. *Diet for a Poisoned Planet.* New York: Harmony Books. 1990.

Triadou, N. and Audron, E. Interaction of the brush border hydrolases of the human small intestine with lectins. *Digestion*, 1983:27:1-7.

Trowbridge, JP and Walker, M. *The Yeast Syndrome.* New York: Bantam Books, 1983.

Waxdal, MJ. Isolation, characterization and biological activities of five mitogens from pokeweed. *Biochemistry*, 1974:13:3671-3675.

Winter, R. *A Consumer's Dictionary of Food Additives.* New York: Crown Publishers, Inc., 1984.

Young, F. *Keeping Drug Residues out of Milk: A Lesson in Industry Education. FDA Consumer*, Mar 1989.

Zafrini, D. et al. Inhibitory activity of cranberry juice on adherence of type1 and type P fimbriated *E. coli* to eucaryotic cells. *Antimicrobial Agents and Chemotherapy*, 1989:33:92-98,

Index

Nutritional Products
Formulated by Dr. Keith DeOrio

ProSana

makes available many of the products recommended by
Dr. Keith DeOrio.
If you would like to receive a catalog, product information, order
products or obtain information on how to purchase products at a
discount please contact the company at:

(877) PROSANA (877-776-7262)

OR

the ProSana website at:

www.prosana.com

OR

Mail or Fax this Information Form to:

ProSana
16932 Gothard, Suite H
Huntington Beach, CA 92647
Fax (714) 841-0630

_____ Please send me a complete product catalog
_____ Please send me further information on how to receive Dr. DeOrio's products at a discount
_____ Please send me information on Dr. DeOrio's newsletter, The New Millennium Medicine
Update

Name_____

Address_____

City_____ State_____ Zip_____

Telephone Number (_____)_____

E-Mail address_____